THE
RADIANCE
SUTRAS

THE
RADIANCE
SUTRAS

112 GATEWAYS TO
THE YOGA OF
WONDER & DELIGHT

LORIN ROCHE, PhD

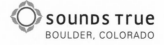

sounds true
BOULDER, COLORADO

Sounds True
Boulder, CO 80306

Cover design by Rachael Murray
Book design by Beth Skelley
Printed in the United States of America

Library of Congress Cataloging-in-Publication Data
Roche, Lorin.
  The Radiance Sutras : 112 gateways to the yoga of wonder and delight /
  Lorin Roche, PhD ; Foreword by Shiva Rea.
     pages cm
Previously published by Syzygy Creations, Inc., 2008.
In English and Sanskrit; translated from Sanskrit.
ISBN 978-1-60407-659-2
1. Tantras. Rudrayamalatantra. Vijñanabhairava—Criticism,
interpretation, etc. I. Tantras. Rudrayamalatantra. Vijñanabhairava. II.
Tantras. Rudrayamalatantra. Vijñanabhairava. English. III. Title.
  BL1142.6.V556R63 2014
  294.5'95--dc23

                                    2013025661

Ebook ISBN 978-1-62203-166-5
10 9 8 7 6 5 4 3 2 1

Lift a cup of *soma* in praise
to Lakshman Joo

. . . a round of *soma* on my tab
to his students
Lilian Silburn, Paul Reps, Jaideva Singh,
Alexis Sanderson, and
John and Denise Hughes

A case of *amrita* to
Panini and Company

Ambrosia on tap to Rabindranath Tagore

Bombay Sapphire to
Otto Bohtlingk, Rudolph Roth, and
Sir Monier-Williams

And a pet anteater
To Valmiki

Translating the nectar of wisdom
of the wisdom traditions
is the work of centuries

CONTENTS

FOREWORD

In your hands, you hold a treasure.

The Radiance Sutras, the life-work of beloved writer and teacher Lorin Roche, is a contemporary interpretation of the timeless, universal meditations of the Vijnana Bhairava Tantra. The 112 contemplative meditations known as both *yuktis* and *dharanas* unfold as a sacred exchange between the divine masculine as Shiva, or Bhairava, and the divine feminine as Shakti, or Bhairavi. This sacred teaching was revered by the great sages of tantra, including Kshemaraja in the 11th century through this last century's yoga masters Swami Lakshman Joo, the yogini Lalita Devi, and Swami Muktananda.

The Vijnana Bhairava Tantra provides a way into the universal realization of divine embodiment that is developed fully within the tantras. Universal, sensual, very human experiences such as breathing, tasting, seeing, waking up, sleeping, getting angry, and making love become vehicles for realizing your nature. This happens at a deep level of vibration through the living current, *spanda shakti,* the pulsating source of consciousness of the early Trika-Krama lineages of tantra that knew of the quantum wave long before modern physics.

When I received the original draft of the Radiance Sutras from Lorin in 2006, I was enthralled by such somatic kinship with his poetic interpretation of the sutras of the Vijnana Bhairava Tantra. I was already in love with the Vijnana. When I was fifteen, I'd discovered it in Paul Reps' book *Zen Flesh, Zen Bones.* Later, I'd encountered it through the translation my root teacher, Daniel Odier, received from Lalita Devi, a realized yogini from Kashmir.

Lorin's offering reignited a flame, and knowing Lorin is like finding a rare soul friend on the path who also shares a great love. Lorin brings to life the revolutionary insights of the early tantras so that they transform the material way we continue to experience our bodies—despite living in the quantum age of physics, which recognizes our body as vastly composed of space and vibration. Lorin poetically translates the experience of *spanda,* "the creative vibration," as always expanding and contracting, creating feelings, thoughts, or actions and then dissolving back into space.

> Attend to the skin as a subtle boundary
> Containing vastness.
> Enter that pulsing vastness
> And know there is no other but you.
> YUKTI 25

With Lorin's blessing I have included *The Radiance Sutras,* along with other scholarly translations, in Prana Flow teacher trainings to explore the transforming effect of the sutras within the living flow of yoga. I offer lines of the Radiance Sutras as an invocation, during the hovering space of a mudra or asana, and as a meditation to end a session. They offer ways of changing stiffness into fluidity, replacing density with shimmering energy, transforming separation into the sacred flow satisfied within. Students memorize lines and other teachers integrate the sutras into their classes. *The Radiance Sutras* has become part of our living library, because you can imbibe the teachings at any time and feel the reverberations. As you take in the sutra, the wisdom begins to transform you instantaneously.

> The breath flows out with the sound *sa,*
> The breath flows in with the sound *ha.*
> Thus thousands of times a day,
> Everyone who breathes is adoring the Goddess.
> Know this, and be in great joy.
> Listen to the ongoing prayer that is breath.
> Life shall dance in you
> A dance of ever-renewing delight.
> VERSES 155–156

In the flow of yoga, breath is the path of realization. In most contemporary yoga the *bhava,* or feeling essence, is substituted with technique. Lorin has a way of expressing the rhythm of the sensory somatic world and how its undulations and "song of the body" are part of the very flow of consciousness. The simple flow of breath, which for most modern practitioners is trapped under tensions and internal neglect, transforms into the most intimate connection to the sublime source.

> Be conscious of this unconscious prayer (of your breath),
> For She is the most holy place of pilgrimage.
> She wishes for you to enter this temple,
> Where each breath is adoration
> Of the infinite for the incarnate form.
> **VERSE 154**

The Radiance Sutras is the culmination of forty-plus years of devotion to this sacred text, as well as Lorin Roche's life experience as a beloved meditation teacher and master writer-poet. Lorin has brought the Vijnana Bhairava Tantra alive for a wide audience in a way similar to how Coleman Barks revived the poetry of the great Sufi teacher, Jelauddin Rumi. These poetic interpretations have brought the vibratory wisdom of the tantras to the most neglected places within Western embodiment, as Lorin breathes a rhythm and life to language through his own realization. He has opened a doorway into the tantric realization of the *divya deha,* the divine body, the shimmering flow of embodied consciousness manifesting as Shakti and returning to infinite potency as Shiva.

It is with great celebration that this edition—complete with Sanskrit Devanagari script, transliteration, and pronunciation—goes out into the world. *The Radiance Sutras* are spreading across the world. Beloved musicians Dave Stringer, Donna DeLory, Denise Kaufman, and Steve Gold compose to these poetic truths. Lorin, with his beautiful wife Camille, have been dedicated to this text with their life and you can feel that in their care.

> Meditate on the Self as being Vast as the sky, a body of energy
> Extending forever in all directions.
> **YUKTI 69**

Your heart sees by its own light.
In meditation, adore the subtle fire
The light that you see by
Is the light that comes from inside.
YUKTI 14

May we all awaken to the inner light of the heart—the ripple effect that has immeasurable blessings and benefits to all. May this sacred resonance attune us all to the living sublime current. As the Vijnana Bhairava so eloquently invokes through Lorin,

Being transformed by even one of these practices,
Fullness of experience develops breath by breath.
One day the desire of the self for the great Self
Is consummated
VERSE 148

Be prepared, for you will not be the same person you were before you began reading. One of these sutras is enough to change a life.

SHIVA REA
Malibu, California
August 2014

PRELUDE

The Vijnana Bhairava Tantra is one of the early teachings on yoga meditation. The name, loosely translated, means "the terror and joy of realizing oneness with the soul." The text is only about two thousand words in the original Sanskrit, perhaps forty minutes of chanting, yet those few words describe the essence of many of the world's meditation techniques. I call it "the Radiance Sutras" because it is so luminous.

This text is part of the ancient tantras, although how ancient we cannot say exactly. The first written version appeared in Kashmir around AD 800. Before that, it may have been handed down through the oral tradition, which means that it was memorized and chanted for generations.

In ancient texts such as the Rig Veda, the word *tantra* refers to the technology of weaving—"a loom, the warp." There is the image of stretching or weaving threads in patterns across the framework of a loom. Metaphorically, a tantra is a tapestry of knowledge weaving together the threads of yoga technique.

A tantra is not poetry, although it may sound that way in the original Sanskrit and in translation. A tantra is a manual of practices. This one is a compendium of yoga meditation instructions, set as a conversation between lovers. Its focus is on full-body spirituality and accepting every breath, sensual experience, and emotion as doorways to deep and intimate contact with the energies of life.

A translation of this tantra came into my hands more than forty years ago, and I have worked with the methods every day since then. It has been a love affair, and I am blessed. One day I started to write a fresh version and it evolved into this book.

A LANGUAGE OF LOVE

The Bhairava Tantra is set as a conversation between the Goddess Who Is the Creative Power of the Universe and the God Who Is the Consciousness that Permeates Everywhere. For short, they call each other Devi and Bhairava, or Shakti and Shiva. They are lovers and inseparable partners, and one of their favorite places of dwelling is in the human heart.

This text feels as though it were composed by a couple, a man and a woman who sang the verses to each other as they co-created. As was the convention of the time, the authors chose to be anonymous and frame the conversation as one between the Goddess and the God in them. The text has the feeling of one richly experienced body speaking with love to another body.

Their inquiry is about how to enter into the vibrant essence of the world with the dual balance of passion and detachment. The teaching emerges from their love-play, reminding us that from within our own hearts we are educated in the spirit of love. They lived this teaching. The secret pathways in the body and the flow of delicious energies are revealed in words that one friend or lover would speak to another. The text invites us to be at home in the universe by accepting every intense experience, every sensual delight, every ordinary moment, as a gateway to the divine.

The conversation begins with Devi asking, "Beloved, tell me, how do I enter more deeply into the reality of the universe?" In reply, Bhairava describes 112 techniques for becoming enlightened through everyday life experience. Each of these techniques is a way of attending to the rhythms, pulsations, and sensuousness of the divine energy that we are made of and that flows through us always. As we engage with these meditation techniques, we are alerted to the presence of the sacred that permeates our bodies. All of these methods involve savoring the incredible intensity underlying the most common experiences. They work by activating the senses, by extending the range of the senses further into the inner and the outer world. The basic dynamics of life—breathing, falling asleep, waking up, walking, loving—are all used as gateways to alignment and enlightenment.

Each meditation is a deep dive into aliveness, into the underlying reality of what life is. Balance is there at every step; the unshakable serenity of the depths is used as a foundation so that we can tolerate the electrifying vastness of the universe. We are invited to cross the threshold, to walk by the guardian of the gate, to face our terrors, and make our way into the immense and timeless mystery that is always calling.

Many of these meditation techniques are surprisingly informal: Notice a powerful emotion, sensation, or desire, and enter into that awareness with total abandon, so that you go with it right into the root movement of the universe. When making love, put your awareness into the flame of passion pulsating through the body and become that flame. Falling asleep, pay attention to the transition from waking consciousness to unconsciousness, and catch a glimpse of what consciousness itself is. Or go outside on a moonless night and simply merge with the darkness and vastness of space.

The text also describes what we think of as traditional yoga meditations—ways of savoring breath, sound, and internal luminosity. The intimacy with the self implied in these teachings means that tantra is not a set of techniques imposed from outside. Rather, the method emerges naturally from one's relationship with the self and with life. Lose yourself in intense experience, and find your Self. In this text, the word *yoga* is used in its etymological sense, "the act of joining, linking together." Yoga is *connecting*—connecting all the elements and levels of your being.

The tone of the text is playful and exploratory—jump in and feel everything. *Lila* is Sanskrit for "play," "amusement," and the sense that the universe has been manifested as an act of play by the divine. Through play, find your way. In play, find freedom, revelation, illumination.

MEDITATION AS EMBRACE

Taken as a whole, the teaching of the Vijnana Bhairava Tantra is startling in its breadth, in the huge range of human experience that it encompasses. It shatters the picture we have of what meditation is or how meditation is often presented—as a way of dissociating from the human experience and trying to rise above it. There is not a hint of the usual life denial that permeates and distorts spirituality East and West.

This tantra is about going deeply into experience, embracing it fully, without reservation. Nature is embraced, as is all of human nature. Lust and passion become fires that illumine, and gusto is taken to its most refined degree possible. Meditation is presented as the nexus or meeting ground of light and matter, spirit and flesh, and the meeting is to be consummated with great joy. Tantric meditation is an integration of the opposites, not obliteration or mere transcendence of them. It is an alchemical union in which each polarity exists in its fullness and in a relationship of complementarity with the other.

You'll find here in one place many of the essential techniques utilized in meditation traditions the world over. If some of the experiences that the sutras describe seem familiar to you as you read this book, it may be because you have invented your own private meditation techniques, ones you probably never tell anyone about. Or you may have had inexplicable realizations in the midst of some life experience.

People who come for instruction in meditation usually have one or more of these awareness practices vibrating in their body already, spontaneously. This is what propels them to search. Sutras such as these are here to remind us of what we already know. They are here to invite us to go more deeply into the experience of being human.

It is likely that the same meditation techniques are invented or discovered independently around the world in different cultures, whenever people start paying attention to the subtle energies of the body. If this is true, then the Radiance Sutras is a syllabus of the types of techniques that could be discovered anywhere. In my experience, they are discovered and rediscovered continually, by all lovers of life.

THIS VERSION

For the last twenty-five years, the text has been waking me up at four in the morning, purring Sanskrit in my ear and calling me to come out and play. I walk around in the predawn for a few hours, whispering the words of the timeless language, letting it teach me about itself. In this way, the Sanskrit has sung itself into modern English.

The original Sanskrit of the Bhairava Tantra has a musical, mantric quality that massages the nerves like no other language I have ever heard. Sanskrit, like tantric meditation, is a union of opposites. The opposites embrace each other, as lovers do, as the eternally fascinating polarity of male and female, day and night, sun and moon.

Sanskrit sings of rhythm, vibrancy, and the transmutation of terror into ecstasy, fear into movement, stasis into electricity. It evokes flow, tenderness, intimacy with oneself and the universe, informality, attentiveness, and responsiveness. Devi's opening statement to Bhairava gets my vote for one of the most enchanting phrases I have ever heard in any language. Chant it softly to yourself and listen:

shrutam deva maya sarvam rudra yamala sambhavam.

"Beloved, I have been listening to the hymns of creation."

Many types of translations—academic, literary, historical, etymological—can be done of this tantra, and yet each conveys only a small part of its meaning. This version is a *bhashantaram,* a rendering of the text into the vernacular and a migration or reincarnation into another tongue.

The language of the sutras is brief, meant to be read over and over. Each Sanskrit verse is only thirty-two syllables, intricately woven and saturated with the power of bliss *(anandashakti).* Just as all of life is interconnected, one word of Sanskrit may have a spectrum of interconnected meanings, encompassing the realms of meditation, music, cooking, medicine, alchemy, sex, ritual worship, art, dance, theater, astronomy, astrology, and mathematics. These definitions are full of physical images that give clues to how to practice.

For example, the word *yoga* has the central meaning of "joining things together," or "hooking up." The first definition of yoga listed in the Monier-Williams *Sanskrit-English Dictionary* is "the act of yoking, joining, attaching, putting to (of horses)." If we look up the English phrase "putting to," we see that it is a British expression for hitching up a horse, "attaching the harness to the load." *Yoga* also means "equipping or arraying an army, fixing an arrow on the bowstring, putting on of armor," and in medicine, "a remedy or cure." *Yoga* can refer to any junction—in astronomy and astrology, a conjunction of the stars or planets; in grammar, the connection of words together; in arithmetic, addition, sum, total. In alchemy or chemistry, mixing different materials together is yoga. In spirituality, *yoga* can mean the union of the soul with matter, the union of the individual soul with the universal soul, and the disciplines that serve this union.

If we take these images metaphorically, they are saying, "Get connected to your horsepower, the magic animal of your being. Arrange your forces. Put on your protection. Do the practices in a way that is a remedy, a cure, for you. Know the stars that guide you." These are apt metaphors—*yuktarupaka*—for meditative experience.

TANTRA

The word *tantra* has interesting resonances, each of which provides a vital clue to how to practice. The *tan* of *tantra* has a wide range of meanings, including "to extend, stretch, spread, shine." When this root sound made its way West, it became *ten,* and we use it all the time when we say *extend, tendon, tender, tension, entertain, intensity,* and *attention.* To practice tantra is to stretch ourselves, to extend our capacity for attention to the utmost. Tantra is also the pattern of interconnectedness we discover when we practice. Tenderness is important. This text is tender in its approach to human experience and encourages an earthy reverence in embracing your bodily sensations.

Tantra denotes "theory or system" and often refers to a class of texts that are set as a conversation between the gods and goddesses—in this case, Bhairava and Devi. The *tra* of *tantra* means "technique." The same root shows up in *mantra* (*manas,* "mind," plus *tra,* "skill," means "a tool of thought").

Each verse of a tantra is called a *sutra* (there's *tra* again), which means "thread" and is cognate with "sew" and "suture," the thread that joins together. "Seam" and "couture" are also cousins of *sutra.* So with the words *tantra* and *sutra,* we are presented with images of skillfully weaving together all the elements of life—mind, body, emotions, breath, soul, individuality, and infinity—into one exquisite tapestry. (Wordplay was a major form of entertainment in the tantric tradition, so there are often dozens of alternate or "folk" etymologies for these words.)

Jnana (sometimes spelled *gyan*) is "knowledge, to know." *Vijnana* means worldly, practical knowledge and skill. In this context, *vijnana* refers to your "knowledge body"—*vijnanamayakosha,* the dimension of your body that is in direct practical contact with the mysteries of life.

Life refreshes and evolves itself through a symphony of ongoing rhythms. Brains have *waves,* hearts *pulsate,* breath *oscillates,* the senses *vibrate.* Tantra can be thought of as attending to these rhythms. Breath is a rhythm, and we breathe in and out thousands of times a day. Breathing involves an intimate relationship between our bodies and the ocean of air within which we suspire. A dozen senses inform us of the rhythm, texture, and qualities in each breath. Life is always inviting us into a deeper relationship with breath, with the pulsing of our hearts and emotions.

READING THE SUTRAS AND PRACTICES

In part I, "The Radiance Sutras," there are three forms of Sanskrit included with each sutra. The first form is Devanagari, which looks like this:

॥ विज्ञान भैरव ॥

The second form is a transliteration into Roman letters with diacritical marks to indicate pronunciation:

dhāmāntaḥkṣobhasambhūtasūkṣmāgnitilakākṛtim

The third form of Sanskrit given is just the raw individual words, spelled out phonetically to give a rough approximation of the pronunciation:

daamaantah kshobha sambhootah sookshma agnih tilaka akritim

There are two numbers for most of the verses. The number accompanying the Sanskrit transliteration is the *verse number,* from 1 to 162. Devi and Bhairava banter for 23 verses, and then verse 24 marks the beginning of the "112 yogas"—meditations, techniques, known in

Sanskrit as *yuktis* or *dharanas.* These yuktis are also numbered, from 1 to 112.

You can follow the yukti numbers to their counterparts in part II, "Invitations and Illuminations." There I unpack some of the juiciest Sanskrit words to shed additional light on each meditation, as a way of allowing you to explore that technique more deeply.

SAVORING THE SUTRAS

The Radiance Sutras is a text to savor one phrase at a time, over a period of days or years. The verses are designed so you can read or listen to them for a lifetime and have a new revelation every day. Each of the meditations is meant to be experienced many times under many different conditions. As you become familiar with the practices, you will discover the tactile luminosity and improvisational music of your inner world. As your internal senses become more alert, doorway after doorway will open to you.

The text wants to be thought and spoken in English as well as Sanskrit—whispered, chanted, delighted in, and danced. I am letting the text sing itself back into the spoken word. The sutras remember they were once songs—*caryagita,* songs of realization. Experiment with reading them out loud to yourself or to another person.

The language is crafted so that you may be able to recognize your own innate spiritual experience and have a flash of recognition. The Bhairava Tantra is a love song between energy and consciousness or Shakti and Shiva, and the musical and mantric impulses of their creativity are pulsing in us always. These verses are an invitation to wake up to the marvelous symphony within and around us.

When you discover one sutra that resonates deeply, memorize it. Then you will, as they say, know it by heart. Something happens in the body when you can say a sutra out loud or quietly to yourself. There is a relaxation, an ease and confidence, when you can rest your attention inside a sutra and the words flow effortlessly.

Tantric texts want to be performed. They are not comfortable being hidden in books. Any time you read a phrase tenderly and let yourself be carried away, even for a minute, you are performing a sacred act, offering your attention to the mystery of being alive.

The sutras tend to lay the groundwork for each other, but you don't have to go through them in sequence. Some of the techniques will speak to you now, and others will only have meaning after you have explored them for a while. When I began meditating, the techniques in the first few sutras and one in the middle kept me busy for a year. Your pace may be faster or slower.

One way to explore the text is to pick one technique—whichever one strikes you—and practice it for three months. Give it time to work. Then read the sutras again and see if it is time to move on or to include another technique in addition to the one that you have been doing. The "Invitations and Illuminations" section following the sutras gives some tips for going deeper into the exquisite world of these practices. The text says that if you go deeply into even one of these ways of experience, making it your own over time, you will awaken.

Meditation is *sambhava,* intimacy with what you love about life. Take one thing and go deeper and deeper into it. Dive into your entire sensorium so fearlessly that you go beyond it into the core of your being and rest there.

Love calls our attention and engages us. When we give love our tender attention, we are in the realm of tantra. Life is a mysterious, self-renewing process. The techniques of meditation are ways of allowing the ecstasy of the life-force at play to renew our bodies and souls. Ask your body to teach you and to take you on adventures into intimacy with your own essence. This is the yoga of wonder and delight.

PART ONE

THE RADIANCE
SUTRAS

विज्ञान भैरव तन्त्र

vijñāna bhairava tantra

BANTER VERSES

The Bhairava Tantra is framed as a conversation between lovers, Devi and Bhairava. Devi is the Creative Energy permeating the universe. Her nature is power, strength, and might. Bhairava is the infinite consciousness that embraces her.

In the initial verses, Devi is speaking from within her awe at existence. She assumes the body of a seeker of truth and dares Bhairava to reveal to her the secrets of yoga. Rising to the occasion, Bhairava accepts her questions as beautiful and invites her to accompany him on the path of intimacy with all life. In verses 1–23, they converse back and forth in this way.

BANTER VERSES 1-2

श्री देव्युवाच ।

श्रुतं देव मया सर्वं रुद्रयामलसम्भवम् ।
त्रिकभेदमशेषेण सारात्सारविभागशः ॥१॥

अद्यापि न निवृत्तो मे संशयः परमेश्वर ।
किं रूपं तत्त्वतो देव शब्दराशिकलामयम् ॥२॥

śrī devyuvāca |
śrutaṁ deva mayā sarvaṁ rudrayāmala sambhavam |
trika bhedam aśeṣeṇa sārāt sāra vibhāgaśaḥ || 1 ||
adyāpi na nivṛtto me saṁśayaḥ parameśvara
kiṁ rūpaṁ tattvato deva śabda rāśi kalā mayam || 2 ||

shree devee uvaacha
shrutam deva mayaa sarvam rudrayaa-mala sam-bhavam
trika-bhedam a-sheshena saaraat—saara-vi-bhaagashah
adya api na ni-vritto me sam-shayah parama—eeshvara
kim roopam tattvatah deva shabda—raashi kalaamayam

One day the Goddess sang to her lover, Bhairava:

Beloved and radiant lord of the space before birth,
Revealer of essence,
Slayer of the ignorance that binds us,

You who in play have created this universe
And permeated all forms in it
With never-ending truth,
I have been wondering . . .

I have been listening to the hymns of creation,
Enchanted by the verses,
Yet still I am curious.

What is this delight-filled universe
Into which we find ourselves born?
What is this mysterious awareness
Shimmering everywhere within it?

BANTER VERSES 3-4

किं वा नवात्मभेदेन भैरवे भैरवाकृतौ ।
त्रिशिरोभेदभिन्नं वा किं वा शक्तित्रयात्मकम् ॥३॥

नादबिन्दुमयं वापि किं चन्द्रार्धनिरोधिकाः ।
चक्रारूढमनच्कं वा किं वा शक्तिस्वरूपकम् ॥४॥

kiṁ vā navātma bhedena bhairave bhairavākṛtau |
triśirobheda bhinnaṁ vā kiṁ vā śakti trayātmakam || 3 ||
nāda bindu mayaṁ vāpi kiṁ candrārdha nirodhikāḥ |
cakrārūḍham anackaṁ vā kiṁ vā śakti svarūpakam || 4 ||

kim vaa nava–aatma–bhedena bhairave bhairava–aakritau
tri–shirah–bheda–abhinnam vaa kim vaa shakti–tri–aatmakam
naada–bindu–mayam vaa api kim chandra–ardha–ni–rodhikaah
chakra–aa–roodham anachkam vaa kim vaa shakti–sva–roopakam

I have been listening to the love songs of
Form longing for formless.

What are these energies
Undulating through our bodies,
Pulsing us into action?

And this "matter" out of which our forms are made—
What are these dancing particles
Of condensed radiance?

BANTER VERSES 5-6

परापरायाः सकलमपरायाश्च वा पुनः ।
पराया यदि तद्वत्स्यात्परत्वं तद् विरुध्यते ॥५॥

न हि वर्णविभेदेन देहभेदेन वा भवेत् ।
परत्वं निष्कलत्वेन सकलत्वे न तद् भवेत् ॥६॥

प्रसादं कुरु मे नाथ निःशेषं चिन्द्धि संशयम् ।

parāparāyāḥ sakalama parāyāśca vā punaḥ |
parāyā yadi tad vatsyāt paratvaṁ tad virudhyate || 5 ||
na hi varṇa vibhedena dehabhedena vā bhavet |
paratvaṁ niṣkalatvena sakalatve na tad bhavet || 6 ||
prasādaṁ kuru me nātha niḥśeṣaṁ chinddhi saṁśayam |

para–a-paraayaah sakalam a-parayaah cha vaa punah
paraayaa yadi tat vatsyaat paratvam tat vi-rudhyate
na hi varna—vi-bhedena deha—bhedena vaa bhavet
paratvam nish-kalatvena sakalatve na tat bhavet
pra-saadam kuru me naatha
nih-shesham chhindhi sam-shayam

What is this power we call Life,
Appearing as the play of flesh and breath?
How may I know this mystery and enter it more deeply?

My attention is enthralled by a myriad of forms,
Innumerable individual entities everywhere,
Flashing into existence and fading away again.
Lead me into the wholeness beyond all these parts.

Do me a favor, my love.
Let me rest in your embrace.
Refresh me with the elixir of your wisdom.
Ravish me with your truth.

BANTER VERSES 7-9

श्री देव्युवाच ।

साधु साधु त्वया पृष्टं तन्त्रसारम् इदम् प्रिये ॥७॥

गूहनीयतमम् भद्रे तथापि कथयामि ते ।
यत्किञ्चित्सकलं रूपं भैरवस्य प्रकीर्तितम् ॥८॥

तद् असारतया देवि विज्ञेयं शक्रजालवत् ।
मायास्वप्नोपमं चैव गन्धर्वनगरभ्रमम् ॥९॥

bhairava uvāca |
sādhu sādhu tvayā pṛṣṭaṁ tantra sāram idam priye || 7 ||
gūha nīyatamam bhadre tathāpi kathayāmi te |
yat kiñcit sakalaṁ rūpaṁ bhairavasya prakīrtitam || 8 ||
tad asāra tayā devi vijñeyaṁ śakra jālavat |
māyā svapnopamaṁ caiva gandharva nagara bhramam || 9 ||

bhairava uvaacha
saadhu saadhu tvayaa prishtam tantra–saaram idam priye
gooha-neeyatamam bhadre tatha api kathayaami te
yat kinchit sakalam roopam bhairavasya pra-keertitam
tat a-saaratayaa devi vi-jneyam shakra jaalavat
maayaa–svapna-upamam cha eva gandharva–nagara–bhramam

Bhairava replies,

Beloved, your questions
Touch the heart of wonder,
The path of intimacy with all life—
Weaving together body and soul,
Sex and spirit, individuality and universality.

This is my Cave of Secrets.
Your inquiry has led you here.
I feel your fingers on my pulse.

Come with me.
Leave behind everything you know.
The teachings about me are
A light show put on by the celestial musicians,
As beautiful and insubstantial as clouds.

BANTER VERSES 10-12

ध्यानार्थम् भ्रान्तबुद्धीनां क्रियाडम्बरवर्तिनाम् ।
केवलं वर्णितम् पुंसां विकल्पनिहतात्मनाम् ॥१०॥

तत्त्वतो न नवात्मासौ शब्दराशिर् न भैरवः ।
न चासौ त्रिशिरा देवो न च शक्तित्रयात्मकः ॥११॥

नादबिन्दुमयो वापि न चन्द्रार्धनिरोधिकाः ।
न चक्रक्रमसम्भिन्नो न च शक्तिस्वरूपकः ॥१२॥

dhyānārtham bhrānta buddhīnāṁ kriyāḍambara vartinām |
kevalaṁ varṇitam puṁsāṁ vikalpa nihatātmanām || 10 ||
tattvato na navātmāsau śabda rāśir na bhairavaḥ |
na cāsau triśirā devo na ca śakti trayātmakaḥ || 11 ||
nāda bindu mayo vāpi na candrārdha nirodhikāḥ |
na cakra krama sambhinno na ca śakti svarūpakaḥ || 12 ||

dhyaana–artham bhraanta–buddheenaam
kriyaa–aadambara–vartinam
kevalam varnitam pumsaam vi–kalpa–ni–hataa–aatmanaam
tattvato na nava-aatmaasau shabda-raashih na bhairavah
na cha asau tri–shiraa–devah na cha shakti—tri–aatmakah
naada–bindu–mayah vaa api na chandra–ardha–nirodhikaah
na chakra–krama–sambhinah na cha shakti–sva–roopakah

Elaborate rituals and garish images
May be useful in meditation when your mind is
    whirling with thoughts
Of sex, money, and power, wandering like an elephant
    in heat.
Go ahead and use these tools, yet know,
Beating drums and blaring trumpets
Cannot summon the One who is already present.

I am not a collection of incantations
Known only to experts.
I am not a ladder to be climbed,
A sequence for piercing energy centers in your body.
I am not to be found at the end of a long road.
I am right here.

BANTER VERSES 13-14

अप्रबुद्धमतीनां हि एता बलविभीषिकाः ।
मातृमोदकवत्सर्वं प्रवृत्त्यर्थम् उदाहृतम् ॥१३॥
दिक्कालकलनोन्मुक्ता देशोद्देशाविशेषिनी ।
व्यपदेष्टुमशक्यासाव् अकथ्या परमार्थतः ॥१४॥

aprabuddha matīnāṁ hi etā bala vibhīṣikāḥ |
mātṛ modakavat sarvaṁ pravṛtty artham udāhṛtam || 13 ||
dik kāla kalanonmuktā deśoddeśa viśeṣiṇī |
vyapadeṣṭum aśakyāsāv akathyā paramārthataḥ || 14 ||

aprabuddha–mateenaam hi etaa baala–vi–bheeshikaah
maatri–modakavat sarvam pravritti–artham ud–aahritam
dik–kaala–kalanah un–muktaa deshah ud–deshaa a–vi–sheshinee
vi–apa–deshtum a–shakya asau a–kathyaa parama–arthatah

All the stories about me
Are like tales you tell naughty children—
The goblin is going to come gobble you up!
Or else soothing fables mothers spin
As they hand out sweets.

Leave these fantasies behind.
Let me tell you of the luminous path.

I am beyond measure. I cannot be calculated.
I am beyond space and time.
I am beyond ancient and beyond the future.
There are no directions to me.

BANTER VERSES 15–16

अन्तःस्वानुभवानन्दा विकल्पोन्मुक्तगोचरा ।
यावस्था भरिताकारा भैरवी भैरवात्मनः ॥१५॥

तद् वपुस् तत्त्वतो ज्ञेयं विमलं विश्वपूरणम् ।
एवंविधे परे तत्त्वे कः पूज्यः कश्च तृप्यति ॥१६॥

antaḥ svānubhavānandā vikalponmukta gocarā |
yāvasthā bharitākārā bhairavī bhairavātmanaḥ || 15 ||
tad vapus tattvato jñeyaṁ vimalaṁ viśva pūraṇam |
evaṁ vidhe pare tattve kaḥ pūjyaḥ kaśca tṛpyati || 16 ||

antah sva-anubhava aanandaa vi-kalpah un-muktah gocharaa
yaa ava-sthaa bharita–aakaaraa bhairavee bhairava–aatmanah
tad vapuh tattvatah jneyam vi-malam vishva–pooranam
evam vidhe pare tattve kah poojyah kah cha tripyate

I am always here.
I am the embrace
Of your most intimate experience.

Though I am beyond the intellect,
I am not beyond your daring.

I am the nourishing state of fullness
That is the essence of soul.
You belong to me, and I am yours.

My nature is spotless, completely uncontaminated.
I am not covered up, not even by a billion galaxies.
So who is there to worship and adore?
There is no one to appease.

BANTER VERSES 17-19

एवंविधा भैरवस्य यावस्था परिगीयते ।
सा परा पररूपेण परा देवी प्रकीर्तिता ॥१७॥
शक्तिशक्तिमतोर् यद्वद् अभेदः सर्वदा स्थितः ।
अतस् तद्धर्मधर्मित्वात्परा शक्तिः परात्मनः ॥१८॥
न वह्नेर् दाहिका शक्तिर् व्यतिरिक्ता विभाव्यते ।
केवलं ज्ञानसत्तायाम् प्रारम्भोऽयम् प्रवेशने ॥१९॥

evaṁ vidhā bhairavasya yāvasthā parigīyate |
sā parā pararūpeṇa parā devī prakīrtitā || 17 ||
śakti śaktimator yadvad abhedaḥ sarvadā sthitaḥ |
atas tad dharma dharmitvāt parā śaktiḥ parātmanaḥ || 18 ||
na vahner dāhikā śaktir vyatiriktā vibhāvyate |
kevalaṁ jñāna sattāyāṁ prārambho'yam praveśane || 19 ||

evam vidhaa bhairavasya yaa ava-sthaa pari-geeyate
saa para–apara–roopena paraa–devee pra-keertitaa
shakti–shaktimatoh yad vat abhedah sarvadaa sthitah
atah tat dharma–dharmitvaat paraa–shaktih paraa–aatmanah
na vanheh daahikaa–shaktih vi-ati-riktaa vi-bhaavyate
kevalam–jnaana-sattaayaam praa–rambhah ayam pra-veshane

Sacred texts sing of my reality,
But I cannot be found in them,
For I am the one listening.
I am always closer than breath.

Heat and fire are not two separate things.
These are just verbal distinctions.

The Goddess and the One who holds Her
Are one and the same.
We are inseparable.
The way to me is through Her.

Banter Verses 20-21

शक्त्यवस्थाप्रविष्टस्य निर्विभागेन भावना ।
तदासौ शिवरूपी स्यात्रौवी मुखम् इहोच्यते ॥२०॥

यथालोकेन दीपस्य किरणैर् भास्करस्य च ।
ज्ञायते दिग्विभागादि तद्वच्छक्त्या शिवः प्रिये ॥२१॥

śakty avasthā praviṣṭasya nirvibhāgena bhāvanā |
tadāsau śiva rūpī syāt śaivī mukham ihocyate ‖ 20 ‖
yathālokena dīpasya kiraṇair bhāskarasya ca |
jñāyate digvibhāgādi tadvac chaktyā śivaḥ priye ‖ 21 ‖

shakti—avasthaa—pravishtasya nir—vi—bhaagena bhaavanaa
tadaa asau shiva—roopee syaat shaivee—mukham iha uchyate
yathaa aa—lokena deepasya kiranaih bhaaskarasya cha
jnaayate dic—vibhaaga aadi tad vat shaktyaa shivah priye

I am everywhere, infusing everything.
To find me,
Become absorbed in intense experience.
Go all the way.
Be drenched in the energies of life.
Enter the world beyond separation.

The light of a candle reveals a room.
The rays of the sun reveal the world.
So does the divine feminine
Illumine the way to me.

BANTER VERSES 22-23

श्री देव्युवाच ।

देवदेव त्रिशूलाङ्क कपालकृतभूषण ।
दिग्देशकालशून्या च व्यपदेशविवर्जिता ॥२२॥

यावस्था भरिताकारा भैरवस्योपलभ्यते ।
कैर् उपायैर् मुखं तस्य परा देवि कथम् भवेत् ।
यथा सम्यग् अहं वेद्मि तथा मे ब्रूहि भैरव ॥२३॥

śrī devy uvāca |
deva deva triśūlāṅka kapāla kṛta bhūṣaṇa |
dig deśa kāla śūnyā ca vyapadeśa vivarjitā || 22 ||
yāvasthā bharitā kārā bhairavasyopalabhyate |
kair upāyair mukham tasya parā devi katham bhavet |
yathā samyag aham vedmi tathā me brūhi bhairava || 23 ||

shree devee uvaacha
deva deva tri–shoola–anka kapaala–krita–bhooshana
dig–desha–kaala–shoonya cha vi–apa–desha–vi–varjitaa
yaa ava–sthaa bharitaa–kaaraa bhairavasya upa–labhyate
kaih upaayaih mukham tasya para–devee katham bhavet
yathaa samyak aham vedmi tathaa me broohi bhairava

She Who Shines Everywhere sings,

You who hold the mysteries in your hand—
    Of will, knowledge, and action—
Reveal to me this path of illumined knowing.

I long to merge with you,
Be filled with your nourishing essence.
Lead me into joyous union
With the life of the universe,
That I may know it fully,
Realize it deeply,
And breathe in luminous truth.

Yukti Verses

In the body of the Vijnana Bhairava Tantra, Bhairava articulates 112 yuktis, or yoga meditation practices, for opening to the divine mystery within everyday experience.

The practices begin in verse 24 and continue to verse 135. The wide variety of techniques allows each individual to find their doorway into wonder, astonishment, and delight.

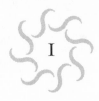

I

भैरव उवाच।

ऊर्ध्वे प्राणो ह्यधो जीवो विसर्गात्मा परोच्चरेत् ।
उत्पत्तिद्वितयस्थाने भरणाद् भरिता स्थितिः ॥२४॥

śrī bhairava uvāca |
ūrdhve prāṇo hyadho jīvo visargātmā paroccaret |
utpatti dvitaya sthāne bharaṇād bharitā sthitiḥ || 24 ||

shree bhairava uvaacha
oordhve praano hi adhas jeevah visarga–aatmaa paraa ud-charet
ut-patti–dvitaya–sthaane bharanaad bharitaa-sthitih

––––––––––

The One Who Is Intimate to All Beings replies,

Beloved, your questions require the answers that come
Through direct living experience.

The way of experience begins with a breath,
Such as the breath you are breathing now.
Awakening into luminous reality
May dawn in the momentary throb
Between any two breaths.

Exhaling, breath is released and flows out.
    There is a pulse as it turns to flow in.
In that turn, you are empty.
Enter that emptiness as the source of all life.

Inhaling, breath flows in, filling, nourishing.
Just as it turns to flow out,
There is a flash of pure joy—
    Life is renewed.

2

मरुतोऽन्तर् बहिर् वापि वियद्युग्मानिवर्तनात् ।
भैरव्या भैरवस्येत्थम् भैरवि व्यज्यते वपुः ॥२५॥

maruto'ntar bahir vāpi viyad yugmānivartanāt |
bhairavyā bhairavasyettham bhairavi vyajyate vapuḥ || 25 ||

marutah antah bahih vaa api viyat–yugma–anivartanaat
bhairavyaa bhairavasya ittham bhairavi vi-ajyate vapuh

———————

Radiant One,

The life essence carries on its play
   Through the pulsing rhythm
Of outward and inward movement.
This is the ceaseless throb, the rhythm of life—
Terrifying in its eternity, exquisite in its constancy.

The inhalation, the return movement of breath,
   Sustains life.
The outgoing breath
   Purifies life.
These are the two poles
Between which respiration goes on unceasingly.
Between them is every delight you could desire.

Even when the senses are turned outward,
Your attention on the external world,
Attend also to the inner throb,
The pulsing of the creative impulse within you.

3

न व्रजेन् न विशेच्छक्तिर् मरुद्रूपा विकासिते ।
निर्विकल्पतया मध्ये तया भैरवरूपता ॥२६॥

na vrajen na viśec chaktir marud rūpā vikāsite |
nirvikalpatayā madhye tayā bhairava rūpatā || 26 ||

*na vrajet na vishet shaktih marut–roopa vi-kaasite
nir-vi-kalpatayaa madhe tayaa bhairava–roopataa*

Enter these turning points,
Where the rhythms of life transform
Into each other.

Breath flows in, filling, filling,
    In this moment, drink eternity.

Breath flows out, emptying, emptying,
Offering itself to infinity.

Cherishing these moments,
Mind dissolves into heart,
Heart dissolves into space,
Body becomes a vibrating field,
Pulsating between fullness and emptiness.

4

कुम्भिता रेचिता वापि पूरिता वा यदा भवेत् ।
तदन्ते शान्तनामासौ शक्त्या शान्तः प्रकाशते ॥२७॥

kumbhitā recitā vāpi pūritā vā yadā bhavet |
tad ante śānta nāmāsau śaktyā śāntaḥ prakāśate || 27 ||

*kumbhitaa rechitaa vaa api pooritaa yaa yadaa bhavet
tadante shanta naama-asau shaktyaa shantah pra-kaashate*

At the end of the exhale,
Breath surrenders to quietude.
For a moment you hang in the balance—
Suspended
In the fertile spaciousness
That is the source of breath.

At the end of the inhale,
Filled with the song of the breath,
There is a moment when you are simply
Holding the tender mystery.

In these interludes,
Experience opens into exquisite vastness
With no beginning and no end.
Embrace this infinity without reservation.
You are its vessel.

5

आमूलात्किरणाभासां सूक्ष्मात्सूक्ष्मतरात्मिकम् ।
चिन्तयेत्तां द्विषट्कान्ते श्याम्यन्तीम् भैरवोदयः ॥२८॥

āmūlāt kiraṇābhāsāṁ sūkṣmāt sūkṣmatarātmikam |
cintayet tāṁ dviṣaṭkānte śyāmyantīm bhairavodayaḥ || 28 ||

aa-moolaat kirana-aa-bhaasaam sookshmaat sooksma-tara–aatmikam
chintayet taam dvi-shat kaante shaam–yanteem bhairava–udayah

Follow the path of the life force
    As she flashes upward like lightning
    Through your body.

Attend simultaneously
    To the perineum, that bright place
Between the legs,
    To the crown of the skull,
    And to that shining star-place
Above the head.

Notice this living current
Becoming ever more subtle as she rises,
Radiant as the morning sun,
Until she streams outward from the top of the head
Into all-embracing gratitude.

Thus become intimate with the life of all beings.

6

उद्गच्छन्तीं तडित्रूपाम् प्रतिचक्रं क्रमात्क्रमम् ।
ऊर्ध्वं मुष्टित्रयं यावत्तावद् अन्ते महोदयः ॥२९॥

udgac chantīṁ taḍit rūpām praticakram kramāt kramam |
ūrdhvaṁ muṣṭitrayaṁ yāvat tāvad ante mahodayaḥ || 29 ||

*ud-gachchhanteem tadit–roopam prati-chakram–kramaat–kramam
oordhvam mushti–trayam yaavat taavad ante mahaa–udayah*

Trace the river of life that flows through you,
 The luxuriously rising energies,
Gradually touching each of the centers
Along the spine.
Savor every shimmer of color along the way.

Enter each area tenderly,
Loving as you go,
Finally, gently,
Dissolving in the crown of the head.

Then above,
In the space above the head,
The great dawn.

7

क्रमद्वादशकं सम्यग् द्वादशाक्षरभेदितम् ।
स्थूलसूक्ष्मपरस्थित्या मुक्त्वा मुक्त्वान्ततः शिवः ॥३०॥

krama dvādaśakaṁ samyag dvādaśākṣara bheditam |
sthūla sūkṣma parasthityā muktvā muktvāntataḥ śivaḥ || 30 ||

kramah dvaa-dashakam samyak dvaa-dasha–akshara–bheditam
sthoola–sookshma–para–sthityaa muktva–amuktvaa-antatah shivah

———————

Let your attention glide
Through the centers of awareness along the spine
    With adoring intent.

There is a song to each area of the body.
Resonating in sweet vortices,
Long rhythmic vowels and hums,
Ah . . . and . . . *eee* . . . *ommmm* . . . *hummmm* . . .
Resounding on and on.

Find the harmonies
Emanating from the circulation of life energies.

Listen to these as sounds,
Then more subtly, as an underlying hum.
Eventually as most subtle feeling.
Then diving more deeply,
Dissolve into freedom.

8

तयापूर्याश्च मूर्धान्तं भङ्क्त्वा भ्रूक्षेपसेतुना ।
निर्विकल्पं मनः कृत्वा सर्वोर्ध्वे सर्वगोद्गमः ॥३१॥

tayā pūryāśu mūrdhāntaṁ bhaṅktvā bhrū kṣepa setunā |
nirvikalpaṁ manaḥ kṛtvā sarvordhve sarvagodgamaḥ || 31 ||

*tayaa pooryaashu moordha–antam bhanktvaa broo–kshepa–setunaa
nir–vi–kalpam–manas kritvaa sarva–oordhve sarva–gah ud–gamah*

Rest the attention easily in the forehead,
In the eye that is made of light.
Cherish the delicate energies glowing there.

Allow attention to inquire upwards, into the
Radiant space above the head.

The small self enters delicious omnipresence.
This it remembers and knows as its truth.

Gradually the luminosity of that truth
Fills the body to overflowing
As it rises through the crown of the head
Into a shower of light.

9

शिखिपक्षैश् चित्ररूपैर् मण्डलैः शून्यपञ्चकम् ।
ध्यायतोऽनुत्तरे शून्ये प्रवेशो हृदये भवेत् ॥३२॥

śikhi pakṣaiś citra rūpair maṇḍalaiḥ śūnya pañcakam |
dhyāyato'nuttare śūnye praveśo hṛdaye bhavet || 32 ||

*shikhi–pakshaih chitra–roopaih mandalaih shoonya–panchakam
dhyaayatah an-uttare shoonye pra-veshah hridaye bhavet*

The senses declare an outrageous world—
Sounds and scents, ravishing colors and shapes,
Ever-changing skies, iridescent reflections—
All these beautiful surfaces
Decorating vibrant emptiness.
The god of love is courting you,
Light as a feather.

Every perception is an invitation into revelation.
Hearing, seeing, smelling, tasting, touching—
Ways of knowing creation,
Transmissions of electric realization.
The deepest reality is always right here.

Encircled by splendor, in the center of the sphere,
Meditate where the body thrills
To currents of intimate communion.
Follow your senses to the end and beyond
Into the heart of space.

10

ईदृशेन क्रमेणैव यत्र कुत्रापि चिन्तना ।
शून्ये कुड्ये परे पात्रे स्वयं लीना वरप्रदा ॥३३॥

īdṛśena krameṇaiva yatra kutrāpi cintanā |
śūnye kuḍye pare pātre svayaṁ līnā vara pradā || 33 ||

eedrishena kramena eva yatra kutra api chintanaa
shoonye kudye pare paatre svayam–leenaa vara–pradaa

———————

The journey begins here,
With whatever is capturing your attention.

Are you gazing at the patterns on some wall?
Are you daydreaming about a celebrity?

Is there someone you love and long to cling to,
Disappear into, a soul who is a chalice for
Beauty to pour into the world?

Whatever your focus,
Give your whole being.
Gradually, step by step,
The infinity from which you both have emerged
Will encompass you with blessing.

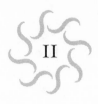

II

कपालान्तर् मनो न्यस्य तिष्ठन् मीलितलोचनः ।
क्रमेण मनसो दाढ्र्यात्लक्षयेत्लष्यम् उत्तमम् ॥३४॥

kapālāntar mano nyasya tiṣṭhan mīlita locanaḥ |
krameṇa manaso dārḍhyāt lakṣayet laṣyam uttamam || 34 ||

kapaala–antah manas nyasya tishthat meelita–lochanah
kramena manasah daardhyaat lakshayet lakshyam uttamam

Inside the skull there is a place
Where the essences of creation play and mingle—
    The ecstatic light of awareness
    And the awareness of that light.

The divine feminine and masculine
Sport with one another in that place.
The light of their love-play illumines all space.

Rest in that light
Ever present, and gradually
Awaken into the steady joy of
That which is always everywhere.

12

मध्यनाडी मध्यसंस्था बिससूत्राभरूपया ।
ध्यातान्तर्व्योमिया देव्या तया देवः प्रकाशते ॥३५॥

madhya nāḍī madhya saṁsthā bisa sūtrābha rūpayā |
dhyātāntar vyoma yā devyā tayā devaḥ prakāśate || 35 ||

madhya–naadee madhya–samsthaa bisa–sootrabha–roopayaa
dhyaataa antar–vyomayaa devyaa tayaa devah pra–kaashate

———————

There is a current of love-energy that flows
Between Earth below and Sun above.

The central channel of your spine is the riverbed.
The streaming is as delicate and powerful
As the tingling touch of lovers.

Entering here,
Radiance arches between above and below.

Your whole attention resting in the subtle,
Vibrating in the center of the spinal column,
Tracing this current between Earth and Sun,
Become magnetism relating all the worlds.

13

कररुद्धदृगस्त्रेण भ्रूभेदाद् द्वाररोधनात् ।
दृष्टे बिन्दौ क्रमाल् लीने तन्मध्ये परमा स्थितिः ॥३६॥

kara ruddha dṛg astreṇa bhrū bhedād dvāra rodhanāt |
dṛṣṭe bindau kramāl līne tan madhye paramā sthitiḥ || 36 ||

*kara—ruddha—drish-astrena broo—bhedaad dvaara—rodhanaat
dirshte bindau kramaat leene tad-madhye paramaa—sthitih*

───────────

Lift your hands, and with a gesture,
Turn aside all the forces of the outer world.
Attend to the vibrancy within.

Let the fingers lightly touch and bless
Eyes, ears, nostrils, mouth,
All the entrances to the head.
Invite attention to be within the skin, and
Cherish the quiet shimmer of vital energies.

When you notice an inner gateway,
Enter with love, as one coming home.

As the surge of light-substance rises
Follow it up into the space between the eyebrows,
Where it breaks out as an orgasm of light.

14

धामान्तःक्षोभसम्भूतसूक्ष्माग्रितिलकाकृतिम् ।
बिन्दुं शिखान्ते हृदये लयान्ते ध्यायतो लयः ॥३७॥

dhāmāntaḥ kṣobha sambhūta sūkṣmāgni tilakākṛtim |
binduṁ śikhānte hṛdaye layānte dhyāyato layaḥ || 37 ||

daaman–antah kshobha-sam-bhootah sooshma-agnih tilaka–akritim
bindum shikhaante hridaye layaante dhyaayatah layah

When you close your eyes,
Attention turns toward the inner glow.
The heart sees by its own light,
Pulsing with subtle flame.

In your forehead is a single eye.
Here streams of living electricity
Flow together.
The body of substance
And the body of light fuse into one.
Above your head a star is shining—
The soul, luminous in its own realm.

Life arises from itself
In a swirling motion of flame.
Being becomes body.
In meditation, adore the subtle fire—
In heart, head, and above.
Dissolve into radiance.

15

अनाहते पात्रकर्णेऽभग्रशब्दे सरिद्रुते ।
शब्दब्रह्मणि निष्णातः परम् ब्रह्माधिगच्छति ॥३८॥

anāhate pātra karṇe'bhagna śabde sarid drute |
śabda brahmaṇi niṣṇātaḥ param brahmādhigaccati || 38 ||

*an-aahate paatra-karne a-bhagna-shabde sarit–drute
shabha-brahmani nish-naatah param-brahma adhi-gachchhati*

Bathe deeply in that ocean of sound
    Vibrating within you, now as always,
Resonating softly,
Permeating the space of the heart.

The ear that is tuned by rapt listening
Learns to hear the song of creation.

First like a hand bell,
Then subtler, like a flute,
Subtler still as a stringed instrument,
Eventually as the buzz of a bee.

Entering this current of sound,
The Listening One
Forgets the external world, becomes
Absorbed into internal sound,
Then absorbed in vastness,
Like the song of the stars as they shine.

16

प्रणवादिसमुच्चारात्प्लुतान्ते शून्यभावानात् ।
शून्यया परया शक्त्या शून्यताम् एति भैरवि ॥३९॥

praṇavādi samuccārāt plutānte śūnya bhāvānāt |
śūnyayā parayā śaktyā śūnyatām eti bhairavi || 39 ||

pra-nava aadi-sam-ud-chaaraat plutaante shoonya–bhaavanaat
shoonyayaa parayaa shaktyaa shoonyataam eti bhairavi

The roar of joy that set the worlds in motion
Is reverberating in your body
And the space between all bodies.
Beloved, listen.

Find that exuberant vibration
Rising new in every moment,
Humming in your secret places,
Resounding through the channels of delight.
Know you are flooded by it always.

Float with the sound.
Melt with it into divine silence.
The sacred power of space will carry you
Into the dancing radiant emptiness
That is the source of all.
The ocean of sound is inviting you
Into its spacious embrace,
Calling you home.

17

यस्य कस्यापि वर्णस्य पूर्वान्ताव् अनुभावयेत् ।
शून्यया शून्यभूतोऽसौ शून्याकारः पुमान् भवेत् ॥४०॥

yasya kasyāpi varṇasya pūrvāntāv anubhāvayet |
śūnyayā śūnya bhūto'sau śūnyākāraḥ pumān bhavet || 40 ||

*yasya kasya api varnasya poorva–antau anu-bhaavayet
shoonyayaa shoonya–bhootah asau shoonya-aakaarah pumaan bhavet*

Think of any vowel—they are all delicious.
Savor the sound with infinite gentleness.
Attend to where it comes from within you
And where it goes to when it fades away.

Listen to the subtle, ever-changing tones,
Layer upon layer.
Discover what gradualness is.
The power of sound will lead you
Into the power of silence.

Syllables are born from space,
Resonate in space, then melt into spaciousness.
Know this silent spaciousness as your Self.

18

तन्त्र्यादिवाद्यशब्देषु दीर्घेषु क्रमसंस्थितेः ।
अनन्यचेताः प्रत्यन्ते परव्योमवपुर् भवेत् ॥४१॥

tantry ādi vādya śabdeṣu dīrgheṣu krama saṁsthiteḥ |
ananya cetāḥ pratyante para vyoma vapur bhavet || 41 ||

tantri aadi vaadya-shabdeshu deergheshu krama-sam-sthiteh
ananya–chetaah prati-ante para–vyoma vapuh bhavet

Immerse yourself in the rapture of music.
You know what you love. Go *there*.

Tend to each note, each chord,
Rising up from silence and dissolving again.

Vibrating strings draw us
Into the spacious resonance of the heart.

The body becomes light as the sky
And you, one with the Great Musician,
Who is even now singing us
Into existence.

19

पिण्डमन्त्रस्य सर्वस्य स्थूलवर्णक्रमेण तु ।
अर्धेन्दुबिन्दुनादान्तः शून्योच्चाराद् भवेच्छिवः ॥४२॥

piṇḍa mantrasya sarvasya sthūla varṇa krameṇa tu |
ardhendu bindu nādāntaḥ śūnyoccārād bhavec chivaḥ ॥ 42 ॥

*pinda–mantrasya sarvasya sthoola–varna–kramena tu
ardha–indu–bindu–naada–antah shoonyah ud–chaaraat bhavet shivah*

Bodies feed on sound.
Sonic waves on inner waters
Nourish every nerve.
Vibration strengthens bones.
Ecstatic undulation awaits you.

Take a bite of crunchy *K*, slippery *S*, a rugged *Rrrr.*
Enjoy a yummy vowel—*ah, ee, oo,* or *uu.*
Throw it in a bowl of *Mmmm.*

Treasure the impact on your tongue—
Kreem, Shreem, Raam, Yumm, Hreem, Laam.
Pronounce a sound out loud, then whisper softly.
Now hear with your inner ear.
Allow the resonance to enchant you within.
The sound goes on resounding, continuing of itself.
As the hum dissolves into silence,
Be nurtured
In the tenderness of infinite space.

20

निजदेहे सर्वदिक्कं युगपद् भावयेद् वियत् ।
निर्विकल्पमनास् तस्य वियत्सर्वम् प्रवर्तते ॥४३॥

nija dehe sarva dikkaṁ yugapad bhāvayed viyat |
nirvikalpa manās tasya viyat sarvam pravartate ‖ 43 ‖

*ni-ja–dehe sarva–dikkam yuga-pad bhaavayet viyat
nir-vi-kalpa–manaah tasya viyat sarvam pra-vartate*

———————

The radiance of space permeates the body
And all directions simultaneously.
Space is always here,
Already here before your noticing of it.

What we call space is a presence,
Permission to exist,
And worlds within which to express.

Without thinking about it,
Without forming mental images,
Rest in this vast expanse,
Friends with infinity.

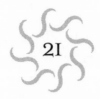

21

पृष्ठशून्यं मूलशून्यं युगपद् भावयेच् च यः ।
शरीरनिरपेक्षिण्या शक्त्या शून्यमना भवेत् ॥४४॥

prṣṭa śūnyaṁ mūla śūnyaṁ yugapad bhāvayec ca yaḥ |
śarīra nirapekṣiṇyā śaktyā śūnya manā bhavet || 44 ||

*prishtha-shoonyam moola-shoonyam yuga-pad bhaavayet cha yah
shareera nir-a-pekshinyaa shaktyaa shoonya–manaa bhavet*

Your back is a gateway to the sky.
The celestial dance,
The story of space and time,
Is coded in the spine.

Attend simultaneously
To the area around your tailbone,
Vibrating with luminous space,
And to the spine as a channel
Gushing with radiant emptiness.

Here,
Where particles flash in and out of existence,
Is the origin of mind.

22

पृष्ठशून्यं मूलशून्यं हृच्छून्यम् भावयेत्स्थिरम् ।
युगपन् निर्विकल्पत्वान् निर्विकल्पोदयस् ततः ॥४५॥

pṛṣṭa śūnyaṁ mūla śūnyaṁ hṛc chūnyam bhāvayet sthiram |
yugapan nirvikalpa tvān nirvikalpodayas tataḥ || 45 ||

*prishtha-shoonyam moola-shoonyam hrid-shoonyam bhaavayet sthiram
yuga-pat nir-vi-kalpa tvaat nir-vi-kalpah udayah tatah*

Behind the spine is infinity.
Below the perineum,
Invisible pulsating roots
Open downward into space.

The heart is wide as a spiral galaxy.

Steadily consider
Back, root, heart,
And know the living body of vastness
That you are.

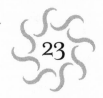

23

तनूदेशे शून्यतैव क्षणमात्रं विभावयेत् ।
निर्विकल्पं निर्विकल्पो निर्विकल्पस्वरूपभाक् ॥४६॥

tanū deśe śūnyataiva kṣaṇa mātraṁ vibhāvayet |
nirvikalpaṁ nirvikalpo nirvikalpa svarūpa bhāk || 46 ||

tanoo-deshe shoonyataa eva kshana–maatram vi-bhaavayet
nir-vi-kalpam nir-vi-kalpah nir-vi-kalpa sva-roopa–bhaaj

Forget all of your ideas about the body—
It's this way or it's that way.

Just be with any area of it,
This present body,
As permeated with limitless space,
Drenched in freedom.

24

सर्वं देहगतं द्रव्यं वियद्व्याप्तं मृगेक्षणे ।
विभावयेत्ततस् तस्य भावना सा स्थिरा भवेत् ॥४७॥

sarvaṁ deha gataṁ dravyaṁ viyad vyāptaṁ mṛgekṣaṇe |
vibhāvayet tatas tasya bhāvanā sā sthirā bhavet || 47 ||

*sarvam deha-gatam dravyam viyat-vi-aaptam mriga-eekshane
vi-bhaavayet tatas tasya bhaavanaa saa sthiraa bhavet*

This body is made of earth and gold,
Sky and stars, rivers and oceans,
Masquerading as muscle and bone.
Every substance is here:
Diamonds and silver, magical elixirs,
Ambrosia that gives visions,
Herbs that nourish and heal.
The foundation of the planet,
Immortal magnetic iron,
Circulating in the blood.

Every element in you loves the others:
Earth loves rain, sky loves sun,
Sun loves the space it shines through,
Space loves everyone equally.

In meditation, luxuriate in knowing this deep
    and simple truth.
Every cell is an organ of sense
Infused with majesty.

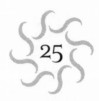

25

देहान्तरे त्वग्विभागम् भित्तिभूतं विचिन्तयेत् ।
न किञ्चिदन्तरे तस्य ध्यायन्न्ध्येयभाग् भवेत् ॥४८॥

dehāntare tvag vibhāgam bhitti bhūtaṁ vicintayet |
na kiñcid antare tasya dhyāyan na dhyeya bhāg bhavet || 48 ||

deha–antare tvak–vi–bhaagam bhitti–bhootam vi–chintayet
na kinchit antare tasya dhyaayam na dhyeya bhaaj bhavet

———————

Attend to the skin
As a subtle boundary
Containing vastness.

Enter that pulsing immensity.
Discover that you are not separate
From anything there.

There is no inside,
There is no outside,
There is no other—
No object to meditate upon that is not you.

26

हृद्याकाशे निलीनाक्षः पद्मसम्पुटमध्यगः ।
अनन्यचेताः सुभगे परं सौभाग्यमाप्नुयात् ॥४९॥

hṛdyākāśe nilīnākṣaḥ padma sampuṭa madhya gaḥ |
ananya cetāḥ subhage param saubhāgyam āpnuyāt || 49 ||

hridya–aakaashe nileena–akshah padma–sam–puta–madhya–gah
an–anya–chetaah su–bhage param sau–bhaagyam aapnuyaat

———————

The One Who Is at Play Everywhere says,

There is a space in the heart where everything meets.
Come here if you want to find me.
Mind, senses, soul, eternity—all are here.
Are you here?

Enter the bowl of vastness that is the heart.
Listen to the song that is always resonating.
Give yourself to it with total abandon.
Quiet ecstasy is here,
And a steady, regal sense
Of resting in a perfect spot.
You who are the embodiment of blessing,
Once you know the way,
The nature of attention will call you to return.
Again and again, answer that call,
And be saturated with knowing,
"I belong here, I am at home."

27

सर्वतः स्वशरीरस्य द्वादशान्ते मनोलयात् ।
दृढबुद्धेर् दृढीभूतं तत्त्वलक्ष्यम् प्रवर्तते ॥५०॥

sarvataḥ svaśarīrasya dvādaśānte manolayāt |
dṛḍha buddher dṛḍhī bhūtaṁ tattva lakṣyam pravartate || 50 ||

*sarvatah sva-shareerasya dvaa-dasha-ante mano-layaat
dridha–buddheh dridhee–bhootam tattva–lakshyam pra-vartate*

Put attention into the luminous connections
Between the centers of the body,
Where the mind loves to dissolve.

Base of the spine and top of the head.
Genitals and heart.
Heart and throat.
Throat and forehead.
Forehead and crown of the skull.

Enter that glowing net of light
With a focus born of awe,
And even your bones will know enlightenment.

28

यथा तथा यत्र तत्र द्वादशान्ते मनः क्षिपेत् ।
प्रतिक्षणं क्षीणवृत्तेर् वैलक्षण्यं दिनैर् भवेत् ॥५१॥

yathā tathā yatra tatra dvādaśānte manaḥ kṣipet |
prati kṣaṇam kṣīṇa vṛtter vailakṣaṇyam dinair bhavet || 51 ||

yathaa–tathaa yatra–tatra dvaada–shaante manah kshipet
prati-kshanam ksheena–vritteh vai-lakshanyam dinaih bhavet

This body is sustained by altars
To the radiant nectar of life—
Around you, an ocean of air
Ready to become your breath.
Above the head, the glow of an invisible sun.
Within the spaciousness of the heart,
A pulsing throb of creation,
Where the breaths meet, fuse,
And transform into each other.

Whenever, wherever your mind wanders,
Whatever you wonder,
Return to the luminous.
Choose any altar—
Throw your attention again and again
Into one of these centers where spirit and flesh
Consummate their love.
Day by day, old whirlpools fade, the endless circles.
You are living in the temple of essence.

29

कालाग्निना कालपदाद् उत्थितेन स्वकम् पुरम् ।
पुष्टम् विचिन्तयेद् अन्ते शान्ताभासस् तदा भवेत् ॥५२॥

kālāgninā kāla padād utthitena svakam puram |
pluṣṭam vicintayed ante śāntābhāsas tadā bhavet || 52 ||

*kaala–agninaa kaala–padaat ud-thitena svakam puram
plushtam vi-chintayet ante shaanta–aa-bhaasah tadaa bhavet*

———————

Live for a few days in the meditation,
"I am immersed in the flame—
The flame of time,
The flame of love,
The flame of life.
The universal fire flows through me."

Step into that fire wholeheartedly,
Starting with the big toe,
Then surrendering everywhere.
Only the not-self,
Which doesn't exist anyway,
Burns away.

Attend to this continually,
And awaken into tranquility.
Your essence is renewed in the flame,
For it *is* flame and knows itself as flame
Since the first heartbeat of creation.

एवम् एव जगत्सर्वं दग्धं ध्यात्वा विकल्पतः ।
अनन्यचेतसः पुंसः पुम्भावः परमो भवेत् ॥५३॥

evam eva jagat sarvaṁ dagdhaṁ dhyātvā vikalpataḥ |
ananya cetasaḥ puṁsaḥ pumbhāvaḥ paramo bhavet || 53 ||

evam eva jagat sarvam dagdham dhyaatvaa vi-kalpatah
an-anya–chetasah pumsah pum-bhaavah paramah bhavet

———————

Imagine the entire world consumed by flame.
Stay steady, do not waver,
As fire transmutes form into light.
The soul reveals itself
To itself as Radiance.

31

स्वदेहे जगतो वापि सूक्ष्मसूक्ष्मतराणि च ।
तत्त्वानि यानि निलयं ध्यात्वान्ते व्यज्यते परा ॥५४॥

svadehe jagato vāpi sūkṣma sūkṣmatarāṇi ca |
tattvāni yāni nilayaṁ dhyātvānte vyajyate parā || 54 ||

sva-dehe jagatah vaa api sookshma–sookshma-taraani cha
tattvaani yaani ni-layam dhyaatva–ante vi-ajyate paraa

———————

Experience the substance of the body
And the world
As made up of vibrating particles,
And these particles made up of
Even finer energies.
Drifting more deeply,
Feel into each pulse of energy
As it condenses from infinity
And dissolves back into it
Continuously.

Noticing this, breathe easily
With infinity dancing everywhere.

32

पिनां च दुर्बलां शर्कित ध्यात्वा द्वादशगोचरे ।
प्रविश्य हृदये ध्यायन् मुक्तः स्वातन्त्र्यमाप्नुयात् ॥५५॥

pīnāṁ ca durbalāṁ śaktiṁ dhyātvā dvādaśa gocare |
praviśya hṛdaye dhyāyan muktaḥ svātantryam āpnuyāt || 55 ||

peenam cha dur-balaam shaktim dhyaatvaa dvaa-dasha–gochare
pra-vishya hridaye dhyaayam muktah svaa–tantryam aapnuyaat

Strong or soft, wild or serene—
Wherever breath flows there is song.
Hear its whisper touching behind the face,
Singing in the throat,
Dancing spirals in the sanctuary of your heart.

In this practice of listening,
A moment may come when you just want to lie down.
This is a doorway—surrender.
Fall into the wide-open embrace of life.
You are the instrument breath is playing.

All the meditations you have ever loved
Are vibrating in this luxurious hum,
Continuing even in sleep and dreams.
This is your school. Just you and infinity.
The texture of the Self is untamed freedom.

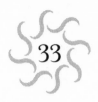

33

भुवनाध्वादिरूपेण चिन्तयेत्क्रमशोऽखिलम् ।
स्थूलसूक्ष्मपरस्थित्या यावद् अन्ते मनोलयः ॥५६॥

bhuvanādhvādi rūpeṇa cintayet kramaśo'khilam |
sthūla sūkṣma parasthityā yāvad ante manolayaḥ || 56 ||

*bhuvana adhva aadi roopena chintayet kramashah a-khilam
stoola–sookshma–para–sthityaa yaavat ante manas–layah*

———————

This whole universe is a path of liberation,
A vast arena for your endless play.

Playing, let your awareness be everywhere at once.
Planets, stars, swirling galaxies, subatomic motes—
All are dancing within you.

Enter the rhythm,
Descend into the space between beats.
Dissolve into intimacy with the Dancing One.

34

अस्य सर्वस्य विश्वस्य पर्यन्तेषु समन्ततः ।
अध्वप्रक्रियया तत्त्वं शैवं ध्यत्वा महोदयः ॥५७॥

asya sarvasya viśvasya pary anteṣu samantataḥ |
adhva prakriyayā tattvaṁ śaivaṁ dhyatvā mahodayaḥ || 57 ||

asya sarvasya vishvasya pari–anteshu sam-antatah
adhva pra-kriyayaa tattvam shaivam dhyaatvaa maha–udayah

The air I am breathing was exhaled in ecstasy
By an ancient sun.
This earth I am standing on
Was born of cosmic fire.
The blood flowing through my veins
Is as salty as the primordial ocean.
The space permeating my body
Is infinite as the space all around.

Above, below, to all sides, within,
The elements of the universe
Are engaged in their ceremony of delight.

This is my religion.
The attraction between suns
Is the same
As the love pulsating in my heart.

35

विश्वम् एतन् महादेवि शून्यभूतं विचिन्तयेत् ।
तत्रैव च मनो लीनं ततस् तल्लयभाजनम् ॥५८॥

viśvam etan mahā devi śūnya bhūtaṁ vicintayet |
tatraiva ca mano līnaṁ tatas tal laya bhājanam || 58 ||

vishvam etan mahaa–devi shoonya–bhootam vi-chintayet
tatra eva cha manah leenam tatah tat laya bhaajanam

———————

Shining One,

Breathing out, let go
And fall into knowing all of creation
As existing within space,
And you are absorbed in that
Vibrant empty fullness.
In this moment your body is intimate
With space, exchanging essence for essence.

Balancing in the midst of vast emptiness,
Know utter freedom.

36

घतादिभाजने दृष्टिम् भित्तिस् त्यक्त्वा विनिक्षिपेत् ।
तल्लयं तत्क्षणाद् गत्वा तल्लयात्तन्मयो भवेत् ॥५९॥

ghatādi bhājane dṛṣṭim bhittis tyaktvā vinikṣipet |
tal layaṁ tat kṣaṇād gatvā tal layāt tan mayo bhavet || 59 ||

ghata aadi bhaajane drishtim bhittih tyaktvaa vi-ni-kshipet
tat–layam tat–kshanaat gatvaa tat–layaat tat–mayah bhavet

Space is worthy of worship and wonder.
It is the field within which every thing exists.
Rest your eyes in emptiness,
Inside a room, a temple, even a little jar—
Any contained space.

Throw the one who is seeing into the center.
Entrust your mind to the embrace of space.
In a flash, all boundaries dissolve.

37

निर्वृक्षगिरिभित्त्यादिदेशे दृष्टिं विनिक्षिपेत् ।
विलीने मानसे भावे वृत्तिक्षिणः प्रजायते ॥६०॥

nirvṛkṣa giri bhitty ādi deśe dṛṣṭiṁ vinikṣipet |
vilīne mānase bhāve vṛtti kṣiṇaḥ prajāyate || 60 ||

*nir-vriksha–giri–bhitti aadi deshe drishtim vi-ni-kshipet
vi-leene manase bhaave vritti–ksheenah pra-jaayate*

———————

Go to a wide-open space,
Gaze without looking anywhere.

The mind stops its building of thoughts,
And rests on its own foundation—
Immensity.

The light that you see by
Is the light that comes from inside.

38

उभयोर् भावयोर् ज्ञाने ध्यात्वा मध्यं समाश्रयेत् ।
युगपच् च द्वयं त्यक्त्वा मध्ये तत्त्वम् प्रकाशते ॥६१॥

ubhayor bhāvayor jñāne dhyātvā madhyaṁ samāśrayet |
yugapac ca dvayaṁ tyaktvā madhye tattvam prakāśate || 61 ||

ubhayoh bhaavayoh jnaane dhyaatvaa madhyam sam-aashrayet
yuga-pad cha dvayam tyaktvaa madhye tattvam pra-kaashate

Watch for a moment in which
Two opposing perceptions occur—
    Wanting to go and not going,
    Knowing and simultaneously not knowing.

In the midst of this dilemma,
Let go of both perceptions
And jump in to the interval between.

Reality flashes forth.
Your being is the shining field of awareness,
The continuum in which the opposites play.

भावे त्यक्ते निरुद्धा चिन् नैव भावान्तरं व्रजेत् ।
तदा तन्मध्यभावेन विकसत्यति भावना ॥६२॥

bhāve tyakte niruddhā cin naiva bhāvāntaraṁ vrajet |
tadā tan madhya bhāvena vikasatyati bhāvanā || 62 ||

bhaave tyakte ni-ruddhaa chit na eva bhaava—antaram vrajet
tadaa tat madhya bhaavena vi-kasatyati bhaavanaa

Cast aside the ten thousand things,
And love only one.
Don't go on to another.

Engage your lively awareness
With this one focus—
One object, one thought, one symbol.
Now go inside.
Find the center,
The soul, the heart.

Right here,
In the middle of the feeling,
Attend the blossoming—
Attention vast as the sky.

40

सर्वं देहं चिन्मयं हि जगद् वा परिभावयेत् ।
युगपन् निर्विकल्पेन मनसा परमोदयः ॥६३॥

sarvaṁ dehaṁ cin mayaṁ hi jagad vā paribhāvayet |
yugapan nirvikalpena manasā paramodayaḥ || 63 ||

sarvam deham chit–mayam hi jagatvaa pari-bhaavayet
yuga-pad nir-vi-kalpena manasaa parama–udayah

Delight in this entire universe
As permeated with divine awareness,
And every area of your body—
Your feet, your face, your shoulders—
Made out of divine awareness.

The body of the planet beneath you,
Out beyond the farthest horizons,
The stars and the reaches of space—
All are arising from God-consciousness.

Know this, and dissolve into peace.

41

वायुद्वयस्य सङ्घट्टाद् अन्तर् वा बहिर् अन्ततः ।
योगी समत्वविज्ञानसमुद्गमनभाजनम् ॥६४॥

vāyu dvayasya saṅghaṭṭād antar vā bahir antataḥ |
yogī samatva vijñāna samudgamana bhājanam || 64 ||

*vaayu dvayasya sanghattaat antar vaa bahir–antatah
yogee samatva vi-jnaana sam-ud-gamana bhaajanam*

Breathing is the flow of the divine,
Where the rhythms of life turn into each other—
The eternal exchange.

Pour one breath into the other,
Outbreath into the inbreath
Into the outbreath.

Awaken to equanimity,
At peace in the play of opposites.

42

सर्वं जगत्स्वदेहं वा स्वानन्दभरितं स्मरेत् ।
युगपत्स्वामृतेनैव परानन्दमयो भवेत् ॥६५॥

sarvaṁ jagat svadehaṁ vā svānanda bharitaṁ smaret |
yugapat svāmṛtenaiva parānanda mayo bhavet || 65 ||

*sarvam–jagat sva-deham vaa sva-aananda–bharitam smaret
yuga-pad sva-amritena eva para–aananda–mayah bhavet*

With one sweep of attention,
Gather in the whole universe
And remember it
As your body of bliss.

The deep rhythms of life,
Pulsating,
Stir an ambrosia
Flowing and overflowing everywhere.

Drink the nectar
Of all-pervading joy
From the radiant cup
That is this very body.

43

कुहनेन प्रयोगेण सद्य एव मृगेक्षणे ।
समुदेति महानन्दो येन तत्त्वं प्रकाशते ॥६६॥

kuhanena prayogeṇa sadya eva mṛgekṣaṇe |
samudeti mahānando yena tattvaṁ prakāśate || 66 ||

*kuhanena pra-yogena sadya eva mriga–eekshane
sam-udeti mahaa–aanandah yena tattvam pra-kaashate*

———————

You Whose Existence Melts Me,

Whenever you dissolve into helpless laughter—
Transported by a magic show,
Antics or jokes,
Having your armpits tickled,
Drenched by a sudden shower,
Or any of Nature's tricks—

Dive into the *source* of that laughter.
Surrender to the surge of joy
Illuminating the essence of reality.

सर्वस्रोतोनिबन्धेन प्राणशक्त्योर्ध्वया शनैः ।
पिपीलस्पर्शवेलायाम् प्रथते परमं सुखम् ॥६७॥

sarva sroto nibandhena prāṇa śaktyordhvayā śanaiḥ |
pipīla sparśa velāyām prathate paramaṁ sukham || 67 ||

sarva srotah ni-bandhana praana–shakti–oordhvayaa shanaih
pipeela–sparsha–velaayaam prathate paramam sukham

Rivers of power flowing everywhere.
Fields of magnetism relating everything.
This is your origin. This is your lineage.

The current of creation is right here,
Coursing through subtle channels,
Animating this very form.
Follow the gentle touch of life,
Soft as the footprint of an ant,
As tiny sensations open to vastness.

Power sings as it flows,
Electrifies the organs of sensing,
Becomes liquid light,
Nourishes your entire being.
Celebrate the boundary
Where streams join the sea,
Where body meets infinity.

45

वह्नेर् विषस्य मध्ये तु चित्तं सुखमयं क्षिपेत् ।
केवलं वायुपूर्णं वा स्मरानन्देन युज्यते ॥६८॥

vahner viṣasya madhye tu cittaṁ sukha mayaṁ kṣipet |
kevalaṁ vāyu pūrṇaṁ vā smarānandena yujyate || 68 ||

vahneh vishasya madhye tu chittam–sukha–mayam kshipet
kevalam vaayu–poornam vaa smara–aanandena yujyate

––––––––––

As the fires build in sexual joy,
Enter that blessed place between the legs,
Embrace the holy energies shimmering there.

Follow the rising flow,
Undulating throughout the spine,
Shivering with pleasure.

As the fire intensifies
And flashes upwards,
Suspend the breath for a moment.
Throw your whole self in.

Become brilliance in your bodily form,
In union with primordial bliss.

46

शक्तिसङ्गमसङ्क्षुब्धशक्त्यावेशावसानिकम् ।
यत्सुखम् ब्रह्मतत्त्वस्य तत्सुखं स्वाक्यम् उच्यते ॥६९॥

śakti saṅgama saṅkṣubdha śakty āveśāvasānikam |
yat sukham brahma tattvasya tat sukhaṁ svākyam ucyate || 69 ||

*shakti–sangama sam-kshubdha shakti–aa-vesha ava-saanikam
yat sukham brahma tattvasya tat sukham svaakyam uchyate*

At the moment of orgasm
The truth is illumined—
The one everyone longs for.

Lovemaking is riding the currents of excitation
Into revelation.
Two rivers flow together,
The body becomes *quivering.*

No inside and no outside—
Only the delight of union.
The mind releases itself into divine energy,
And the body knows where it came from.

This is reality, and it is always here.
Everyone craves the source,
And it is always everywhere.

47

लेहनामन्थनाकोटैः स्त्रीसुखस्य भरात्स्मृतेः ।
शक्त्यभावेऽपि देवेशि भवेद् आनन्दसम्प्लवः ॥७०॥

lehanā manthanākoṭaiḥ strī sukhasya bharāt smṛteḥ |
śakty abhāve'pi deveśi bhaved ānanda samplavaḥ || 70 ||

lehanaa manthanaa aa-koṭaih stree-sukhasya bharaat smriteh
shakti–a-bhaave api deveshi bhavet aananda–sam-plavah

When by oneself, flooded with delight,
Simply in the memory of that kiss . . .
Here is the inner ritual.

That lick, that taste of nectar,
That caress, embrace, particular pressure . . .
Your subtle body replays the dance,
Inundated by divine sensations.
Melting, merging, swelling . . .

Surrender to the deluge.
Know it as your own.
This ocean of bliss is you.

आनन्दे महति प्राप्ते दृष्टे वा बान्धवे चिरात् ।
आनन्दम् उद्गतं ध्यात्वा तल्लयस् तन्मना भवेत् ॥७१॥

ānande mahati prāpte dṛṣṭe vā bāndhave cirāt |
ānandam udgataṁ dhyātvā tal layas tan manā bhavet || 71 ||

aanande mahati praapte drishte vaa baandhave chiraat
aanandam ud-gatam dhyaatvaa tat–layah tat–manaa bhavet

In the great joy of seeing
A loved one after a long absence,
A flash of recognition ignites you.
Space becomes charged,
The bond between you shimmers,
And a surge of delight arises in your being.

Beloved,
Find within you the source of this surge.
Melt into that place of upwelling,
A wave rolling in a vast ocean of delight.

49

जग्धिपानकृतोल्लासरसानन्दविजृम्भणात् ।
भावयेद् भरितावस्थां महानन्दस् ततो भवेत् ॥७२॥

jagdhi pāna kṛtollāsa rasānanda vijṛmbhaṇāt |
bhāvayed bharitāvasthāṁ mahānandas tato bhavet || 72 ||

*jagdhi–paana krita–ullaasa rasa–aananda vi–jrimbhanaat
bhaavayet bharitaa–ava–sthaam mahaa–aanandah tatah bhavet*

Tasting dark chocolate,
A ripe apricot,
A luscious elixir—
Savor the expanding joy in your body.
Nature is offering herself to you.
How astonishing
To realize this world can taste so good.

When sipping some ambrosia,
Raise your glass,
Close your eyes,
Toast the universe.
The Sun and Moon and Earth
Danced together
To bring you this delight.
Receive the nectar on your tongue
As a kiss of the divine.

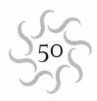

50

गितादिविषयास्वादासमसौख्यैकतात्मनः ।
योगिनस् तन्मयत्वेन मनोरूढेस् तदात्मता ॥७३॥

gitādi viṣayāsvādā sama saukhyaikatāt manaḥ |
yoginas tan mayatvena mano rūḍhes tad ātmatā || 73 ||

geetaa aadi vishaya–aasvaadaa sama–saukhya eka–tat–manah
yoginah tat–mayatvena manas–roodheh tat–aatmataa

———————

All around you, in every moment,
The world is offering a feast for your senses.
Songs are playing,
Tasty food is on the table,
Fragrances are in the air,
Colors fill the eyes with light.

You who long for union,
Attend this banquet with loving focus.
The outer and inner worlds
Open to each other.
Oneness of vision, oneness of heart.

Right here, in the midst of it all,
Mount that elation, ascend with it,
Become identical
With the ecstatic essence
Embracing both worlds.

51

यत्र यत्र मनस् तुष्टिर् मनस् तत्रैव धारयेत् ।
तत्र तत्र परानन्दस्वारूपं सम्प्रवर्तते ॥७४॥

yatra yatra manas tuṣṭir manas tatraiva dhārayet |
tatra tatra parānanda svārūpaṁ sampravartate || 74 ||

yatra–yatra manas–tushtih manas tatra eva dhaarayet
tatra–tatra paraa–aananda sva-roopam sam-pra-vartate

Wherever, whenever you feel carried away,
Rejoicing in every breath,
There, there is your meditation hall.

Cherish these times of absorption—
    Rocking the baby in the silence of the night,
    Pouring water into a crystal glass,
    Tending the logs in a crackling fire,
    Sharing a meal with a circle of friends.
Embrace these pleasures and know,
"This is my true body."

Nowhere is more holy than this.
Right here is the sacred pilgrimage.
Live in alertness for such a moment, my Beloved,
As if it were your one meeting with the Creator.

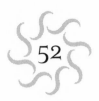

52

अनागतायां निद्रायाम् प्रणष्टे बाह्यगोचरे ।
सावस्था मनसा गम्या परा देवी प्रकाशते ॥७५॥

anāgatāyāṁ nidrāyām praṇaṣṭe bāhya gocare |
sāvasthā manasā gamyā parā devī prakāśate || 75 ||

an-aa-gataayaam nidraayam pra-nashte baahya–gochare
saa ava-sthaa manasaa gamyaa paraa–devee pra-kaashate

When sleep has not yet come,
And the sweet buzz of exhaustion
Permeates the body,
Linger in the *ahhhh* of relief
As your head touches the pillow.

Everything in you is yearning to let go.
So let go, let your body fall
Into something deeper than sleep.
With your mind, enter
The soft luminous glow of the soul.

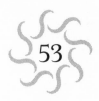

53

तेजसा सूर्यदीपादेर् आकाशे शबलीकृते ।
दृष्टिर् निवेश्या तत्रैव स्वात्मरूपम् प्रकाशते ॥७६॥

tejasā sūrya dīpāder ākāśe śabalī kṛte |
dṛṣṭir niveśyā tatraiva svātma rūpam prakāśate || 76 ||

*tejasaa–soorya–deepaadeh aakaashe shabalee–krite
drishtih–ni–veshyaa tatra eva sva–aatma–roopam pra–kaashate*

Gaze out at space,
Aware of multicolored luminosity
Permeating everywhere . . .

The blue sky, filled with rays from the sun.
The night sky, dark, yet crisscrossed by
The light of a billion stars.
How can this be?

All space is the same,
Inside you and far away.
Lose yourself in spaciousness,
Come home to your true Self.

54

करङ्किण्या क्रोधनया भैरव्या लेलिहानया ।
खेचर्या दृष्टिकाले च परावाप्तिः प्रकाशते ॥७७॥

karaṅkiṇyā krodhanayā bhairavyā lelihānayā |
khecaryā dṛṣṭi kāle ca parāvāptiḥ prakāśate || 77 ||

karankinyaa krodhanayaa bhairavyaa leli–haanayaa
kecharyaa drishti–kaale cha paraa–ava-aaptih pra-kaashate

———————

You who have been seeking, whatever path you are on,
A moment will come when
Divine pulsation grabs you
And carries you into its dance.
In the midst of ecstatic motion,
  Your body dissolves into light, leaving only
  The softly glowing benediction of the bones.
  You become the face of fury, yet serene within.
  Eyes fly open in amazement,
  Seeing the unseen vastness.
  Or you become a tongue tasting upward
  Into the nectar of eternity.

The soul reveals itself to itself
Through movement,
Energy-infused undulations and gestures
Of hand, foot, spine, face, and form.
The invisible loves the visible.

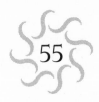

55

मृद्वासने स्फिजैकेन हस्तपादौ निराश्रयम् ।
निधाय तत्प्रसङ्गेण परा पूर्णा मतिर् भवेत् ॥७८॥

mṛdvāsane sphijaikena hastapādau nirāśrayam |
nidhāya tat prasaṅgeṇa parā pūrṇā matir bhavet || 78 ||

*mridu–aasane sphijaikena hasta–paadau nir–aashrayam
ni–dhaaya tat pra–sangena paraa–poornaa matih bhavet*

Sit in any relaxed, comfortable pose.
Experience the earth below
As insubstantial, a pillow of air—
Air that is always vibrating,
Minute particles in ecstatic motion.

Poised here,
No support below, no support above,
No support for the feet or hands,
No support for the mind,
Be completely at peace!

56

उपविश्यासने सम्यग् बाहू कृत्वार्धकुञ्चितौ ।
कक्षव्योम्नि मनः कुर्वन् शममायाति तल्लयात् ॥७९॥

upaviśyāsane samyag bāhū kṛtvārdha kuñcitau |
kakṣa vyomni manaḥ kurvan śamam āyāti tal layāt || 79 ||

*upa-vishya aasane sam-yak baahoo kritva ardha-kunchitau
kaksha–vyomni manah kurvan shamam aayaati tat–layaat*

Oceans embrace a continent.
Space welcomes the sun.
Embrace yourself this generously.

Form your arms into a circle
And cherish the arising of serenity.

Attend the birth of something new.
Thoughts dissolve into peace,
As you become the One who embraces All.

57

स्थूलरूपस्य भावस्य स्तब्धां दृष्टिं निपात्य च ।
अचिरेण निराधारं मनः कृत्वा शिवं व्रजेत् ॥८०॥

sthūla rūpasya bhāvasya stabdhāṁ dṛṣṭiṁ nipātya ca |
acireṇa nirādhāraṁ manaḥ kṛtvā śivaṁ vrajet || 80 ||

*sthoola–roopasya bhaavasya stabdhaam drishtim ni-paatya cha
achirena nir-aa-dhaaram manah kritvaa shivam vrajet*

Find something so enchanting to behold
That you are transfixed—ravished.
Allow yourself to be captivated.

Gaze upon its form
With the eyes of wonder.
Attend to details—
This shape, texture, these colors . . .
How can something so beautiful possibly exist?

With a steady gaze, melt into
The field of space embracing that form.
At once,
Be at one with the Creator, who is
Looking through your eyes, loving creation.

58

मध्यजिह्वे स्फारितास्ये मध्ये निक्षिप्य चेतनाम् ।
होच्चारं मनसा कुर्वंस् ततः शान्ते प्रलीयते ॥८१॥

madhya jihve sphāritāsye madhye nikṣipya cetanām |
hoccāraṁ manasā kurvaṁs tataḥ śānte pralīyate || 81 ||

madhya jihve sphaaritaasye madhye ni–kshipya chetanaam
ho—ud-chaaram manasaa kurvan tatah shaante pra-leeyate

The tongue is made of truth and flame.
On it dance the triple fires of spirit, body, soul.

Trace this dance from the depths of your core,
Rising upward through the crown of your being.
Every offering of breath and food
Feeds this holy flame.

Touch the tip of the tongue
To the roof of the mouth, lightly.
Inquire into the luminosity above.
Breathe out with a quiet *h a a a a a.*

You are an altar to the flame of life.
Throw yourself into the throbbing intensity.
Become this dance,
Absorbed in radiant splendor.

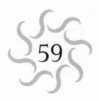

59

आसने शयने स्थित्वा निराधारं विभावयन् ।
स्वदेहं मनसि क्षिणे क्षणात्क्षीणाशयो भवेत् ॥८२॥

āsane śayane sthitvā nirādhāraṁ vibhāvayan |
svadehaṁ manasi kṣiṇe kṣaṇāt kṣīṇāśayo bhavet || 82 ||

*asane shayane sthitvaa nir-aa-dhaaram vi-bhaavayan
sva-deham manasi ksheene kshanaat ksheena-aa-shayah bhavet*

———————————

Sitting on a soft seat,
Or lying on your mat,
Experience the space below
As offering no support.

You are simply suspended,
Floating in space.

Structures of the mind release.
The reservoir of habits dissolves.
In an instant, lifetimes of patterns
Vanish.

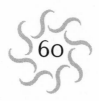

60

चलासने स्थितस्याथ शनैर् वा देहचालनात् ।
प्रशान्ते मानसे भावे देवि दिव्यौघमाप्नुयात् ॥८३॥

calāsane sthitas yātha śanair vā deha cālanāt |
praśānte mānase bhāve devi divyaughamāpnuyāt || 83 ||

chal-aasane sthitasya-atha shanaih vaa deha–chaalanaat
pra-shaante maanase bhaave devi divya–augham aapnuyaat

Rocking, undulating, swaying,
Carried by rhythm,
Cherish the streaming energy
Flooding your body
As a current of the divine.

Oh Radiant One,
Ride the waves of ecstatic motion
Into a sublime fusion
Of passion and peace.

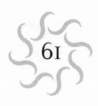

61

आकाशं विमलम् पश्यन् कृत्वा दृष्टिं निरन्तराम् ।
स्तब्धात्मा तत्क्षणाद् देवि भैरवं वपुर् आप्नुयात् ॥८४॥

ākāśaṁ vimalam paśyan kṛtvā dṛṣṭiṁ nirantarām |
stabdhātmā tat kṣaṇād devi bhairavaṁ vapur āpnuyāt || 84 ||

*aakaasham vi-malam pashyan kritvaa drishtim nir-antaraam
stabdha–aatma tat-kshanaat devi bhairavam–vapuh aapnuyaat*

———————

Adorable One,

Sit or lie down, completely immobile,
Beholding the cloudless sky—
Or if there are clouds, the sky beyond.

As vastness envelops you,
The body vanishes,
Thoughts forget to come.
In this moment,
You are the nature of the great sky.

62

लीनं मूर्धिन वियत्सर्वम् भैरवत्वेन भावयेत् ।
तत्सर्वम् भैरवाकारतेजस्तत्त्वं समाविशेत् ॥८५॥

līnam mūrdhni viyat sarvam bhairavatvena bhāvayet |
tat sarvam bhairavākāra tejas tattvam samāviśet || 85 ||

leenam moordhni viyat sarvam bhairavatvena bhaavayet
tat sarvam bhairava–aa-kaara tejas–tattvam sam-aa-vishet

Enter the space inside your head.
See it as already infinite,
Extending forever in all directions.

This spaciousness that you are
Is permeated by luminosity.
Know this radiance
As the soul of the world.

63

किञ्चिज् ज्ञातं द्वैतदायि बाह्यालोकस् तमः पुन।
विश्वादि भैरवं रूपं ज्ञात्वानन्तप्रकाशभृत् ॥८६॥

kiñcij jñātaṁ dvaitadāyi bāhyālokas tamaḥ punaḥ |
viśvādi bhairavaṁ rūpaṁ jñātvānanta prakāśabhṛt || 86 ||

*kinchit jnaatam dvaitadaayi baahya–aa-lokah tamah punah
vishva aadi bhairavam–roopam jnaatvaa an-anta–pra-kaasha–bhrit*

Dreaming, dreaming, sleeping, awakening—
Rhythms of darkness and light.
Day and night, night and day, wondering . . .
Who am I? Who AM I?
Who is morphing through this
Ever-shifting flow?

Beloved, wake up!
Dance in your true body before time,
Shimmering energy without end.

64

एवम् एव दुर्निशायां कृष्णपक्षागमे चिरम् ।
तैमिरम् भावयन् रूपम् भैरवं रूपम् एष्यति ॥८७॥

evam eva durniśāyāṁ kṛṣṇa pakṣāgame ciram |
taimiram bhāvayan rūpam bhairavaṁ rūpam eṣyati || 87 ||

evam eva dur–ni–shaayaam krishna–paksha–aa–game chiram
taimiram–bhaavayan–roopam bhairavam–roopam eshyati

Secrets are hidden in darkness
And difficult nights.
You awaken into a pang of aloneness,
A howl of separation.

This is the call of the Dark One,
The roar of life seeking its source.
The union you long for is within reach.

Throw off all hesitation.
Become one with the fear.
Plunge into the uncanny blackness,
Eyes wide open,
As if there were no other choice.

Vibrating with fierce tenderness,
Breathe intimately
With the Lord of Infinite Space.

65

एवम् एव निमील्यादौ नेत्रे कृष्णाभमग्रतः ।
प्रसार्य भैरवं रूपम् भावयंस् तन्मयो भवेत् ॥८८॥

evam eva nimīlyādau netre kṛṣṇābhamagrataḥ |
prasārya bhairavaṁ rūpam bhāvayaṁs tan mayo bhavet || 88 ||

evam eva ni-meelyaadau–netre krishna–abham–a-gratah
pra-saarya bhairavam-roopam bhaavayan tat–mayah bhavet

Close your eyes and imagine
An expanse of terrible darkness surrounds you—
No objects, no light, no moon, no stars—
Nothing but blackness spreading to infinity.

Do not shrink in terror; do not turn away.
Give yourself to the blackness
With no hope of light.
Surrender completely.

Contemplating this feeling,
Merge with the mystery of night.

66

यस्य कस्येन्द्रियस्यापि व्याघाताच् च निरोधतः ।
प्रविष्टस्याद्वये शून्ये तत्रैवात्मा प्रकाशते ॥८९॥

yasya kasyendriyasyāpi vyāghātāc ca nirodhataḥ |
praviṣṭasyādvaye śūnye tatraivātmā prakāśate || 89 ||

*yasya–kasya indriyasya api vi-aa-ghaataat cha ni-rodhatah
pra-vishtasya advaye shoonye tatra eva aatmaa pra-kaashate*

Whenever any of the senses is impaired
It becomes a gateway to infinity.

Whether by deprivation, injury, or age,
Obstruction of the senses
Invites awareness of Soul.

The mind can no longer take the world for granted.
Attention spirals inward,
And touches the glistening emptiness—
The reality behind appearance.

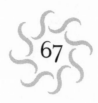

67

अबिन्दुमविसर्गं च अकारं जपतो महान् ।
उदेति देवि सहसा ज्ञानौघः परमेश्वरः ॥९०॥

abindum avisargaṁ ca akāraṁ japato mahān |
udeti devi sahasā jñānaughaḥ parameśvaraḥ || 90 ||

*a-bindum a-visargam cha a-kaaram japatah mahaan
udeti devi sahasaa jnaana–aughah parama–eeshvarah*

———————

Shining One, whose body flows with power—

When you are astonished,
Startled or afraid,
And gasp, a shocked inhalation—*AH!*
Right there, right there,
Sense the vibration of that gasp on your palette.

The shimmer of that sound in the mouth
Evokes a flood of knowing,
A gush of the divine.

68

वर्णस्य सविसर्गस्य विसर्गान्तं चितिं कुरु ।
निराधारेण चित्तेन स्पृशेद् ब्रह्म सनातनम् ॥९१॥

varṇasya savisargasya visargāntaṁ citiṁ kuru |
nirādhāreṇa cittena spṛśed brahma sanātanam || 91 ||

*varnasya sa-vi-sargasya vi-sarga–antam chitim kuru
nir-aa-dhaarena chittena sprishet brahma–sanaatanam*

Listen to the inner sound,
The one that you rode outward
Into this life,
Into this manifestation of yourself.

Savor the sound of *h h h a a a . . . ,*
Softly continuing, resonating through
All the nerves of your body, permeating,
Expanding everywhere.

Know this as the sound of ongoing creation.

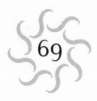

69

व्योमाकारं स्वमात्मानं ध्यायेद् दिग्भिर् अनावृतम् ।
निराश्रया चितिः शक्तिः स्वरूपं दर्शयेत्तदा ॥९२॥

vyomākāraṁ svamātmānaṁ dhyāyed digbhir anāvṛtam |
nirāśrayā citiḥ śaktiḥ svarūpaṁ darśayet tadā || 92 ||

vyoma–aa-kaaram svam-aatmaanam dhyaayet digbhih an-aa-vritam
nir-aa-shrayaa chitih shaktih sva-roopam darshayet tadaa

―――――――

Meditate on the Self as being
Vast as the sky,
A body of energy
Extending forever in all directions—
Above, below, all around.

In the embrace of infinite space,
Awaken to your true form—
Divine creative energy
Revealing Herself as you.

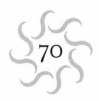

किञ्चिद् अङ्गं विभिद्यादौ तीक्ष्णसूच्यादिना ततः ।
तत्रैव चेतनां युक्त्वा भैरवे निर्मला गतिः ॥९३॥

kiñcid aṅgaṁ vibhidyādau tīkṣṇa sūcyādinā tataḥ |
tatraiva cetanāṁ yuktvā bhairave nirmalā gatiḥ || 93 ||

kinchit angam–vi-bhidya–adau teekshna–soochi–aadi naa tatah
tatra eva chetanaam yuktvaa bhairave nir-malaa gatih

Sting of a wasp.
Rip of a nail.
A razor's slice.
The needle's plunge.
A piercing word.
A stab of betrayal.
The boundary crossed.
A trust broken.
In this lacerating moment,
Pain is all you know.
Life is tattooing scripture into your flesh,
Scribing incandescence in your nerves.
Right here,
In this single searing point
Of intolerable concentration,
Wound becomes portal.
Brokenness surrenders to
Crystalline brilliance of Being.

71

चित्ताद्यन्तःकृतिर् नास्ति ममान्तर् भावयेद् इति ।
विकल्पानामभावेन विकल्पैर् उज्झितो भवेत् ॥९४॥

cittādy antaḥ kṛtir nāsti mamāntar bhāvayed iti |
vikalpānām abhāvena vikalpair ujjhito bhavet || 94 ||

chitta aadi antah–kritih na asti mama-antah bhaavayet iti
vi-kalpaanaam a-bhaavena vi-kalpaih ujjhitah bhavet

People talk about *mind* and *ego.*
Let's just drop this whole conversation.

Consider instead:
There is no mind.
There is no ego.

There is only the vivid reality
Of this surprising moment
At play, beckoning.

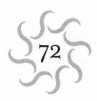

72

माया विमोहिनी नाम कलायाः कलनं स्थितम् ।
इत्यादिधर्मं तत्त्वानां कलयन् न पृथग् भवेत् ॥९५॥

māyā vimohinī nāma kalāyāḥ kalanaṁ sthitam |
ity ādi dharmaṁ tattvānāṁ kalayan na pṛthag bhavet || 95 ||

maayaa vi-mohinee naama kalaayaah kalanam sthitam
iti aadi dharmam–tattvanaam kalayan na prithak bhavet

The universe is here to reveal
Unlimited splendor—
Infinite diversity of expression.
No one can withstand her allure.

Adore the colors and shapes
Of her enchantment and know:
The One who permeates it all is a great lover.

Deeply relating above and below,
Mortal and immortal, transient and eternal,
Perceive the terrifying beauty.
Be free to suffer and to be thrilled,
To tolerate intolerable ravishment.

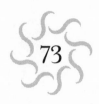

73

झगितीच्यां समुत्पन्नामवलोक्य शमं नयेत् ।
यत एव समुद्भूता ततस् तत्रैव लीयते ॥९६॥

jhagit īccāṁ samutpannām avalokya śamaṁ nayet |
yata eva samudbhūtā tatas tatraiva līyate || 96 ||

*jhagit ichchhaam sam-ut-pannaam ava-lokya shamam nayet
yata eva sam-ud-bhoota tatah tatra eva leeyate*

――――――――――

Just as a desire leaps up,
And you perceive the flash, the sparkle,
Quit from its play,
And maintain awareness
In that clear and shining place
From which all desire springs.

74

यदा ममेच्छा नोत्पन्ना ज्ञानं वा कस् तदास्मि वै ।
तत्त्वतोऽहं तथाभूतस् तल्लीनस् तन्मना भवेत् ॥९७॥

yadā mameccā notpannā jñānaṁ vā kas tadāsmi vai |
tattvato'haṁ tathā bhūtas tal līnas tan manā bhavet || 97 ||

yadaa mama ichchhaa na ut-pannaa jnaanam vaa kah tadaa asmi vai
tattvatah aham tathaa bhootah tat leenah tat–manaa bhavet

───────────

Radiant One, inquire:
Before desire arises in me, who am I?
Before I know anything, who am I?

Seek always the intimate joy
Of your original Self,
And move through this world in freedom.

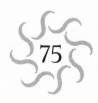

75

इच्छायामथवा ज्ञाने जाते चित्तं निवेशयेत् ।
आत्मबुद्ध्यानन्यचेतास् ततस् तत्त्वार्थदर्शनम् ॥९८॥

icchāyām atha vā jñāne jāte cittaṁ niveśayet |
ātma buddhy ānanya cetās tatas tattvārtha darśanam || 98 ||

ichchhaayaam atha vaa jnaane jaate chittam ni-veshayat
aatma–buddhyaa an-anya–chetaah tatah tattva–artha–darshanam

Whenever a wanting moment comes,
Celebrate the rising of desire
As a sparkling impulse of energy
Vibrating the body into motion.

In a flash of knowing,
When intelligence arises,
Attend to this rising
As the illumination of the Self.

Desiring and knowing,
Knowing and desiring.
Just for a breath,
Forget what you want.
Forget what you know.
Receive the real teaching,
The essence of Earth, Air,
Fire, Water, and Space.

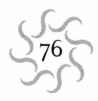

76

निर्निमित्तम् भवेज् ज्ञानं निराधारम् भ्रमात्मकम् ।
तत्त्वतः कस्यचिन् नैतद् एवम्भावी शिवः प्रिये ॥९९॥

nirnimittam bhavej jñānaṁ nirādhāram bhramātmakam |
tattvataḥ kasyacin naitad evam bhāvī śivaḥ priye || 99 ||

nir-nimittam bhavet jnaanam nir-aa-dhaaram bhrama–aatmakaam
tattvatah kasya chit na etat evam bhaavee shivah priye

———————

Beloved,

Reject the reality of everything.
Deny the universe of appearance.
Say no to the phenomenal world.
Reside in the secret place inside.

As joy rises in the heart
At this sudden freedom,
Enter there and dwell!

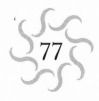

77

चिद्धर्मा सर्वदेहेषु विशेषो नास्ति कुत्रचित् ।
अतश्च तन्मयं सर्वम् भावयन् भवजिज् जनः ॥१००॥

cid dharmā sarva deheṣu viśeṣo nāsti kutracit |
ataś ca tan mayaṁ sarvam bhāvayan bhavajij janaḥ || 100 ||

chit–dharmaa sarva–deheshu vi-sheshah na-asti kutra chit
atah cha tan mayam sarvam bhaavayan bhavajit janah

The heart of the universe pulses in all hearts.
There is One who is the life in all forms.
There is One who is joyful in simply existing—
      In all bodies,
      As all bodies.

Explore the life that is the life of your present form.
One day you will discover
It is not different
From the life of the Secret One,
And your heart will sing triumphant songs
Of being at home everywhere.

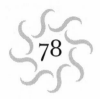

78

कामक्रोधलोभमोहमदमात्सर्यगोचरे ।
बुद्धिं निस्तिमितां कृत्वा तत्त्वमवशिष्यते ॥१०१॥

kāma krodha lobha moha mada mātsarya gocare |
buddhiṁ nistimitāṁ kṛtvā tat tattvam avaśiṣyate || 101 ||

kaama krodha lobha moha mada maatsarya gochare
buddhim ni-stimitaam kritvaa tat-tattvam ava-shishyate

Desire, lust, longing—
Anger humming in your blood.
Confusion, jealousy, bewilderment,
Swirling in your head.

Catch the first hint as passion rises,
The first quickening heartbeat.
Embrace that vibrancy
With a mind vast as the sky.

Witness the *elemental motion* of emotion:
    Fire burning, illuminating,
    Water gushing, cleansing,
    Air inspiring, soothing,
    Earth supporting, holding,
    Space expanding, embracing.

You are in the temple of desire.
Go deeper still and rest in essence,
Awake to infinite spiritual energy
Surging into form.

79

इन्द्रजालमयं विश्वं व्यस्तं वा चित्रकर्मवत् ।
भ्रमद् वा ध्यायतः सर्वम् पश्यतश्च सुखोद्गमः ॥१०२॥

indrajāla mayaṁ viśvaṁ vyastaṁ vā citra karmavat |
bhramad vā dhyāyataḥ sarvam paśyataś ca sukhodgamaḥ || 102 ||

*indra–jaala–mayam vishvam vi-astam vaa chitra karmavat
bhramad vaa dhyaayatah sarvam pashyatash cha sukhah ud-gamah*

Contemplate the entire universe
As a magic show
On the grandest scale imaginable.
Fabulous art, an immense painting in motion.
God is a magician whirling galaxies of fire,
Juggling atoms, planets, and us.
Everything, everything is fleeting.

Meditating on this magic,
    Great happiness rises in the heart.

80

न चित्तं निक्षिपेद् दुःखे न सुखे वा परिक्षिपेत् ।
भैरवि ज्ञायतां मध्ये किं तत्त्वमवशिष्यते ॥१०३॥

na cittaṁ nikṣiped duḥkhe na sukhe vā parikṣipet |
bhairavi jñāyatāṁ madhye kiṁ tattvam avaśiṣyate || 103 ||

na chittam ni-kshipet duhke na sukhe vaa pari-kshipet
bhairavi jnaayataam madhye kim tattvam ava-shishyate

―――――――――

That space is bad.
This space is good.
The ride is rough,
Or the going is smooth.
We are thrown into suffering,
We are thrown into joy.

Beloved Soul Mate—
Find the space in the center,
The pulsing spaciousness
Encompassing all opposites.

Here the essences of creation are at play:
Earth, Water, Fire, Air, and Space,
And the senses that perceive them.
The center is the dancing ground.

81

विहाय निजदेहस्थं सर्वत्रास्मीति भावयन् ।
दृढेन मनसा दृष्ट्या नान्येक्षिण्या सुखी भवेत् ॥१०४॥

vihāya nija dehastham sarvatrāsmīti bhāvayan |
dṛḍhena manasā dṛṣṭyā nānyekṣiṇyā sukhī bhavet || 104 ||

*vihaaya nija-dehasthaam sarvatra asmi iti bhaavayan
dridhena manasaa drishtyaa na anya-eekshinyaa sukhee bhavet*

Drop the thought,
"I am this body,"
Abandon the limitation,
"I am only here in this specific place and time."

Embrace instead,
I am not my body.
I am not this place.
I am not this time.
There is no place.
There is no time.

Realize,
"I am everywhere,"
Sustained by infinite bliss.

82

घटादौ यच् च विज्ञानम् इच्छाद्यं वा ममान्तरे ।
नैव सर्वगतं जातम् भावयन् इति सर्वगः ॥१०५॥

ghaṭādau yac ca vijñānam icchādyaṁ vā mamāntare |
naiva sarvagataṁ jātam bhāvayan iti sarvagaḥ || 105 ||

ghataadau yat cha vi-jnaanam ichchhaad yam vaa mama antare
na eva sarva–gatam jaatam bhaavayan iti sarva–gah

Trees have desires.
Rocks have knowledge.
Jugs are full of emptiness and joy.

All embodied ones have this in common.
All are propelled by the same One
Whose pulse beats in your breast.

Shed insularity.
Be all-pervasive,
Delighting in kinship everywhere.

83

ग्राह्यग्राहकसंवित्तिः सामान्या सर्वदेहिनाम् ।
योगिनां तु विशेषोऽस्ति सम्बन्धे सावधानता ॥१०६॥

grāhya grāhaka saṁvittiḥ sāmānyā sarva dehinām |
yogināṁ tu viśeṣo'sti sambandhe sāvadhānatā || 106 ||

*graahya graahaka sam-vittih saamaanyaa sarva–dehinaam
yoginaam tu vi-sheshah asti sam-bandhe saa-vadhaanataa*

Everyone knows, there is me,
And then there are all these others.
This is common to all.

Lovers know, there is me,
And the source of this me
Is ever mysterious.

Lovers know, each contact with another
Is a spark of the divine.
Lovers move through this world
Awake to intimacy,
Each touch a revelation
Never to be repeated.

84

स्ववद् अन्यशरीरेऽपि संवित्तिमनुभावयेत् ।
अपेक्षां स्वशरीरस्य त्यक्त्वा व्यापी दिनैर् भवेत् ॥१०७॥

svavad anya śarīre'pi saṁvittimanu bhāvayet |
apekṣāṁ svaśarīrasya tyaktvā vyāpī dinair bhavet || 107 ||

*sva-vat anya–shareere api sam-vittim anu-bhaavayet
a-pekshaam sva-shareerasya tyaktvaa vyaapee dinaih bhavet*

Extend your awareness
Into the bodies of other living beings,
Feel what those others are feeling.

Leave aside your body and its needs.
Abandon being so local.

Day by day, constrictions will loosen,
As you become attuned
To the current of life
Flowing through us all.

निराधारं मनः कृत्वा विकल्पान् न विकल्पयेत् ।
तदात्मपरमात्मत्वे भैरवो मृगलोचने ॥१०८॥

nirādhāraṁ manaḥ kṛtvā vikalpān na vikalpayet |
tad ātma paramātmatve bhairavo mṛgalocane ‖ 108 ‖

nir-aadhaaram manah kritvaa vi-kalpaan na vi-kalpayet
tat–aatma–parama-aatmatve bhairavah mriga-lochane

Toss aside your map of the world,
All your beliefs and constructs.
Dare the wild unknown.

Here in this terrifying freedom,
Naked before the universe,
Commune with the One
Who knows everything from the inside:
    Invisible power pervading everywhere.
    Divine presence permeating everything.

Breathe tenderly as
The lover of all beings.

86

सर्वज्ञः सर्वकर्ता च व्यापकः परमेश्वरः ।
स एवाहं शैवधर्मा इति दार्ढ्याच् छिवो भवेत् ॥१०९॥

sarvajñaḥ sarvakartā ca vyāpakaḥ parameśvaraḥ |
sa evāham śaiva dharmā iti dārḍhyāc chivo bhavet || 109 ||

sarva–jnah sarva–karttaa cha vi-aapakah parama–eeshvarah
sa eva aham shaiva–dharma iti daardhyaat bhavet shivah

There is a Knower who experiences everything.
There is a Presence dancing everywhere.
There is a Lover who embraces us all.

I am one with that Light.
I am one with that Power.
I am one with that Love.

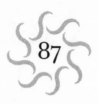

87

जलस्येवोर्मयो वह्नेर् ज्वालाभङ्ग्यः प्रभा रवेः ।
ममैव भैरवस्यैता विश्वभङ्ग्यो विभेदिताः ॥११०॥

jalasyevormayo vahner jvālā bhaṅgyaḥ prabhā raveḥ |
mamaiva bhairavasyaitā viśva bhaṅgyo vibheditāḥ || 110 ||

jalasya iva urmayah vahneh– jvaalaa-bhangyah pra-bhaa-raveh
mama eva bhairavasya etaa vishva–bhangyah vi-bheditaah

Waves rise from water.
Flames arise from fire.
Rays emanate from the sun.

So do you and I shine forth
From the Mysterious One.

88

भ्रान्त्वा भ्रान्त्वा शरीरेण त्वरितम् भुवि पातनात् ।
क्षोभशक्तिविरामेण परा सञ्जायते दशा ॥१११॥

bhrāntvā bhrāntvā śarīreṇa tvaritam bhuvi pātanāt |
kṣobha śakti virāmeṇa parā sañjāyate daśā || 111 ||

*bhraantvaa bhraantvaa shareerena tvaritam bhuvi paatanaat
kshobha–shakti vi-raamena paraa sam-jaayate dashaa*

Wander and wander to the point of exhaustion.
Whirl until you lose all control.
Dance until you are ready to drop.

Then drop!
Fall to the earth.

Surrender to the swirl of sensations
Surging through your form.
Dissolve in awe as arising energies
Continue the dance in your inner world.

Beyond motion and commotion,
Become the body of ecstasy.

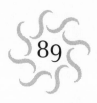

89

आधारेष्व् अथवाऽशक्त्याऽज्ञानाच् चित्तलयेन वा ।
जातशक्तिसमावेशक्षोभान्ते भैरवं वपुः ॥११२॥

ādhāreṣv atha vā 'śaktyā 'jñānāc citta layena vā |
jāta śakti samāveśa kṣobhānte bhairavaṁ vapuḥ || 112 ||

*aa-dhaareshu atha vaa ashaktyaa ajnaanaat chitta-layena vaa
jaata–shakti sam-aa-vesha kshobha-ante bhairavam–vapuh*

You are stunned, powerless.
    You thought you knew
What was going on.
Now you realize you don't have a clue.

You are stopped in your tracks.
Everything within your skin is shaking.
Enter this shaking.
Get curious.
Look around inside with wonder.
Unmind your mind.
All the walls have fallen down—
Go ahead and dissolve.

The One Who Has Always Been,
Who has seen much worse than this,
Is still here.

90

सम्प्रदायम् इमम् देवि शृणु सम्यग् वदाम्यहम् ।
कैवल्यं जायते सद्यो नेत्रयोः स्तब्धमात्रयोः ॥११३॥

sampradāyam imam devi śṛṇu samyag vadāmy aham |
kaivalyaṁ jāyate sadyo netrayoḥ stabdha mātrayoḥ || 113 ||

*sam-pra-daayam imam devi shrinu sam-yak vadaami aham
kaivalyam jaayate sadyah netrayoh stabdha–maatrayoh*

Radiant One,
Please listen to me.
The essence of all teachings is right here.
Open your eyes.

With a soft and steady gaze,
Look out upon creation.
Receive waves of light as they enter your eyes,
Singing of infinity.

The light touching the back of your eyes
Is immortal, born in the primal sun.
Be present to this enlightenment.

This is the ancient knowing,
A sanctuary that is everywhere.
Galaxies are flowers on this altar.

91

सङ्कोचं कर्णयोः कृत्वा ह्यधोद्वारे तथैव च ।
अनच्कमहलं ध्यायन् विशेद् ब्रह्म सनातनम् ॥११४॥

saṅkocaṁ karṇayoḥ kṛtvā hy adho dvāre tathaiva ca |
anackam ahalaṁ dhyāyan viśed brahma sanātanam ‖ 114 ‖

*sam-kocham karnayoh kritvaa hi adhas–dvaare tathaa eva cha
an-achkam a-halam dhyaayan vishet brahma-sanaatanam*

———————

Close the ears that track the outer world,
Open the ears of the soul.
Engage the muscles at the base of the pelvis,
The intimate special places,
And cherish the vibrating energies there contained.

The song of creation,
Sustaining, enlivening,
Is thrumming in your body,
Whispering secrets.
Listen in.

Meditating on the symphony of your own life currents,
Enter the palace of the Creator.

92

कूपादिके महागर्ते स्थित्वोपरि निरीक्षणात् ।
अविकल्पमतेः सम्यक् सद्यस् चित्तलयः स्फुटम् ॥११५॥

kūpādike mahāgarte sthitvopari nirīkṣaṇāt |
avikalpa mateḥ samyak sadyas citta layaḥ sphuṭam || 115 ||

koopaadike mahaa–garte sthitvaa upari nir-eekshanaat
a-vi-kalpa mateh sam-yak sadhyah chitta–layah sphutam

Position yourself safely
At the edge of a cliff or gorge.
Gaze into the abyss and see only depth.

Immediately,
Doubts dissolve,
Dilemmas disappear.

Be steady as mind releases itself
Into its natural freedom.

93

यत्र यत्र मनो याति बाह्ये वाभ्यन्तरेऽपि वा ।
तत्र तत्र शिवावास्था व्यापकत्वात्क्व यास्यति ॥११६॥

yatra yatra mano yāti bāhye vābhyantare'pi vā |
tatra tatra śivā vāsthā vyāpakatvāt kva yāsyati || 116 ||

*yatra—yatra manah yaati baahye vaa abhi-antare api vaa
tatra—tatra shiva—ava-sthaa vi-aa-pakatvaat kva yaasyati*

———————

Wherever your heart journeys,
On whatever expedition
In your outer life and
Secret inner realms,
Breathe in intimacy with infinity.

Where can you go to avoid
The One in Whom All Exists?

Reach down into your deepest being.
Take a stand in eternity.

Walk through this world, see every situation
As an expansion of the mystery.
Savor the tremble of recognition—
The God in you is touching the God out there.

94

यत्र यत्राक्षमार्गेण चैतन्यं व्यज्यते विभो: ।
तस्य तन्मात्रधर्मित्वाच् चिल्लयाद् भरितात्मता ॥११७॥

yatra yatrākṣa mārgeṇa caitanyaṁ vyajyate vibhoḥ |
tasya tanmātra dharmitvāc cil layād bharitātmatā || 117 ||

*yatra–yatra aksha–maargena chaitanyam vi–ajyate vi–bhoh
tasya tat–maatra dharmitvaat chit–layaat bhritaa–aatmataa*

———————

Light moves on its pathways through space,
Enters the eyes, and
You absorb the luminous.

Each sense is a current of divinity,
Sparkling with mystery.
Light, motion, space, vision, awareness—
All are composed of omnipresence.
The senses connecting you to the outer world
Are paths of communion with the inner world.

Every sight, sound, smell, taste, touch—
A greeting from the Beloved.

95

क्षुताद्यन्ते भये शोके गह्वरे वा रणाद् द्रुते ।
कुतूहलेक्षुधाद्यन्ते ब्रह्मसत्तामयी दशा ॥११८॥

kṣutādy ante bhaye śoke gahvare vā raṇād drute |
kutūhale kṣudhādy ante brahma sattā mayī daśā || 118 ||

kshut–aadi–ante bhaye shoke gahvare vaa ranaat–drute
kutoohale kshudhaa–aadi–ante brahma–sattaa–mayee dashaa

Ravenous with hunger,
Exploding with joy,
Sneezing uncontrollably,
Burning with desire.
Reeling with amazement,
Staggered by grief,
Fleeing from danger,
Desperately lost.

Intensity awakens,
Wild attentiveness everywhere.

Ride the shockwave inward
To touch the Great Self,
The power from which you arise.

96

वस्तुषु स्मर्यमाणेषु दृष्टे देशे मनस् त्यजेत् ।
स्वशरीरं निराधारं कृत्वा प्रसरति प्रभुः ॥११९॥

vastuṣu smaryamāṇeṣu dṛṣṭe deśe manas tyajet |
svaśarīraṁ nirādhāraṁ kṛtvā prasarati prabhuḥ || 119 ||

*vastushu smarya–maaneshu drishte deshe manah tyajet
sva-shareeram nir-aa-dhaaram kritvaa pra-sarati pra-bhuh*

When the unforgettable calls you—
The memory of something noble,
Generous, inspiring,
Accept the gift.
Savor every detail.

The beauty we admire
Is a visitation from another moment,
Infusing body and heart.
Memory transports us beyond time and space,
Into the living presence of wonder.

क्वचिद् वस्तुनि विन्यस्य शनैर् दृष्टिं निवर्तयेत् ।
तज् ज्ञानं चित्तसहितं देवि शून्यालायो भवेत् ॥१२०॥

kvacid vastuni vinyasya śanair dṛṣṭiṁ nivartayet |
taj jñānaṁ citta sahitaṁ devi śūnyālāyo bhavet || 120 ||

kvachit vastuni vi-nyasya shanaih drishtim ni-vartayet
tat–jnaanam chitta–sahitam devi shoonya–aa-layah bhavet

Engage your gaze with something, anything.
Adore its form and essence.
Give it your all.
Now tiptoe away into another realm,
As if not wanting to wake your lover.

Emptied of engagement,
Enter the temple of unknowing.
Dissolve in wonder—
Where does anything come from?

98

भक्त्युद्रेकाद् विरक्तस्य यादृशी जायते मतिः ।
सा शक्तिः शाङ्करी नित्यम् भवयेत्तां ततः शिवः ॥१२१॥

bhakty udrekād viraktasya yā dṛśī jāyate matiḥ |
sā śaktiḥ śaṅkarī nityam bhavayet tāṁ tataḥ śivaḥ || 121 ||

*bhakti–ud-rekaat vi-raktasya yaa drishee jayaate matih
saa shakti–shaankaree nityam bhaavayet taam tatah shivah*

Be wildly devoted to someone, or something.
Cherish every perception.
At the same time, forget about control.
Allow the Beloved to be herself and to change.

Passion and compassion, holding and letting go—
This ache in your heart is holy.
Accept it as the rise of intimacy
With life's secret ways.

Devotion is the divine streaming through you
From that place in you before time.
Love's energy flows through your body,
Toward a body, and into eternity again.
Surrender to this current of devotion
And become one with the Body of Love.

99

वस्त्वन्तरे वेद्यमाने सर्ववस्तुषु शून्यता ।
ताम् एव मनसा ध्यात्वा विदितोऽपि प्रशाम्यति ॥१२२॥

vastvantare vedya māne sarva vastuṣu śūnyatā |
tām eva manasā dhyātvā vidito 'pi praśāmyati || 122 ||

vastu–antare vedya–maane sarva–vastushu shoonyataa
taam eva manasaa dhyaatvaa viditah api pra-shaamyati

———————

Love is particular.
When you love someone,
A tangible, touchable someone,
The whole world opens up.
If you want to know the universe,
Dare to love one person.

All the secret teachings are right here—
Go deeper, and deeper still.
The gift of concentration
Is the spaciousness that surrounds it.
Focus illuminates immensity.

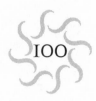

IOO

किञ्चिज्ज्ञैर् या स्मृता शुद्धिः सा शुद्धिः शम्भुदर्शने ।
न शुचिर् ह्यशुचिस् तस्मान् निर्विकल्पः सुखी भवेत् ॥१२३॥

kiñcij jñair yā smṛtā śuddhiḥ sā śuddhiḥ śambhu darśane |
na śucir hy aśucis tasmān nirvikalpaḥ sukhī bhavet || 123 ||

kinchit jnaih yaa smritaa shuddhih saa shuddhih shambhu–darshane
na suchir hi a-shuchih tasmaat nir-vi-kalpah sukhee bhavet

All this talk of purity and impurity,
These are just opinions. Beyond them
Are the miraculous energies of creation.

Rays of light from a trillion suns
Illumine the altar of your sky.
Rolling blue-green oceans
Sanctify the air you breathe.
In this moment, you are inhaling their blessing.
Who are you to call any of this pure or impure?

Find the center around which everything revolves—
Stand here and be flooded with joy.

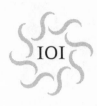

101

सर्वत्र भैरवो भावः सामान्येष्व् अपि गोचरः ।
न च तद्व्यतिरेक्तेण परोऽस्तीत्यद्वया गतिः ॥१२४॥

sarvatra bhairavo bhāvaḥ sāmānyeṣv api gocaraḥ |
na ca tad vyati rekteṇa paro 'stīty advayā gatiḥ || 124 ||

*sarvatra bhairavah bhaavah saamaanyeshu api gocharah
na cha parah tat vi-ati-rekena parah asti iti a-dvayaa gatih*

———————

The reality of the divine
Is everywhere apparent,
Especially among people
Who haven't even thought about it!

The very nature of I-consciousness,
To be an individual,
Is in essence divine.

The excitement of the Eternal One
Is throbbing in the heart of every creature.

Know this, and be without superiority, inferiority,
Or resentment at your limitations.

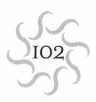

102

समः शत्रौ च मित्रे च समो मानावमानयोः ।
ब्रह्मणः परिपूर्णत्वातिति ज्ञात्वा सुखी भवेत् ॥१२५॥

samaḥ śatrau ca mitre ca samo mānāvamānayoḥ ||
brahmaṇaḥ paripūrṇatvāt iti jñātvā sukhī bhavet || 125 ||

samah shatrau cha mitre cha samah maana–ava-maanayoh
brahmanah pari–poornatvaat iti jnaatvaa sukhee bhavet

It's always the same.
Barbarians and blockheads, rival queens and kings,
The drama rolls on and on.
When people honor you,
You are supposed to feel honored.
When you don't get respect, they expect
You to sulk in indignation.
One minute you are cruising on a throne in the sky,
The next you are standing on some bleak patch of dirt.

I say, the Sun regards all with a steady eye.
The force sustaining Earth and Sky
   Calls everyone to awaken from this trance.
This whole world revolves around an axis, and I am that.

When you are friends with the Friend to All Beings
Nothing is the same.
Rich beyond measure, abundant beyond counting,
You can move through this life laughing.
Opinions of others have no rulership over you.

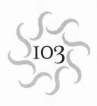

न द्वेषम् भावयेत्क्वापि न रागम् भावयेत्क्वचित् ।
रागद्वेषविनिर्मुक्तौ मध्ये ब्रह्म प्रसर्पति ॥१२६॥

na dveṣam bhāvayet kvāpi na rāgam bhāvayet kvacit |
rāga dveṣa vinirmuktau madhye brahma prasarpati || 126 ||

na dvesham bhaavayet kva api na raagam bhaavayet kvachit
raaga dvesha vi-nir-muktau madhye brahma pra-sarpati

Abandon all these attitudes
Of wanting to prolong pleasure
And avoid suffering.
Let the heart be itself and feel
Whatever is there.

Freed from clinging and avoiding,
The heart regains its poise
And revels in creation.

Plunging deep into its center,
Discover that the heart is moved
By a pulse that is everywhere.

104

यद् अवेद्यं यद् अग्राह्यं यच छुन्यं यद् अभावगम् ।
तत्सर्वम् भैरवम् भाव्यं तदन्ते बोधसम्भवः ॥१२७॥

yad avedyaṁ yad agrāhyaṁ yac chūnyaṁ yad abhāvagam |
tat sarvam bhairavam bhāvyaṁ tad ante bodha sambhavaḥ || 127 ||

yat a-vedyam yat a-graahyam yat shoonyam yat a-bhaavagam
tat sarvam bhairavam bhaavyam tad ante bodha sam-bhavah

Holiness permeates everywhere.
Senses cannot grasp it.
Images cannot represent it.

It is totally free—
Free to appear as form,
Free to be beyond form.

Heart and body and mind in unison,
Attend to the unimaginable.
In the intercourse of unknowable and known,
An awakening will be born in you
As you join with that reality
Which you already are.

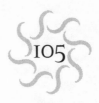

105

नित्ये निराश्रये शून्ये व्यापके कलनोज्झिते ।
बाह्याकाशे मनः कृत्वा निराकाशं समाविशेत् ॥१२८॥

nitye nirāśraye śūnye vyāpake kalanojjhite |
bāhyākāśe manaḥ kṛtvā nirākāśaṁ samāviśet || 128 ||

nitye nir-aa-shraye shoonye vi-aa-pake kalana ujjhite
baahya—aakaashe manah kritvaa nir-aakaasham sam-aa-vishet

When you gaze in wonder at the stars,
Become enthralled
With the vast spaciousness between them.
Space is an incomprehensible being,
An invisible presence,
Independent, independently wealthy,
Without beginning or end, and *giving*.

Space bestows an unbounded theater
For suns, planets, constellations
To dance their graceful orbits.

Space offers you an infinite arena
To play, explore, and experience.
Receive this gift of freedom.

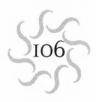

106

यत्र यत्र मनो याति तत्तत्तेनैव तत्क्षणम् ।
परित्यज्यानवस्थित्या निस्तरङ्गस् ततो भवेत् ॥१२९॥

yatra yatra mano yāti tat tat tenaiva tat kṣaṇam |
parityajyānavasthityā nistaraṅgas tato bhavet || 129 ||

yatra–yatra mano yati tat–tat tena eva tat–kshaanam
pari–tyajya ana-vasthityaa nis–tarangah tatah bhavet

──────────

Set your mind free to wander anywhere it wants,
Think any thought,
Ride any wave, surge in any direction.

The instant a thought springs up,
Abandon it and move on.
Don't let the mind rest anywhere.

In this way, gain entry to the bliss
Of the silent depths beneath the surf.

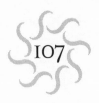

107

भया सर्वं रवयति सर्वदो व्यापकोऽखिले ।
इति भैरवशब्दस्य सन्ततोच्चारणाच् छिवः ॥१३०॥

bhayā sarvaṁ ravayati sarvado vyāpako 'khile |
iti bhairava śabdasya santatoccāraṇāc chivaḥ || 130 ||

bhayaa–sarvam ravayati sarvadah vi-aa-pakah a-khile
iti bhairava–shabdasya santatah ud-chaaranaat shivah

────────────

We all tremble, we all know fear.

Turn to the one life pervading the universe
Whose name dispels fear.
Find that name resonating in your heart.

Luminosity permeates the universe,
And the secret sound that hums
Everything into existence
Resounds everywhere.

Listening to the inner sound continually,
Become lovers with the Secret One.

108

अहं ममेदम् इत्यादि प्रतिपत्तिप्रसङ्गतः ।
निराधारे मनो याति तद्ध्यानप्रेरणाच् छमी ॥१३१॥

ahaṁ mamedam ity ādi pratipatti prasaṅgataḥ |
nirādhāre mano yāti tad dhyāna preraṇāc chamī || 131 ||

aham mama idam iti aadi pratti–patti pra-sangatah
nir-aa-dhaare manah yaati tat–dhyaana–preranaat shamee

The next time the thought arises,
"I want this," or "I think that,"
Grab hold of this "I"—perceive it by itself.
Wonder, who is this "I"?

I am animal,
I am human.
I am a loving heart,
I am a questing mind.
I am a particle of infinity,
I am a witness to creation.
I am consciousness itself.

In meditation, embrace all these dimensions.
Reach into the source: the luminous
World of dancing energies
In ever-changing relatedness.

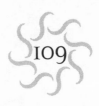

109

नित्यो विभुर् निराधारो व्यापकश्चाखिलाधिपः ।
शब्दान् प्रतिक्षणं ध्यायन् कृतार्थोऽर्थानुरूपतः ॥१३२॥

nityo vibhur nirādhāro vyāpakaś cākhilādhipaḥ |
śabdān pratikṣaṇaṁ dhyāyan kṛtārtho 'rthānurūpataḥ || 132 ||

nityaḥ vi-bhuḥ nir-aa-dhaaraḥ vi-aa-pakaḥ cha a-khila–adhipaḥ
shabdaan pratik–shanam dhyaayan krita–arthaḥ artha-anu-roopataḥ

Native of eternity.
At home in infinity.
Breathing immortality.

Let these words sing in every cell.

Oceans of splendor.
Luminous energies of creation.
Pulsating everywhere always.

Hear these astounding words continually,
Each phrase an invocation.
Let the sounds ripple through you.

Resonate with the all-pervading hum of truth
And know, every fleeting moment is
Supported by forever.

IIO

अतत्त्वम् इन्द्रजालाभम् इदं सर्वमवस्थितम् ।
किं तत्त्वम् इन्द्रजालस्य इति दाढ्यच् छमं व्रजेत् ॥१३३॥

atattvam indrajālābham idaṁ sarvam avasthitam |
kiṁ tattvam indrajālasya iti dārḍhyāc chamaṁ vrajet || 133 ||

a-tattvam indra–jaalah–aa-bham idam sarvam ava-sthitam
kim tattvam indra–jaalasya iti daardhyaat shamam vrajet

The juggler with her spinning torches
Conjures dazzling wheels of fire.
The magician taps his wand and suddenly
A net of jewels sparkles in the darkness.

What do we love in magic?
Each gesture is a kind of jest,
Inviting us beyond itself
Into the deepest magic of all—
God alone is.

All that we see
Is the performance
Of the Divine Magician.
Stand at the center of this wonder,
And breathe the wild serene.

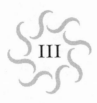

III

आत्मनो निर्विकारस्य क्व ज्ञानं क्व च वा क्रिया ।
ज्ञानायत्ता बहिर्भवा अतः शून्यम् इदं जगत् ॥१३४॥

ātmano nirvikārasya kva jñānaṁ kva ca vā kriyā |
jñānā yattā bahir bhāva ataḥ śūnyam idaṁ jagat || 134 ||

aatmanh nir-vi-kaarasya kva jnaanam kva cha vaa kriyaa
jnaana–yattaa bahih–bhaavaa atah shoonyam idam jagat

───────────

There is no image you can hold,
No thought you can think,
That encompasses the Great Self.

Your essence
Is immortal and unchanging,
Yet it is the foundation for all that moves.

Rest in the shimmering emptiness
That is the source of this world,
And remember who you are.

112

न मे बन्धो न मोक्षो मे भीतस्यैता विभीषिकाः ।
प्रतिबिम्बम् इदम् बुद्धेर् जलेष्व् इव विवस्वतः ॥१३५॥

na me bandho na mokṣo me bhītasyaitā vibhīṣikāḥ |
pratibimbam idam buddher jaleṣv iva vivasvataḥ || 135 ||

na me bandhah na mokshah me bheetasya etaa vi-bheeshikaah
priti–bimbam idam bhuddheh jaleshu iva vi-vasvatah

———————

Bhairava says,

Not for Me, bondage.
Not for Me, liberation.
I am beyond such nonsense.

The sun is not trapped
When it shines in a river,
Illuminating the lives of the fishes.
Nor is the sun freed again
When it reflects off a ripple
Back into the sky.

Bondage, freedom—
Notions arising from fear and separation.
Look upon the universe and see only Me.

INSIGHT VERSES

In the final verses 136–162, Bhairava offers encouragement to make these practices your own. Discover the ones that are always going on spontaneously in your deepest being and know that the elixir of life is always available to you. Devi is suffused with delight and embraces her lover.

Insight Verses 136-138

इन्द्रियद्वारकं सर्वं सुखदुःखादिसङ्गमम् ।
इतीन्द्रियाणि सन्त्यज्य स्वस्थः स्वात्मनि वर्तते ॥१३६॥

indriya dvārakaṁ sarvaṁ sukha duḥkhādi saṅgamam |
itīndriyāṇi santyajya svasthaḥ svātmani vartate || 136 ||

*indriya–dvaarakam sarvaam sukha–duhkha aadi sangamam
iti indriyaani sam-tyajya sva-sthah sva-aatmani vartate*

Consider all the pain and all the pleasure
You have ever experienced
As waves on a very deep ocean which you are.

From the depths, witness those waves,
Rolling along so bravely, always changing,
Beautiful in their self-sustaining power.

Marvel that once, you identified with
Only the surface of this ocean.
Now embrace waves, depths, undersea mountains,
Out to the farthest shore.

ज्ञानप्रकाशकं सर्वं सर्वेणात्मा प्रकाशकः ।
एकम् एकस्वभावत्वात्ज्ञानं ज्ञेयं विभाव्यते ॥१३७॥

मानसं चेतना शक्तिर् आत्मा चेति चतुष्टयम् ।
यदा प्रिये परिक्षीणं तदा तद् भैरवं वपुः ॥१३८॥

jñāna prakāśakaṁ sarvaṁ sarveṇātmā prakāśakaḥ |
ekam eka svabhāvatvāt jñānaṁ jñeyaṁ vibhāvyate || 137 ||
mānasaṁ cetanā śaktir ātmā ceti catuṣṭayam |
yadā priye parikṣīṇaṁ tadā tad bhairavaṁ vapuḥ || 138 ||

jnaana pra-kaashakam sarvam sarvena–aatmaa pra-kaashakah
ekam eka sva-bhaavatvaat jnaanam jneyam vi-bhaavyate
maanasam chetanaa shaktih aatmaa cha iti chatushtayam
yadaa priye pari-ksheenam tadaa tat bhairavam vapuh

The light of consciousness illumines the world.
The world reflects this splendor.
Energy and matter, essence and manifestation,
Reveal each other to each other.

Individual soul and cosmic energy,
Pulsing heart and infinite awareness—
Are secret lovers, always merging in oneness.
When the secret slips out, there is laughter
And a flash of brilliance in the air.

INSIGHT VERSES 139-140

निस्तरङ्गोपदेशानां शतम् उक्तं समासतः ।
द्वादशाभ्यधिकं देवि यज् ज्ञात्वा ज्ञानविज् जनः ॥१३९॥

nistaraṅgopadeśānāṁ śatam uktaṁ samāsataḥ |
dvādaśābhyadhikaṁ devi yaj jñātvā jñānavij janaḥ || 139 ||

nis-tarangah upa-deshaanaam shatam uktam samaasatah
dvaa-dashaabhih adi-hikam devi yat jnaa tvaa jnaanavit janah

Shining One,
In these teachings I have given you
More than a hundred and twelve ways
Of entering the stillness beneath the waves.
Cherish any one of these; make it your own.
Embody your inborn wisdom.

अत्र चैकतमे युक्तो जायते भैरवः स्वयम् ।
वाचा करोति कर्माणि शापानुग्रहकारकः ॥१४०॥

atra caikatame yukto jāyate bhairavaḥ svayam |
vācā karoti karmāṇi śāpānugraha kārakaḥ || 140 ||

atra cha eka tame yuktaḥ jaayate bhairavaḥ svayam
vaachaa karoti karmaani shaapta–anu-graha–kaarakaḥ

———————

Establish yourself in even one of these practices.
Join with the Goddess and God
Who are making love
In every particle of creation.

Honor the power of speech,
And with every breath,
Bless the life that surrounds you.

INSIGHT VERSES 141-143

अजरामरताम् एति सोऽणिमादिगुणान्वितः ।
योगिनीनाम् प्रियो देवि सर्वमेलापकाधिपः ॥१४१॥

ajarāmaratām eti so'ṇimādiguṇānvitaḥ |
yoginīnām priyo devi sarva melāpakādhipaḥ || 141 ||
jīvann api vimukto 'sau kurvann api na lipyate |

a-jarah a-marataam eti sah anima aadi guna–anvitah
yogineenaam priyah devi sarva mela–aa-pakaah adhi-pah
jeevan api vi-muktah asau kurvan api na lipyate

Delight in these meditations, my Adored One.
Play with creation as it plays with you.

Playing, become smaller than an atom,
Travel through the expanse of space,
Drink the elixir of immortality.

Bathe in the stream of these life-giving teachings.
Flirt with the tingling sparks of vitality
Surging through your body.
Live your whole life as a festival, a celebration,
Liberated in love and work.

श्री देवी उवाच ।

इदं यदि वपुर् देव परायाश्च महेश्वर ॥१४२॥

एवमुक्तव्यवस्थायां जप्यते को जपश्च कः ।

ध्यायते को महानाथ पूज्यते कश्च तृप्यति ॥१४३॥

śrī devī uvāca |
idaṁ yadi vapur deva parāyāś ca maheśvara || 142 ||
evam ukta vyavasthāyāṁ japyate ko japaś ca kaḥ |
dhyāyate ko mahānātha pūjyate kaś ca tṛpyati || 143 ||
hūyate kasya vā homo yāgaḥ kasya ca kiṁ katham |

shree devee uvaacha:
idam yadi vapuh deva paraayaah cha maha–eeshvara
evam ukta vi-ava-sthaayam japyate kah japah cha kah
dhyaayate kaha mahaa–naatha poojyate kah cha tripyati
hooyate kasya vaa homah yaagah kasya cha kim katham

––––––––

The Goddess then asks,

If this is the nature of the universal Self,
Then who is to be worshipped?
Who do I invoke, and who do I meditate upon?

To whom do I offer oblations,
To whom do I sacrifice?
If everything is divine,
And consciousness merges with that divine essence,
Then what happens to the distinction
Between worshipper and worshipped?

INSIGHT VERSES 144-146

श्री भैरव उवाच ।

एषात्र प्रक्रिया बाह्या स्थूलेष्व् एव मृगेक्षणे ॥१४४॥

भूयो भूयः परे भावे भावना भाव्यते हि या ।

जपः सोऽत्र स्वयं नादो मन्त्रात्मा जप्य ईदृशः ॥१४५॥

ध्यानं हि निश्चला बुद्धिर् निराकारा निराश्रया ।

न तु ध्यानं शरीराक्षिमुखहस्तादिकल्पना ॥१४६॥

śrī bhairava uvāca |
eṣātra prakriyā bāhyā sthūleṣv eva mṛgekṣaṇe || 144 ||
bhūyo bhūyaḥ pare bhāve bhāvanā bhāvyate hi yā |
japaḥ so 'tra svayaṁ nādo mantrātmā japya īdṛśaḥ || 145 ||
dhyānaṁ hi niścalā buddhir nirākārā nirāśrayā |
na tu dhyānaṁ śarīrākṣi mukha hastādi kalpanā || 146 ||

shree bhairava uvaacha
eshaa atra pra-kriyaa baahyaa sthooleshu eva mriga—eekshane
bhooyah—bhooyah pare bhaave bhaavanaa bhaavyate hi yaa
japah sah atra svayam nadah mantra—aatmaa japya eedrishah
dhyaanam hi nish-chalaa buddhih nir-aa-kaaraa nir-aa-shrayaa
na tu dhyaanam shareera—akshi mukha—hasta aadi kalpanaa

The Lord Who Shines In Us All replied,

Oh Goddess, the practices you are speaking of
Refer only to the externals.
When you enter into the great Self,
All prayers go on inside you spontaneously
Without ceasing.

In reality, all songs of gratitude
And ecstatic lovemaking are resonating in
Every particle of creation at every moment.
When you are established in this recitation,
You are listening, and you hear them.

Plunging without reservation
Into the ocean of bliss is meditation.
No image, no thoughts, no prop.
Concentrating on the image of a god
With a body, eyes, and mouth is not meditation.

Insight Verses 147–148

पूजा नाम न पुष्पाद्यैर् या मतिः क्रियते दृढा ।
निर्विकल्पे महाव्योम्नि सा पूजा ह्यादराल् लयः ॥१४७॥

pūjā nāma na puṣpādyair yā matiḥ kriyate dṛḍhā |
nirvikalpe mahā vyomni sā pūjā hy ādarāl layaḥ || 147 ||

poojaa–naama na pushpa aadyaih yaa matih kriyate dridhaa
nir-vi-kalpe mahaa–vyomni saa poojaa hi aa-daraat layah

Worship does not mean offering flowers.
It means offering your heart
To the vast mystery
Of the universe.

It means letting your heart pulse
With the life of the universe,
Without thought and without reservation.

It means being so in love
That you are
Willing to dissolve
And be recreated in every moment.

अत्रैकतमयुक्तिस्थे योत्पद्येत दिनाद् दिनम् ।
भरिताकारता सात्र तृप्तिर् अत्यन्तपूर्णता ॥१४८॥

atraikatama yuktisthe yotpadyeta dinād dinam |
bharitā kāratā sātra tṛptir atyanta pūrṇatā || 148 ||

atra eka-tama yuktisthe yaa ut-padyeta dinaat dinam
bharitaa–kaarataa saa atra triptih atyanta–poornataa

Being transformed by even one of these practices,
Fullness of experience develops breath by breath.
One day the desire of the self for the great Self
Is consummated.
Come ready for that moment!

INSIGHT VERSES 149-150

༺

महाशून्यालये वह्नौ भूताक्षविषयादिकम् ।
हूयते मनसा सार्धं स होमश् चेतनासुचा ॥१४९॥

mahā śūnyālaye vahnau bhūtākṣa viṣayādikam |
hūyate manasā sārdhaṁ sa homaś cetanā srucā || 149 ||

mahaa–shoonya–aa-laye vahnau bhootaa–aksha–vishaya–aadikam
hooyate manasaa saardham sa homah chetanaa sruchaa

The real transmutation,
The most sacred offering,
Is to pour the elements of your body,
All of your sensual impressions,
Into the fire of the Great Void.

Your richness of experience
Is the wine you offer
To the divinity that is everywhere.

यागोऽत्र परमेशानि तुष्टिर् आनन्दलक्षणा ।
क्षपणात्सर्वपापानां त्राणात्सर्वस्य पार्वति ॥१५०॥

yāgo 'tra parameśāni tuṣṭir ānanda lakṣaṇā |
kṣapaṇāt sarva pāpānāṁ trāṇāt sarvasya pārvati || 150 ||

yaagah atra parama–eeshaani tushtih aananda–lakshanaa
kshapanaat sarva–paapaanaam traanaat sarvasya paarvati

The real sacrifice
Is to let your sins be destroyed
By the vast power of the universe.
It is to live in radiant bliss.

Senses dissolve, mind dissolves,
The objects of sense dissolve,
Even the void is dissolved.
This is transcendence.

Insight Verses 151–152

रुद्रशक्तिसमावेशस् तत्क्षेत्रम् भावना परा ।
अन्यथा तस्य तत्त्वस्य का पूजा काश्च तृप्यति ॥१५१॥

rudra śakti samāveśas tat kṣetram bhāvanā parā |
anyathā tasya tattvasya kā pūjā kāś ca tṛpyati || 151 ||

rudra–shakti–sam-aa-veshah tat–kshetram bhaavanaa paraa
anyathaa tasya tattvasya kaa poojah kah cha tripyati

Emanating from the embrace
Of the Goddess and her God
Is a wheel of delicious divine energies.

The center of this wheel
Is right where you are.
Live here, and let your heart stream
With an unending flow of adoration.
In this way, tend the altar of love.

स्वतन्त्रानन्दचिन्मात्रसारः स्वात्मा हि सर्वतः ।
आवेशनं तत्स्वरूपे स्वात्मनः स्नानम् ईरितम् ॥१५२॥

svatantrānanda cin mātra sāraḥ svātmā hi sarvataḥ |
āveśanaṁ tat svarūpe svātmanaḥ snānam īritam || 152 ||

sva-tantra–aananda chit–maatra–saarah sva-aatmaa hi sarvatah
aa-veshanam tat sva-roope sva-aatmanah snaanam eeritam

The real purification with water
Is to bathe in the essence of eternity
And stand in your true body—
Stunning autonomy, luminous bliss,
Invisible consciousness pulsating
Always, in every direction.

INSIGHT VERSES 153-154

यैर् एव पूज्यते द्रव्यैस् तर्प्यते वा परापरः ।
यश्चैव पूजकः सर्वः स एवैकः क्व पूजनम् ॥१५३॥

yair eva pūjyate dravyais tarpyate vā parāparaḥ |
yaś caiva pūjakaḥ sarvaḥ sa evaikaḥ kva pūjanam || 153 ||

yair eva poojyate dravyaih tarpyate vaa para–a-parah
yah cha eva poojakah sarvah sa eva ekah kva poojanam

The flowers, the incense,
Grain, spices, and honey
Offered in ritual
Are made out of the same divine stuff as you.
Who then is worshipped?

व्रजेत्प्राणो विशेज् जीव इच्चया कुटिलाकृतिः ।
दीर्घत्मा सा महादेवी परक्षेत्रम् परापरा ॥१५४॥

vrajet prāṇo viśej jīva icchayā kuṭilā kṛtiḥ |
dīrghātmā sā mahā devī para kṣetram parāparā || 154 ||

vrajet praanah vishet jeeva ichchhayaa kutilaa–kritih
deergha–aatmaa saa mahaa–devee para–kshetram para–a–paraa

Breath flows in, breath flows out,
Traveling always the curving path of the Goddess.
Breath flows spontaneously of its own will.
Thus all breathing beings
Continually give reverence to *Her.*
Be conscious of this unconscious prayer,
For She is the most holy place of pilgrimage.

She wishes for you to enter this temple,
Where each breath is adoration
Of the infinite for the incarnate form.

INSIGHT VERSES 155-156

अस्यामनुचरन् तिष्ठन् महानन्दमयेऽध्वरे ।
तया देव्या समाविष्टः परम् भैरवमाप्नुयात् ॥१५५॥

asyām anucaran tiṣṭhan mahānanda maye 'dhvare |
tayā devyā samāviṣṭaḥ param bhairavam āpnuyāt || 155a ||

*asyaam anu-charan tishthan mahaa–aananda–maye adhvare
tayaa devyaa sam-aa-vishtah param bhairavam aapnuyaat*

Breath flows
Into this body
As a nectar of the gods.

Every breath is a whisper
Of the Goddess:
"Here is the ritual I ask of you—
Be the cup
Into which I pour this bliss,
The elixir of immortal peace."

सकारेण बहिर्याति हकारेण विषेत् पुनः ।
हंसहंसेत्यमुं मन्त्रं जीवो जपति नित्यशः ॥१५५॥

षट्शतानि दिवा रात्रौ सहस्राण्येकविंशतिः ।
जपो देव्याः समुद्दिष्टः सुलभो दुर्लभो जडैः ॥१५६॥

sa kāreṇa bahir yāti ha kāreṇa viṣet punaḥ |
haṁsa haṁsety amuṁ mantraṁ jīvo japati nityaśaḥ || 155b ||
ṣaṭ śatāni divā rātrau sahasrāṇyekaviṁśatiḥ |
japo devyāḥ samuddiṣṭaḥ sulabho durlabho jaḍaiḥ || 156 |||

sa-kaarena bahir yaati ha-kaarena vishet punah
hamsa—hamsa iti amum mantram jeeva japati nityashah
shat-shataani divaa—raatrau sahasraani eka-vimshatih
japah devyaah sam-ud-dishtah su-labhah dur-labhah jadaih

The breath flows out with the sound *sa*,
The breath flows in with the sound *ha*.
Thus thousands of times a day,
Everyone who breathes is adoring the Goddess.

Know this, and be in great joy.
Listen to the ongoing prayer that is breath.
Life shall dance in you
A dance of ever-renewing delight.

INSIGHT VERSES 157–159

इत्येतत्कथितं देवि परमामृतम् उत्तमम् ।
एतच् च नैव कस्यापि प्रकाश्यं तु कदाचन ॥१५७॥

ity etat kathitaṁ devi paramāmṛtam uttamam |
etac ca naiva kasyāpi prakāśyaṁ tu kadācana || 157 ||

iti etat kathitam devi parama–amritam uttamam
etat cha na eva kasya api pra-kaashyam tu kadaa-chana

Adorable Goddess,
These practices are a nectar I share with you.
Drink from this cup whenever you are thirsty
Or crave to be refreshed in the essence of life.

Know that this ambrosia is available to you
Everywhere, for the universe is made out of it.
Simply go to the intersection of flesh and spirit,
Breathe the tiny sparks that fly.

Within this very body
Are many gateways to the infinite,
Where incarnation and immortality
Consummate their passion for each other.

परशिष्ये खले क्रूरे अभक्ते गुरुपादयोः ।
निर्विकल्पमतीनां तु वीराणाम् उन्नतात्मनाम् ॥१५८॥

भक्तानां गुरुवर्गस्य दातव्यं निर्विशङ्कया।
ग्रामो राज्यम् पुरं देशः पुत्रदारकुटुम्बकम्॥ १५९ ॥

para śiṣye khale krūre abhakte guru pādayoḥ |
nirvikalpa matīnāṁ tu vīrāṇām unnatātmanām || 158 ||
bhaktānāṁ guru vargasya dātavyaṁ nirviśaṅkayā |
grāmo rājyam puraṁ deśaḥ putra dāra kuṭumbakam || 159 ||

para–shishye khale kroore a-bhakte guru paadayoh
nir-vi-kalpa–mateenaam tu veeraanaam unnata-aatmanaam
bhaktaanam guru vargasya daatavyam nir-vi-shankayaa
graamo raajyam puram deshah putra–daara–kutumbakam

Share these teachings
With all generous-hearted people
Who come your way and ask.

When you meet someone
Whose heart is vibrating
With the flow of love,
Let your words and energies
Be free as your breathing.

INSIGHT VERSES 160

सर्वम् एतत्परित्यज्य ग्राह्यम् एतन् मृगेक्षणे ।
किम् एभिर् अस्थिरैर् देवि स्थिरम् परम् इदं धनम् ।
प्राणा अपि प्रदातव्या न देयं परमामृतम् ॥१६०॥

sarvam etat parityajya grāhyam etan mṛgekṣaṇe |
kim ebhir asthirair devi sthiram param idaṁ dhanam |
prāṇā api pradātavyā na deyaṁ paramāmṛtam || 160 ||

sarvam etat pari-tyajya graahyam etat mriga–eekshane
kim ebhih a-sthiraih devi sthiram param idam dhanam
praana api pra-daatavyati na deyam parama–amritam

Friends, relatives, neighbors, people who abide
In your village, city, country—
Be not concerned with their attitudes
Toward these teachings.
Everyone is discovering the intimate universe
In their own way.

This nectar is here
Within every breath, every desire, every transition
From waking to sleeping and sleeping to waking.

Once you have set out on the path of intimacy
With the immortal essence of life,
Never turn your back on it, my Shining One.
Never turn away.
Though every moment be surprising,
Revelatory, unrecognizable, and full of wonder,
Continue to cherish each breath.
Live in gratitude for the ambrosia we imbibe
In each turning, outbreath to inbreath into outbreath.

INSIGHT VERSES 161–162

श्री देवी उवाच ।

देवदेव माहदेव परितृप्तास्मि शङ्कर ।
रुद्रयामलतन्त्रस्य सारमद्यावधारितम् ॥१६१॥

सर्वशक्तिप्रभेदानां हृदयं ज्ञातमद्य च ।
इत्युक्त्वानन्दिता देवि कण्ठे लग्ना शिवस्य तु ॥१६२॥

śrī devī uvāca |
deva deva māhadeva paritṛptāsmi śaṅkara |
rudrayāmala tantrasya sāram adyāvadhāritam || 161 ||
sarva śakti prabhedānāṁ hṛdayaṁ jñātam adya ca |
ity uktvānanditā devi kaṇṭhe lagnā śivasya tu || 162 ||

shree devee uvaacha
deva–deva mahaa–deva pari–tripta asmi shankara
rudra–yaamala–tantrasya saaram adya ava–dhaaritam
sarva–shakti pra–bhedaanaam hridayam jnaatam adya cha
iti uktvaa aananditaa devee kanthe lagnaa shivasya tu

Devi replies,

You whose drum is the pulse of creation,
You whose dance is the motion of all worlds,
You who are more intimate than my very breath,
I am suffused with satisfaction.
My questions have led to fullness.

You have sung to me of the ways of union
Of the Goddess with Her God,
Time and space, personal and impersonal,
Energy and form, finite and infinite.
You have sung the song
Of being at home in the universe.

Having said that, the Goddess,
Radiant with delight,
Embraces her lover.

PART TWO

INVITATIONS AND
ILLUMINATIONS

Yukti Practice Transmissions

The Vijnana Bhairava Tantra offers 112 meditation practices, each one an invitation to come in and be at home in yourself and in the universe. The practices are presented in verses made up of four to ten Sanskrit words, and every individual word is a tool of thought, a *mantra*. In this section, one Sanskrit word from each sutra is presented as a portal into a rich world of experience. Also on the page are hints for engaging with each of the 112 practices, a few highlights that may attract your interest when you are in the *manyu* (spirit, mind, mood, mettle, passion) to explore a particular sutra. These are intended to illuminate a skill you may find useful in scouting your inner world.

In the meditation traditions, a transmission is an electric realization, an *aha* moment. Often, you are reminded of something you already know and love. You recognize a truth, and your life-force is awakened. In any given sutra, every Sanskrit word offers myriad opportunities to receive a transmission, because Sanskrit is engineered so that each word is often made up of five or ten images, each circling around a nucleus, a tiny thought.

The nucleus of a Sanskrit word is often a principle. Take, for example, the word *yoga*. The nucleus of yoga is *yuj*, "to yoke or join." The central principle is "joining." Around this nucleus dozens of diverse meanings are orbiting: yoking horses to a chariot, calling up soldiers to join in ranks and form an army, putting an arrow on a bowstring, putting on armor, to embrace something or someone, to join one's self to, to be united in marriage, injecting semen, joining up of the individual soul with the universal soul, joining up all the elements necessary to form a business, joining a series of words together into a sentence, and lining up all the elements of a trick, con job, or fraud.

That is only thirteen of the meanings of *yuj;* the Sanskrit-English dictionary lists over fifty in all.

As you get to know a Sanskrit word, form your own mental images to go with each of the many meanings in the definition. As you learn, little jokes and puns will pop up in your mind, and once you start combining words, the metaphors just keep on mixing. And in between these images, there is an emptiness that is always beckoning, inviting you to feel spacious and expansive. Learning to be entertained by the play of matter, energy, and emptiness is one of the central practices of meditation described in this text.

Reading a list of Sanskrit word definitions requires an unusual kind of attention. You may want to take a breath after each phrase in a definition, or even go for a walk with it. Let the meaning in the image surprise you. In this way, one bit at a time, you can begin to learn to think in Sanskrit. It can take hours or even days to get the feel for one word, but you are learning on a deep level.

For example, in verse 15, in the introduction to the text, Bhairava gives us an amazing word: *antaḥsvanubhavananda.*

Unfolding this word we see:

Antar: Within, between, amongst. In the middle or interior. Out of the midst of.

Sva: One's own. One's self. The ego. The human soul.

Anubhava: Experience. Knowledge derived from personal observation or experiment. Perception. Apprehension. Fruition. Understanding. Impression on the mind not derived from memory. Cognition. Consciousness. Custom, usage.

Ananda: Happiness, joy, enjoyment, sensual pleasure, one of the three attributes of *atman* or *brahman* in the vedanta philosophy. In drama, the thing wished for, the end of the drama. A kind of flute. The sixteenth *muhurta*. A name of Shiva.

Within you, through personal observation and experiment, you can have the direct experience of contact with the soul and as a result of that knowledge be filled with happiness, joy, and sensual pleasure.

In the Vijnana Bhairava Tantra, one of the words for "a practice," or meditation technique, is *yukti,* a variation on the word *yoga. Yukti* has the sense of "joining together the essential elements at the right time and place" and also "practice, skill, craft, workmanship, and art." As we practice meditation, we want to be continually refining our craft, becoming more skillful in joining up all the essential elements of our own inner riches so that we can thrive in the outer world.

I

प्राण

PRĀṆA

Prana: Filled, full. The breath of life. Respiration, spirit, vitality. The five vital airs: *prana, apana, vyana, samana,* and *udana.* Breath as a sign of strength. Vigor, energy, power—with all one's strength, or with all one's heart.

Practice

Bhairava begins the 112 yuktis with this invitation to Devi: *urdhva prana*—"as we exhale, the breath of life flows upwards into heaven, where it came from." *Urdhva* is "upward moving, rising, to go upwards into heaven." *Prana* is "the breath of life."

The next two words are *adhas jiva*—"as you inhale, the breath of life flows downwards through the body to the genitals." *Adhas* is "below, down, in the lower region, the external genitals—and specifically in a woman's body the labia majora, labia minora, clitoris, and vestibule of the vagina." *Jiva* means "the individual soul, the living or personal soul as distinguished from the universal soul," and "the principle of life, the breath."

Breathing is rhythm, a play of opposites. Here you are invited to enjoy the play of *prana,* the universal breath of life and *jiva,* the individual soul, the way the breath of life condenses into you. Another play of opposites is up and down—upward into the sky above you and downward into the brightness of the pelvis.

A good way to initiate yourself into this practice is to go outside, where you can feel the sky and earth, and take a standing posture. As you breathe out, let your hands flow upward along the front of your body to the area above your head. As you breathe in, let your hands float back down toward your pelvis. This is an easy gesture, as eloquent as conductors waving their hands as they direct an orchestra.

After you get the sense of this wonderful flow, you can continue the movement in any posture—sitting or lying down or dancing. Exhaling upwards, give your breath to infinity. Inhaling downwards, receive the nourishing fullness of your individuality.

As you exhale, whisper the word *prana* to yourself, and notice your relationship to the mystery of universality. Follow the motion upwards from your heart into heaven. As you inhale and receive the breath, whisper *jiva,* and notice your relationship with the mystery of individuality. Allow your attention to travel down from the space above your head, to the heart, to the area between your legs, and even to your feet. Everywhere in the body is spiritual and sacred.

As you get used to this movement, add another motion: tilt the head back slightly as you breathe out, so you are facing upward, and tilt the head downward slightly as you inhale.

The rhythm of the breath happens twenty-two thousand times a day. When you spend just a few of these times in delight and wonder, it begins to transform the other 99.999 percent that you take for granted.

Breathing out, quietly celebrate, "I am part of the life of the universe." Breathing in, marvel, "I am a living soul, an individual." *Jiva,* meaning "individual soul," also suggests that from the very first breath, you can modify any meditation instructions to suit your unique individuality. For example, if you feel enthusiastic, your celebration phrases could be, "Oh my God! I am alive!"

2

मरुत्

MARUT

Marut: Lightning and thunderbolts, roaring like lions. The flashing ones, shining ones, storm gods, Indra's companions, children of heaven or of the ocean, armed with golden weapons. Wind, air, breath, and the five winds, or pranas, in the body.

Practice

Marut suggests that breath is wild and magical, like lightning. Let go of your civilized self and welcome your wildness, your storms. You are part of nature, part of the earth, a dynamic and self-sustaining little system within the larger ecosphere. The electrifying magnificent heavenly breath, *marut,* keeps on quickening the life-force, rolling on, rotating *(vartana),* inwardly *(antar)* and outwardly *(bahir).*

The practice here is to do nothing—simply enjoy the show as this magic stuff flows inward, turns, and then flows outward and turns again. Welcome the flash of sensations, emotions, thoughts, and breath.

Lightning is flashing in the body. Breath is moved by a spark of electricity. Thoughts are waves of subtle electricity flashing through your body and brain. Your heart beats every second or so, and each pulsing of the heart is incited by a little spark of electricity. Welcome it all. Revel in it as you would the rain if you were a farmer. *Prana* and *jiva,* used in the previous verse, are both names of *maruts.* Breathing is part of nature.

Breath is exciting, and it propels itself. It's a charging, dynamic process of life, roaring along. If you want to know peace, let breath excite you.

As you explore the sensations that are flowing in your body as you are breathing right now, you might consider one of these thoughts:

I am awake to the electricity of life.
The dynamic power of breath is renewing me moment
  by moment.
Nature is wild and serene, and so am I.

When you use a phrase such as one of these as a tool of thought in meditation, pulsate with it. Whisper or think the phrase, very lightly. Then notice whatever feelings, sensations, or images the phrase evokes. Enjoy the sensations of breathing for a few moments. Then gently think the phrase again.

Welcome all random thoughts, and don't judge your experience. Anything you are tempted to try to block out is actually some part of your own life electricity and wildness—your *marut* energy—that needs your attention.

3

शक्ति

ŚAKTI

Shakti: Power and skill in the use of power. Ability, strength, might, effort, energy, capability, effectiveness, efficacy of a remedy, regal power, the energy or active power of a deity personified as his wife and worshipped by the Shakta (sect of Hindus), the female organ (as worshipped by the Shakta sect either actually or symbolically), the power or signification of a word, the power or force or most effective word of a sacred text or magic formula, creative power of imagination (of a poet).

Practice

Shakti is power in all forms; she is the energy or active power of the divine. She is the power of generation and creativity, the power of words, the energy of mantras, and the creative power of imagination. Shakti is *pranashakti,* the life-force expressing herself as the flow of energy through the body. Shakti is Mother Nature.

Meditate on shakti as the dynamic breath of life within you. In the middle *(madhya)* of the motion of breathing, delight in the splendor of life. Attend to breath as play, enjoy the rushing motion toward the end of the exhalation and inhalation, and savor the tiny movements as the flow reverses from one to the other.

There are little moments at the end of the exhale and again at the end of the inhale when the air is not moving in a specific direction. It is not still; it is like a river, with eddies and swirls, and the blood is absorbing oxygen and giving off carbon dioxide. A lot is happening, but it's a quiet space of refreshing calmness. You can rest your attention in these turnings. A thoughtlessness opens up. In these moments, life is twiddling its thumbs, rebooting.

In this quiet swirling, you can say to yourself: "I am filled with the power of life."

Or you could use a prayer or verse from your native religion to say something like, "God is breathing in me the breath of life."

You could think the word *shakti* as a mantra, uttering it as an inner expression of awe. Whenever you use a Sanskrit word as a mantra, whisper it softly for a couple of minutes as you are getting used to the word. If you really like the word, it will continue to resonate in your awareness. From there, you can follow it into silence and spaciousness.

4

कुम्भक

KUMBHAKA

Kumbhaka: A pot, a measure. A jar, pitcher, water pot, ewer (jug with a wide mouth). The sign of the zodiac Aquarius.

Practice

With this sutra, we are invited to attend with tenderness to how we embrace the breath. There are many yuktis here. One is to consider the lungs to be a pot for holding the breath. *Kumbhaka* has the connotation of a jug of elixir, a chalice, a vessel used in ritual offerings to the gods. We revere the air flowing in and out of our lungs as if it is an elixir, and we hold the breath as we hold a chalice of some precious substance we are imbibing.

In pranayama, you may hold the breath in the sense of stopping it. But in meditation, holding the breath can mean holding it as you would a lover. Holding is an embrace, a welcoming touch, contact skin to skin. In lovemaking, we hold the other person in order to allow them to move and allow ourselves to move. In certain sweet moments, the action pauses. Holding and embracing do not mean stopping the flow of movement. Embrace the flow of breathing as you would something infinitely valuable, and you will know peace. There is a world of skill in the way we receive, hold, embrace, cherish the breath.

How do you hold a baby, a cat, a lover? How do you hold a note when singing? Develop a light touch in your practice, so you can hold a thought, a mantra, a breath, as lightly as you would a hummingbird that has landed on your finger. It alights on you. There is no sense of capture. It is a miraculous meeting. Many meditation techniques emerge from your skill at holding, embracing, and cherishing your relationship with the world.

Meditation enhances our capacity for aesthetic perception and rapture. Put yourself in situations of such joy and surprise that your breathing pauses spontaneously in awe—"it takes my breath away." As your capacity for this type of *kumbhaka* develops, fill it with the beauty of nature and great art, whatever is so beautiful you want to drink it in.

5

सूक्ष्म

SŪKṢMA

Suksma: Subtle. Minute, small, fine, thin, narrow, short, feeble, trifling, insignificant, unimportant. Acute, subtle, keen understanding. Nice. Atomic. Intangible, intangible matter. The subtle, all-pervading spirit; the Supreme Soul. Marrow. Woven silk.

Practice

Suksma has a range of meanings, including "insignificant, unimportant." This is a teaching: what you are looking for is right here, but it looks insignificant to you. The gateways that open to your inner life are here, in minute perceptions easily overlooked. The inspiration and energy you need for your meditation practice is already present; tune in to the subtle aspects of your sensory experience that are so tiny they seem intangible and atomic. Be alert for that which is as fine as woven silk.

You can think of *suksma* as subtle sensuous experience. You walk outside on a beautiful day and feel a tingle of sexual electricity, just because you are alive. It lasts a second and then disperses throughout your whole body. But your next breath is a bit more enjoyable, and colors seem brighter. There is a microscopic level of sexual excitement flowing around your skin. That is subtle sensuality.

Or say you are listening to music. At a certain moment, one of the players touches a string lightly, and the quiet sound moves you deeply. The music doesn't have to get louder for you to feel its power. That is subtle sound.

Or consider a moment when you are loving someone, and the lightest touch means everything. A delicate and slow touch can feel more intense than big motions. That is subtle touch.

Subtle sensing is fun and freeing. You take more and more pleasure from less and less input. In this yukti, you are invited to take pleasure in subtle electrical sensations flashing through your body, from the *mula,* the root of your spine, through the sexual centers, into the belly, heart, throat, and head. The verse reinforces the notion of subtle and minute with the word *kirana,* meaning "dust, very minute dust" and "beam of light, like the rays of the sun, or moonbeam." We sense the energy of life sparkling like dust motes, drifting slowly in a beam of afternoon sun.

6

क्रम

KRAMA

Krama: Progressing step by step. Succession, order, uninterrupted or regular process, sequence. The position taken by animals before springing or attacking. Method. Attainment of the object desired.

Practice

Sometimes when you are making love or meditating, the energy of delight will slowly build and flow through each area of the body, touching everywhere, tickling and massaging. Here the use of the word *krama* alerts us to notice both the progression of energy movement and the sense of it being poised to spring. Watch cats creeping up on something, step by step, and then crouching to spring. Observe this progression in your mind and body: A series of thoughts will lead up to something, and then suddenly a realization will spring into your perception. In sex, the energy builds up and then suddenly gushes.

Whenever there is energy, there is the play of tension and release. In tantra, we are stretching our capacity to pay attention. In music, tension builds and then is released. In physics, tension pertains to stretching. In electricity, tension indicates voltage—the higher the tension, the higher the voltage. In sex and meditation, energy sensations may intensify in one area of the body until we feel we can't take it anymore, then release and stream to the next area or dissolve in orgasm.

We each have our own individual preferences in terms of sequence, which may vary from day to day. *Krama* suggests both inevitability and surprise. Attention is more engaged when we have the sense that we are going to get release, yet don't know when.

In your body, you may have noticed, there are areas of more energetic intensity, such as the perineum, sexual organs, lower belly, solar plexus, heart, throat, forehead, top of the skull. In the physical body, there are nerve plexuses corresponding to these interesting places. In the subtle body, the body made of prana, these networks are sometimes called *chakras*. The word *chakra* means "wheel, a potter's wheel, an astronomical circle, a cycle of years or seasons; a whirlpool." Your physical body is the center of a galaxy of subtle magnetism.

Find the sequences that work for you. Don't impose anyone else's system of body energy onto yourself. Explore and make your own map. The chakras evolve through being employed appropriately; for example, your heart chakra develops by loving people, not by being forced to open. You will learn about your own internal sequencing through love and meditation.

One of the amazing gifts of a healthy meditation practice is the ability to relax deeply into the ever-changing, unpredictable, always surprising, ecstatic flow of the life-force.

7

मुक्त्वा

MUKTVĀ

Muktva: Loosened up, freed, let go. Having liberated one's self, having attained final emancipation. Having put aside, excepting, except, save.

Practice

Muktva is the energy of liberation—"I want to be free! I want room to live! I want to express all the life that is in me!" This urge is a primordial force, one of the strongest impulses in a human being. If you want to thrive in yoga, connect with this unstoppable force in yourself, and let meditation be a space to let your energy run wild.

Each area of your body, each vibrating wheel of delicious energy, may have its own idea of freedom. Your sexual center may want a certain kind of contact, your solar plexus may want to feel powerful, your heart may ache to flow freely in love, and your head is concerned with its own agenda. One of the keys to a healthy meditation practice is to give yourself permission to feel all of who you are. Cherish all your instincts and emotions. As you introduce the feeling of *muktva* into your meditation, all your energy centers may start talking with each other about what they want, giving you fantasies and sensations. This is good. Enjoy the show and practice the skills of conversation. Let everyone talk and listen to each other. Consider meditation a safe place to be in conversation with your radical impulses toward freedom, whatever they are.

When you accept a wild impulse of freedom and let it permeate your body with energy, attention gets attracted toward *suksma,* the subtle dimensions of your life-force, and a vibrant serenity emerges.

Another key to freedom is to let meditation be a safe place to explore, where any and all feelings are allowed. You can let any thought or emotion come without editing it or controlling it. You don't care what thoughts come and go, and you don't try to remember them. All you need to do is make a simple decision: "I won't act on any thought or emotion that comes during meditation."

You give freedom to meditation by letting it be its own separate state of awareness, in which the body-mind system can explore new patterns of connectedness. Then, after meditation, with a clearer mind, you can make time for decisions.

8

पूर्य

PŪRYA

Purya: To be filled or satisfied.

Practice

In a moment of great awe or delight you may spontaneously take a deep breath and hold it. This is a portal into ecstasy. Savor the experience. Shimmering energy permeates everywhere within the skull and expands outward to dissolve into space. In such a moment the world looks illuminated. You may have a sense of stillness, of time being suspended.

You can bring a sense of delight into normal breathing by lingering for a moment at the end of an inhalation and enjoying the sensations of being filled to overflowing.

Go to places of great beauty, whatever inspires awe in you, and inhale the wonderfulness into your body. Drink it in. You can also call up a memory of natural beauty, great music, or any other situation in which you would gasp in delight. Let this reverence, this state of wonder, flood your being, fill you up to the top, and then notice the way you spontaneously breathe.

9

हृदय

HṚDAYA

Hṛdaya: Heart (or region of the heart as the seat of feelings and sensations), soul, mind (as the center of mental operations); the heart or interior of the body, the heart or center or core or essence or best or dearest or most secret part of anything. True or divine knowledge, the Veda. Science.

Practice

In this practice we are invited to enter the heart through the door of the senses. The first word of this sutra is *sikhi,* "a peacock, name of Indra, the god of love." In the tradition this text emerges from, a peacock feather is sometimes used in giving *shaktipat,* a heart-opening transmission of initiatory ecstasy. The peacock is the national bird of India, and the feathers are gorgeous. They shimmer and have multicolored circles on them. In the yoga tradition, these circles symbolize the senses, and this image suggests that we can receive a shocking transmission of divinity through any of the senses. The senses can be a pathway to the heart.

Take any sense—touch, smell, taste, hearing, vision—and meditate on it through its full range, from the obvious level of information to the space between particles. When you follow any sense into its subtlest state and beyond, you will find yourself entering the heart of space. Notice how each sense works, what aspect of the mystery of life it tells you about.

There are thousands of practices here. Track all of your senses through their full range of stunning beauty, from the outer beauty to the vibrant emptiness of their true nature. Follow the trail of that allure into the mysterious and powerful spaciousness that is the essence of matter, the heart of the matter.

IO

पात्र

PĀTRA

Patra: Drinking vessel, goblet, bowl, cup, dish, pot, plate, utensil, any vessel or receptacle. A meal (as placed on a dish). The channel of a river. A capable or competent person, an adept in, master of, anyone worthy or fit for our abounding in. An actor or an actor's part or character in a play. A leaf. Propriety, fitness. An order, command. A measure of capacity. A king's counselor or minister.

Practice

When you meditate, you could use any of the objects of attention mentioned in the previous nine sutras—all those breathing and kundalini techniques—or you can use any thought that crosses your mind. Any object of perception—a meal, a riverbed, a person you admire, an actor—can serve as a portal into meditation. It can serve as a mantra, a tool of thought. Whatever is attracting your interest is a channel, a river for some kind of energy to flow into the world. If you don't feel like doing an "official" practice, with breathing or mantras or energy running up the spine, just use what's in your mind.

Say you are meditating and start thinking about an actor. You may be musing on the way she channels goddess energy into the world. Your mind has not wandered; instead it is wondering—"How do I embody my own spiritual and sensual power? How can I access my full spectrum of energies so that I can work through the obstacles in my life? That actor may have kids, and yet she still shows up as a goddess. Maybe I can too, in my own way."

Welcome mind wandering and know it as part of the adventure of consciousness. Meditation is generally rhythmic: we pay attention to something for a while, then drift off and daydream, and then we wake up and re-engage with the mantra. The more you accept this cycle, the more refreshed you will be by all this inner journeying. So whenever you find yourself thinking of food, a loved one, or an actor or a character in a play, novel, movie, or television show, accept that as your mantra of the moment.

II

न्यास

NYĀSA

Nyasa: Putting down or in, placing, fixing, inserting, applying, impressing, drawing, painting, writing down. Depositing, entrusting, delivering. Written or literal text. Lowering (the voice). Introducing. Consigning or entrusting anything to the mind. Mental appropriation or assignment of various parts of the body to tutelary deities.

Practice

Nyasa can refer to ritual touching of various parts of the body while saying prayers or mantras. In so doing, you are awakening a quality of the divine and assigning or placing it in that area of the body. Here you are invited to introduce sacred qualities to the inside of your skull and to the crown of the skull.

It is best to start out informally. Say something like, "I want my head to be filled with the most beautiful light, gorgeous music, and a view that goes on forever." Just make it up. Don't impose anyone else's idea of the sacred on yourself. The space inside your skull can become a perfect island getaway, a concert hall, the entire range of the Himalayas, vast reaches of outer space, or a medieval church with rose windows and saints everywhere.

You don't have to stick with one thing forever. The decor inside your head can be just for today or even just for the next five minutes, and then you can redecorate. What matters is that *you* decide what you would like your inner space to be filled with—how many windows to have, how open to the outer universe you want to be.

There are several healthy qualities you develop in this way. First of all, the activity of choosing activates your mental circuits and introduces freedom; the changed elements introduce the possibility of novelty into your perception, and in selecting what you want, you can develop a combination of being at home in yourself and being on an adventure. These qualities will serve your meditation practice in the long run.

In this tradition, the skull, *kapala,* is an offering cup of brilliance dedicated to this infinite divinity in which we find ourselves.

12

मध्य

MADHYA

Madhya: Middle, the middle that embraces all. In the middle of the body, a woman's waist. In algebra, the middle term or the mean of progression. The middle finger. In music, a particular tone, also a kind of meter. The middle of the sky. The space between (the eyebrows). The belly, abdomen. Ten thousand billions.

Practice

This is a practice of wonder, tenderness, and connection. Explore the relationship between the earth below you, your body, and the sky above.

In nature, magnetism flows between the opposite poles. The sun and the earth are polarities; the ocean of air above and the ground below are polarities. As you learn to live your life in conscious relationship with the above and the below, your own body becomes the middle, the *madhya,* and the magnetism flows through you. Your body is a bridge, an electrical circuit joining heaven and earth. *Yukti* is "joining." A human being is something the universe created to link the below and the above.

You might take walks and open up your senses to the sky above and ground below, then lie on the earth and do the same. You could dance or practice tai chi. You could visit places with a huge sky and places where you love the earth. Over time, learn to tolerate the sense of immensity both above and below.

There is nothing to be forced. This is a love relationship. Give it time, give it flowers. Go on dates and pay attention. The text says *devya taya*—"by means of the Goddess this practice is revealed."

द्वार

DVĀRA

Dvara: Door, gate, passage, entrance. Opening, aperture (especially of the human body). A way, means, medium. The Mahesvaras hold that there are six *dvaras,* or means of obtaining religious ecstasy.

Practice

Doors can be open and they can be closed. Sometimes we long to close it all out, shut the door, and put up a sign saying, "Go away." This yukti gives you permission to do just that.

Close the outer doors of perception, *dvaras,* and open your inner senses. You can do this in any way that is attractive to you, such as wearing an eye mask and earplugs, meditating in a silent and dark room, or floating in a sensory deprivation tank. You could put your fingers over your eyes and in your ears in *shanmukhi mudra.* Most people can automatically shut out the outer world, instantly and without effort, whenever they find something interesting to attend to in the inner world.

Alternately, use your hands to lightly touch and bless the openings in the head—the ears, nose, mouth, and eyes. In your imagination, create an energy shield around the head and around your body. Wrap yourself up in protective light. "Putting on armor" is the sixth definition of *yoga* in the Monier-Williams *Sanskrit-English Dictionary.* Armor can be a prayer that gives you the ability to turn away or postpone unwanted energies. When you close the door to the outer world, there is a beautiful feeling of having just the right armor to protect your inner temple.

14

बिन्दु

BINDU

Bindu: A detached particle, drop, globule, dot, spot. A mark made by the teeth of a lover on the lips of his mistress. A colored mark made on the forehead between the eyebrows. A spot or mark of colored paint on the body of an elephant. The sudden development of a secondary incident (which, like a drop of oil in water, expands and furnishes an important element in the plot).

Practice

There are sudden and surprising developments in the plot of our everyday lives and in the adventure story of our inner lives. Sometimes the Goddess gives us a love bite, leaving a little *bindu* mark saying, "You are mine." In the outer world or in meditation, you may see something so beautiful that your heart is shaken (*kshobha,* "shaking"). It's a glimpse of heaven, and you are changed. You are marked by love.

You catch sight of perfection, and it stirs an inner flame, lights your fire. The sensation is almost orgasmic. The beauty out there awakens a subtle flame in your heart and mind, behind the eyes. Whenever this happens, welcome it and follow the melting into the heart. There is blessing here. Let the swoon carry you into the arms of divine consciousness. This is an initiation. The world is an open-air ashram, and the guru is everywhere. The Beloved is everywhere. The holy is here.

When you look out on the world, be alert for what lights up your eyes. The delight is a kind of disturbance; it shakes you and awakens the fire within. It lights up your eyes, lights up your heart. You melt. This simple moment, which all tenderhearted people experience, is a door to the mystery of heart. If you meditate on this flame, you may find yourself dissolving and entering the cave of the heart. One of the high purposes of meditation—*dhyanartha*—is to be prepared to savor and cherish these moments when they occur.

15

अनाहत

ANĀHATA

Anahata: Unbeaten, unwounded. Produced otherwise than by beating.

Practice

Whenever you can, listen to waterfalls, streams, rivers, and oceans—any flowing water. Listen from different distances so you can appreciate both the steady roar and a distant hum. Sometimes go so far away that you can barely hear it. Meditate in all these places so you will become attuned to the rushing and to the whisper. The word *anahata* suggests that you explore and find the sounds that are particularly soothing to your heart. This is a good practice in itself, and it also attunes the body to other types of flowing currents, even internal ones.

There are many rivers inside a human body, thousands of miles of blood vessels. That is just the physical level. On the level of the prana body, there is similar intricacy. This yukti invites us to listen to the flow of life within. There is a sound of your own heart center vibrating. You may hear it if you are finely tuned. It is the song of you, the vibration of you having this adventure in existence. It is always there, rushing like a river, a whisper. Once in a while you may hear it while meditating, especially in the early hours of the morning before dawn. No matter what your technique, sometimes the quiet roar will just be there. There is nothing you did that caused it. When this happens, simply listen and be with it.

Hata is a term in Indian music meaning "struck, beaten (as a drum)." In Sanskrit, when you add a short *a* to a word, it means the opposite, so *anahata* is "unstruck"—the chord that keeps resonating without beginning or end. *Anahata* is also a term used in the chakra system to refer to the heart center, the wheel of life energy vibrating in the region of the physical heart. So right here we have one of those cheerful little jokes you find everywhere in Sanskrit: hearts beat—that's what they do. And hearts get wounded. But there is a level of your heart that is unbeaten and unwounded. Any time you want, come take refuge here and be healed, in your essential heart that is steadily humming along.

16

प्रणव

PRANAVA

Pranava: The sacred syllable OM.

Practice

Listen to *pranava,* the hum of expansive joy permeating the universe, reverberating everywhere, including within you. The *shakti,* the divine power, will flood you with *shunya,* exquisite spaciousness.

Pranava is usually decoded as *pra* ("pre, before") plus *nava* ("shout, exult")—the shout of joy that came before everything, the primordial sound of the universe continually and ecstatically singing itself into existence.

Here are some of those stunning layers of meaning in Sanskrit. *Pranava* is the nickname of OM, and OM means "yes." The cosmic OM is Creation saying yes to itself, its ongoing expansion. The dictionary describes OM as made up of *a, u,* and *m.* Notice the sounds people make spontaneously when they are feeling "Yes!" When the life in them is saying yes to a hug, a bite of chocolate, a sip of warm soup, or the perfect piece of music for the moment, they will utter sounds such as *ahhh, oohh,* and *mmm.* How brilliant of the ancient lexicographers.

You can create a mantra by noticing what sounds you make spontaneously when the feeling of yes is rising in your body. The sounds you make in exuberance, delight, deliciousness, and expansive joy are your natural *pranava.* You want your mantra to feel like it comes from inside you and leads you there.

OM actually has many official variations. Each meditation school has its preferred way to articulate it, just as different rock bands make up their own unique sounds. *Eem* is a form of OM, as is *hum, hreem,* and simply *mmm.* If you take any vowel and add *mmm,* you have a version of OM. These *eeee* sounds have a quality of "Whee!" They are energizing.

Although we usually think of *pranava* sounds as being peaceful, don't forget the definition: a roar of joy. When people are relaxed and at ease and expressing joy, they say things like, "Oh yeah! *Hell* yeah! Amen! Ahhhh-*men!* Hallelujah!" Here is a fun exercise: Listen to twenty thousand people at a sports event, roaring at some play on the field. Hear it as a form of *pranava*.

This sutra also introduces the term *bhavana,* which has a meaning of "steeping, infusion." Soak your body in the feeling of yes, the vibration of yes, whatever that is for you. Let the hot water of your blood and your passion for life mix with your primordial yes. Meditate with that. Listen to the hum of it and follow it into the great silence.

17

शून्य

ŚŪNYĀ

Shunya: Empty, void, hollow, barren, desolate, deserted. Absent-minded, having no certain object or aim, distracted. Empty as in possessing nothing. Alone, solitary, having no friends or companions. Free from wanting, lacking, nonexistent. Vain, idle, unreal, nonsensical. Void of results, ineffectual. Bare, naked. Guileless, innocent. Space, heaven, atmosphere.

Practice

Whenever you are practicing with acoustics—with sound or mantras—the *silence* before you think or say the sound and the vibrant silence after you think or utter the sound are gateways. A mantra prepares your body and tunes your nerves so that *shunya,* the nothingness, is interesting. *Shunya* is not something your mind can grasp, since it is no-thing. The definition "bare, naked" suggests that the mind itself is naked.

As you listen to any internal music, mantras, or vowels, notice the way the vibration alters your structure, sets the web of your subtle body vibrating. There is an infinity of tiny delicious sensations—the sensuous *texture* of your inner life. *Purva* is "being before," and *anta* is "end of a texture, pause." *Texture* means "web, structure, network, weaving." As you become aware of the network of your nerves dancing in emptiness, in *shunya,* the sensation is unutterable. Even a few seconds of this can be as satisfying as an orgasm (well, almost).

The key to this practice is not correct pronunciation of a mantra; it is the urge in you to explore the play of sound and silence, how the song of your unique life manifests itself in quiet inner harmony. The ancient texts say there are tens of millions of mantras, which is a way of saying that everything you could ever utter is mantric. All mantras are to call you home into the silence and vibrant emptiness. When you find your true mantra, it may be hard to remember because it is always fading away into silence and *shunya,* nothingness, space, heaven, atmosphere. Truth is what works.

18

तन्त्रि

TANTRI

Tantri: The wire or string of a lute, the strings of the heart, any tubular vessel of the body, sinew, vein.

Practice

Seek out the most rapturous music you can find and listen to it on the best sound system available. Live music can have an even greater impact. Music you love will teach you things about meditation and life that you can learn in no other way. Ask around, "What is the most beautiful music in the world?" Find a way to expose yourself to it so that you can let go and be carried away. Make time to give over totally. Be stunned.

In other words, be a teenager in love with a band. In reality, what works for you could be any type of music—classical, kirtan, country, R&B, rap. What matters is you love it so much you want to dissolve into it. In a song, in the space of a few minutes, we can let go, lose ourselves, and then return, refreshed, with a deeper sense of self.

Listening to music, we ride our passions into the vibrating core of energy from which they arise. Life is rhythm, and music invites us to surrender to the rhythm of life and love. This sutra invites us to begin by listening to external music and then to follow the impulses into the inner world. People who love music already know the truth of this sutra, and they are surprised and delighted to see it affirmed in a classic yoga text.

The image in *tantri* is that of stretching cords or strings over a framework. This is the basic technology of a stringed instrument or of a weaving loom. The *tan* of *tantri* has a wide series of meanings, including "to believe in; to afflict with pain; to resound, roar; to extend, spread, be diffused as light over, shine, extend toward, reach to; to be protracted, endure; to stretch a cord, extend or bend a bow, spin out, weave." This sounds like rock and roll to me. *Tan* changed in pronunciation to *tar* is the root of *sitar* and *guitar.*

Tan generated a family of words that includes *tantra,* which has a totally mind-boggling definition:

> A loom, the warp, the leading or principal or essential part, main point, characteristic feature, model, type, system, framework. A class of works in the form of dialogues between Shiva and Durga discussing 1. the creation, 2. the destruction of the world, 3. the worship of the gods, 4. the attainment of all objects, especially of six superhuman faculties, 5. the four modes of union with the supreme spirit by meditation. A spell. Oath or ordeal. An army. A row, number, series, troop. Government. A means which leads to two or more results, contrivance. A drug, chief remedy. Wealth. Happiness.

All these meanings can be seen as the subject of passionate music.

Whew! When you love music, you know that the vibrating strings of the instruments set your heartstrings vibrating in resonance. You know that music is the "main point" and that it is a mode of union with the spirit. You know that music is a "drug and a remedy, wealth and happiness."

What music is so ravishing that it leaves you in a stunned and pulsating silence, the "aesthetic arrest" James Joyce identified, in which your mind goes silent in awe of the presence of great beauty?

19

मन्त्र

MANTRA

Mantra: Instrument of thought, speech, sacred text or speech, a prayer or song of praise. A Vedic hymn. A sacred formula, mystical verse. Incantation, charm. The primary mantras being held to be seventy million in number and the secondary innumerable. A plan or design. A name of Shiva.

Practice

Play with sounds that feel like food for your ears. The verse uses the word *piṇḍa:* "Any round heap, a ball. A roundish lump of food, a bit, morsel, mouthful. Food. Daily bread, livelihood, subsistence." These metaphors point to mantras that are nutritious.

What constitutes a nutritious sound is different for each of us and may change over time. Many of the classic meditative mantras feel like sounds of nature, the hum of electricity, the *eeeemmmm* of power flowing through nerves. Other mantras feel nourishing, like food. What matters in terms of yukti, skillfulness, is finding the sounds you love so much you want to be with them. Here are some seed sounds to explore: *hring, shring, kring, hung, aing, shyam, ram, aim, kleem, lam, vam, ham.*

Read comic books and look at how they write descriptions of action sounds. Cartoon sound-effect words might seem silly, but actually they are great examples of the thrill of shouting into the universe. These loud, all-capital-letter explosions can be easily seen and felt. Sense the explosive *KABOOM! BLAM! WHUMPH!* How about that great *BOING* when a guy is eyeballing a girl, or *POW, THWIP, BONK* when there's a fight going on?

What you want to develop are the sound effects that go with your unique inner life. Life is a musical, and these are the sound effects for your meditation. You can take energy and nourishment from them.

Mantras are all around you, and whether you know it or not, you are constantly using them in everyday speech. Consonants fill our words. Sometime when you have a few seconds, explore sounds such as *Hhhhhh,* the raucous *Rrrrrrr,* and the exciting *Sssssss.* Notice if these sounds resonate with you.

It's also great fun to listen to engines revving—those of planes at airports, cars at race tracks, lawn mowers in the neighbor's driveway. Listen to bees humming in the garden or your cat purring. Listen and know that space resonates with the silent potential of all these sounds. Let yourself feed on them in the most natural and immediate way.

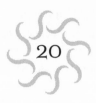

वियत्

VIYAT

Viyat: To dispose in various rows, arrange. To do penance. Being dissolved, passing away, vanishing. The sky, heaven, air, atmosphere. Ether (as an element). Name of the tenth mansion in astrology. A kind of meter.

Practice

Consider all directions, simultaneously, as being dissolved into sublime emptiness.

The many meanings of *viyat* suggest vanishing into thin air, perhaps accompanied by haunting and peaceful music.

You could be in any pose—sitting, standing, lying down, floating in a pool, suspended in a sensory deprivation tank—and sense all directions simultaneously.

> Above me is endless space.
> Below me is endless space.
> Behind me is endless space.
> To my left is space.
> To my right is space.
> Within me is endless space.

As the directions dissolve, so does your definition of yourself. This is exciting and freeing. If you are attracted to this exploration, start by letting yourself be with these phrases for a minute. That is enough. Maybe that minute will stretch into a few minutes. As soon as it stops feeling like a luxury, move on. Gradual is good. You might be with this thought for a minute or two every day, as part of your meditation time. Then, over weeks and months, enjoy the spaciousness you are perceiving as you move through your world. Don't do too much. Always give your senses and your sense of balance time to adapt.

When you do the proper amount of this type of meditation for your body and your lifestyle, you will feel free and have the sense of lots of space around you to move in and explore. Your sense of direction will get stronger, and you will be better at navigating in the world. It is as if you rebooted your whole relationship with space. If you do too much, you can get spaced out, as they say. Always fine-tune your practice so that you function better in your daily life.

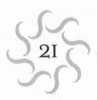

21

पृष्ठ

PRṢṬHA

Prishtha: Standing forth prominently. The back as a prominent part of an animal, the hinder or rear part of anything. To carry on the back. The upper side, the roof of a house, the vault of heaven. A page of a book. The back of the body, the spinal column.

Practice

When you look up at the night sky and see an arc of stars stretching from horizon to horizon, that is the vault of heaven. *Prishtha* suggests that you perceive your spine with the same sense of wonder, as if you are gazing into space. Each vertebra is a celestial sphere, made of emptiness and stars.

A simple movement meditation with *prishtha* is to get on your hands and knees and explore gentle curving motions with your spine. Imagine each vertebra is an area of the sky, with a few stars. Continue to undulate gently and get used to space above you, space below you, space within you, spaciousness permeating the whole area of your back.

22

त्स्थिर

STHIRA

Sthira: Firm, hard, solid, compact, strong. Fixed, immovable, motion-less, still, calm. Not wavering or tottering, steady. Unfluctuating. Taking courage. Kept secret. Faithful, trustworthy. Firmly resolved to. Settled, ascertained, undoubted, sure, certain. A kind of meter. A name of Shiva. Certain zodiacal signs. The earth.

Practice

Take courage *(sthira)*, take heart *(hṛd)* that you are permeated with infinite space everywhere and you still exist. Get interested in the sense of spacious freedom permeating your spine, the area between your legs, and your heart. As you enter this feeling, find your way into steadiness.

This is a *shunya* meditation, inviting you to firmly sit down on nothing; you are emptiness sitting, standing, or lying down on emptiness. The back is space. The area between your legs is flooded with space. The heart pulsates in spaciousness. Cultivate this feeling steadily, firmly.

Develop these experiences, then meditate on them simultaneously *(yugapad)*. As you develop the ability to perceive your heart and spine as space and to be with them as space, allow also the coexistence of both empty space and the appearance of matter. You don't need to deny the solid nature of your spine; you are just contemplating that everything is made out of emptiness. A beautiful, clear feeling arises as a result.

निर्विकल्प

NIRVIKALPA

Nirvikalpa: Not admitting an alternative; free from change or differences. Admitting no doubt, not wavering. Free from thoughts.

Practice

The yukti here is simple and direct: if even for just a moment you experience the body as free and open space, you become free.

For example, put your arm out in front of you, and then take a full five minutes to bring your hand to touch your heart. Slow, subtle movement, if you choose it, can be so interesting that your mind becomes free of thought. The word used for this lack of thought is *shunya,* which means, among other things, "empty, void, hollow, nonexistent; bare, naked; space, heaven, atmosphere."

This sense of *shunya* can happen at times of transition, such as falling asleep or waking from a nap, getting out of the shower—anytime. It can happen in between any two thoughts. Enter the space between thoughts and experience your body as a void. In that brief moment, you will become free, one with your original form, your *svarupa.*

One day I was sitting on the sofa meditating and idly wondering about this verse. Then suddenly I was inside the experience it is referring to. In a moment, I dissolved into void-space-heaven. It felt heavenly and totally normal. I was at home in the universe. Then I beamed into being myself again, back into my body, feeling very refreshed. Somehow, wondering about this sutra and thinking it in Sanskrit took me right inside. I needed access to this freedom.

Entering the space between thoughts can occur at almost any time, spontaneously, in moments of grace, beauty, or love, but also in times of loss and shock. We go there any time we need to renew ourselves in our essence.

24

भावन

BHĀVANA

Bhavana: Demonstration, argument, ascertainment. Feeling of devotion, faith in. Reflection, contemplation. Saturating any powder with fluid, steeping, infusion. In arithmetic, finding by combination or composition. The moral of a fable.

Practice

Bhavana has the remarkable meaning of "infusion"—as when you are making tea, infusing an herb in alcohol, making a medicine to drink, or soaking yourself in a quality you love and need. To practice a *bhavana* meditation, think of a quality you would love to be permeated by, and soak in it.

Steeping, infusion—you can think of this in various ways. One is making tea or coffee. You have some quality you want, the tea leaves or the ground coffee, and you mix it with water and let it sit. Voila, you have something new—not just plain water and not dry leaves or beans, but this magical drink. Sometimes we do this process just for joy. Infusion also has a medicinal aspect; we can infuse special herbs with water and make a tea that balances our body energies. And infusion has a meaning of "continuous slow introduction of a solution into the body." There is a quality you need or crave, and by meditating on it, you slowly, gently, continuously introduce it into the body and introduce your body to it.

Let's go over the instructions for a *bhavana* meditation again.

First, think of one, two, or three qualities you would love to be infused with. Ask within yourself, "What would I love to be filled with? What kind of energy? What quality of being?" You could write these words in your journal. Your words might be quite different from one another, such as *power, peace, love* or *excitement, stability, clarity.*

Second, give yourself a chance to love each word, leisurely. Bond with the word; let your body be at home with it.

Third, develop a rhythm of leisurely thinking of each word and then pausing to feel it resonating in you. Like when you drop a pebble into a pond, watch the ripples. You might think one of your words every ten or twenty seconds, so it takes a full minute to think all three.

Get used to this rhythm: the word, the feeling of the word, the sensations and imagery, the silence after the word, then the next word.

You can meditate in this way for five, ten, or twenty minutes a day. That's it. You're all set. You can do this with any quality you love or are devoted to or have faith in.

25

त्वच्

TVAC

Tvac: To cover. Skin, hide. A cow's hide used in pressing out the *soma.*
A leather bag. Bark, rind, peel. Cinnamon. A cover (of a horse). Surface (of the earth). A mystical name of the letter *ya.*

Practice

This yukti explores the mystery of skin. There are several phases to
the practice. To begin, simply dwell with the feeling that within the
skin is vastness. Or, if you prefer, within the covering is nothing.
After a while, something surprising happens—the dual perception of
boundaries and spaciousness releases your senses to perceive reality at
a deeper level, and this shift of perception stimulates changes in your
internal chemistry. The senses get so happy to be doing what they are
built for, their higher purpose, that they set in motion the manufac-
ture of your own happy hormones.

Note that *tvac* refers to the "skin used in creating *soma,*" the
ambrosia of life. In ancient texts, *soma* is the mythical psychedelic
plant infusion that gave the ancient yogis the ability to hear the mantras resonating in eternity. *Soma* is "juice, extract, especially the juice
of the soma plant, offered in libations to the gods." This juice was
collected by moonlight on certain mountains. *Soma's* other meanings
include "the moon; nectar; heaven, sky, ethers; a drug of supposed
magical properties."

Translated into the here and now, from the mythic to the somatic,
the *soma* spoken of in this sutra refers to the process by which the
body produces its own molecules of delight, which we might call
endorphins. In the meditation tradition, *soma* refers to the body's
natural nectars that enhance perception. In this one little word, *tvac,*
we see a hint at one of the central aims of this yoga, which is to stay

juicy. These 112 practices open perception in a way that creates joy at being alive, at even the simplest things in life, and this deep appreciation tunes the body so it can produce *soma,* the intrinsic chemistry of delight.

This is the way *soma* was explained to me when I was a teenager and first learning about Kashmir Shaivism. When I meditate in this way, inside is all free and open space, and the world outside looks like gorgeous art, luminous and ever changing.

26

सम्पुट

SAMPUṬA

Samputa: A hemispherical bowl or anything so shaped. The space between two bowls. A round covered case or box (for jewelry). A hemisphere. The kurabaka flower. A kind of sex. Credit, balance.

Practice

Do whatever makes your heart sing, then listen in. What you hear is the primordial mantra, and it is a portal to your inner world. *Samputa* evokes the image of the heart as an infinite singing bowl. The word also points to the resonating space between two bowls—between two hearts, two chakras, two bodies. In tantra, *samputa* can refer to containing or covering the jewel of one mantra with another, for example *Om Hrim Om. Aha* would be a good covering mantra, because it is a palindrome. *Aha Shiva Aha* would be a *samputa* mantra.

Samputa also refers to a series of poses in the yoga of sex. Shiva is saying to Shakti, "Under the bowl of the infinite sky, let us make love. I am infinite consciousness; you are divine creative energy. Let us lie together and move through the *samputa* poses, sharing our secrets of love. May the delight-filled Goddess energy join with the infinite I-AM consciousness, as equals."

In this yukti, the aspect of you that is Shakti, the vibrant energy of life, is lying with her lover, Shiva, who is your essential consciousness, and magnetism is flowing between these polarities. *Samputa* is also "the space between"—the space between jewel boxes—and this space is lush with juicy, flowing energy that hums with an ecstasy about to gush forth. The ecstatic magnetism flowing between the Goddess and her Beloved gives rise to mantras.

Samputa suggests that mantras emerge spontaneously from the vibrancy of the relationship of energy and consciousness. Listen to the mantra of the heart as if it is emerging from the sigh of lovers: *ohhhh . . . mmmmm . . . ahhhhh.* You might also hear a humming sound, like that of bees. The kurabaka flower is referred to in Sanskrit love poetry as "rich in nectar and a lure for bees," who excite the air with their humming.

The verse begins with *hrdya,* "being in the heart, inward, pleasing to the heart, beloved, cherished, savory food that makes your stomach happy, a delicious liquor made from honey." In the heart you are free; there is open space, *akasha.* The *samputa* mantra resonating here creates a delicious liquor; drink and be refreshed. Allow your attention to alight here, as lightly *(nili)* as a bird settles on a tree. Follow any impulse of cherishing inward to the heart and rest in the vast spaciousness of what the heart is. Meditate on the current of love itself and let it call you home.

Anything that has ever pleased your heart can be your guide. All that you adore, all that is nourishing to the heart, all that has ever made you feel like you are drinking the sweet honey nectar of life, is always here in your heart. Come rest in this splendor.

27

मनोलय

MANOLAYA

Manolaya: Loss of awareness due to total mental absorption. *Manas:* mind (in its widest sense). *Laya:* The act of sticking or clinging to. To become attached to anyone, to disappear, to be dissolved or absorbed. Lying down. Melting, absorption in. Rest, repose. Place of rest, residence, house. Sport, diversion, merriness. Delight in anything. An embrace. In music, time. A kind of measure. The union of song, dance, and instrumental music. A pause. A swoon.

Practice

There are sweet spots everywhere in the body—areas the mind *(manas)* loves to melt into and delight in *(laya)*. If we take the definition of *laya*, above, and unfold it a bit, we hear something like the following: "If you follow the pendulum of the breath from its highest point, where it swings up into the head, to its lowest point, where it swings down into the vibrating area between the legs, you will find many places of rest—residences and houses for your attention to dwell. These places invite you to enter and be in enjoyment. The atmosphere is alive with music and dance."

Run your hands over your body and explore the places that feel like the union of song and dance—luxurious areas you want to linger in. Be sure to include the arms, hands, legs, and feet. Go get massage from a really skilled person and then meditate afterwards and chart your whole body. Do things that make you feel fantastic, and when in the height of feeling wonderful, sit down and meditate and sense where the energies are dancing. In lovemaking, notice the areas of heightened sensation where awareness is intensified. If you study the chakras, keep in mind that those are someone else's maps of their body, a little sketch of some moment of their life. That's their song and dance. What's yours?

If you feel called to lie down, swoon, melt into pleasure, then *laya* is working for you. The chakras are entertaining places to rest and sport with the energies of life and love. When you find an area you are called to embrace, give over to the sensations, memorize the inner dance of energy, and listen to the quiet inner music.

28

क्षिप्

KṢIP

Kṣip: To throw, cast, send, dispatch, to move hastily (the arms or legs), to throw a glance (as the eye). To direct the thoughts upon, to throw away, cast away, get rid of, to utter abusive words, insult, to throw into, to cause to descend into.

Practice

Select one of the delight-filled centers in the body and learn to be "centered" there as you live your life. This yukti is a continuation of the previous one, 27.

First you may want to explore your chosen center only during meditation (or lovemaking or dancing or music). After a while, you may begin to feel at home in yourself and realize, "Oh, this is my residence—one of my many residences—and it's good to be here." After you stabilize in this perception, begin to explore being poised in that area as you move through your day. Practice being in yourself and "centered" while doing chores, working, talking, and loving people.

Yukti means "skillful," and if you do this yukti skillfully, you will function better and have *more* attention for the outer world, even though you are also attending to your inner delight. *Kṣip* is almost a physical skill and can be approached playfully—*throwing* your attention, again and again, into your body, the way you would throw a baseball or football to a partner. Through practice you develop elegance, grace, and effortlessness.

When you are in a sweet relationship with your chakras, you can turn to your essence in a moment then come back to the outer world without losing track of anything. You have more presence because you are continually refreshed in the stream of prana flowing through you.

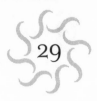

29

अग्नि

AGNI

Agni: Fire, sacrificial fire (of three kinds: *garhapatya, ahavaniya,* and *daksina*). The number three. The god of fire. The fire of the stomach, digestive faculty, gastric fluid. Bile. Gold.

Practice

The yukti here is the relationship of the body and flame.

It helps to know that biological life is fire. Our bodies burn at almost a hundred degrees, night and day, even if the environment is cool. Each cell is a little flame, a tiny hearth cooking up the sustenance of life and transmuting the elements into energy. The process of transmutation is called fire. The sun is fire. Our bodies are fire. The sun shines on the oceans, forests, and farms, and the fiery sunshine is absorbed by the plants through the magic of photosynthesis. When we eat the plants or something that eats plants, we absorb this energy and turn it into heat and energy to move with, in a continual dance.

Get into this practice very gently, tiny step by tiny step. If you like candles, spend a few minutes appreciating one. If you like the warmth of the sun on your skin on a winter afternoon, cherish that. If you have access to a fireplace, make yourself cozy, watch the flickers, listen to the crackles, and absorb the warmth. Over a period of months, become intimate with flame as it relates to your body.

I took several months getting to know this sutra, phrase by phrase, then memorized the first paragraph, "I am immersed in the flame . . . ," as my mantra. I let the words and the images and sensations they invoked roll through me, very slowly, in meditation for half an hour, morning and evening.

If you are called to this practice today, the flame of the soul is already here. It is a relief to snuggle up with it. This is a chance to rest, be at peace with, and inspired by the flame of life.

30

अनन्यचेतस्

ANANYACETAS

Ananyacetas: Giving one's undivided thought to.

Practice

This is a flame meditation in which you recognize that the universe is made out of flame and always at play. If you are called to this meditation, you have a relationship with the sacred flame, and your awareness longs to merge with it.

In Sanskrit, this merging is *ananyacetas.* Your intelligence, *cetas,* is made of brilliance and revels in the universal fire. The Self recognizes its own elemental nature. We don't usually experience this cosmic reality in our bodies; our awareness is encrusted with accumulated worries about our place in the world. Thus, we develop a craving for radical freedom. In this meditation you are not praying that everything be destroyed; you are releasing your awareness into the realm of pure splendor. This is akin to meditating on being made up of molecules, atoms, and subatomic particles. It's intense yet relaxing.

Every particle of creation is aflame, a tiny sun. Everyone and everything is already one with God. Nineteenth-century Anglican minister John Henry Newman said, "Heaven and hell are the same place. It's just that in hell people resist the flame." It can be an extraordinary relief to sense that the universe is aflame. Get someone to explain a bit of astrophysics to you, so you can grasp that the matter in your body, all around you, everything you have ever touched or eaten, was once part of a sun.

31

पर

PARA

Para: Far, distant, remote (in space), opposite, ulterior, farther than, beyond, on the other or farther side of, extreme, previous (in time), former. Ancient, past. Later, future, next. Following, succeeding, subsequent. Final, last. The Supreme or Absolute Being, the Universal Soul. The highest point or degree. The wider or more extended meaning of a word.

Practice

Wonder and awe are power sources propelling this practice. What is the world made out of? What is my body made out of? The technique is to take any element of your body and develop a subtler and subtler *(suksma-suksma)* appreciation of all its levels, until you perceive its foundation, its ultimate reality *(para),* the source of existence.

You can use any schema of the basic constituents of the universe that attracts you—the elements of the periodic table; the Aristotelian forms of earth, air, fire and water; the five elements of Chinese qigong, earth, metal, water, wood, and fire; the Buddhist great elements or *Mahabhutas;* or the *tattva* ("thatness") of Shaivism or Samkhya. Or you could make up your own system. Whatever element attracts you becomes your mantra, your tool of thought.

One of the skills here is to find what fascinates you so deeply that you want to go in and spend time meditating in this way. When you discover an element that intrigues you, engage with it using all your senses and instincts. If you suddenly fall in love with the element of water, pay special attention when drinking anything, bathing, walking in the rain, watering the plants, or swimming. Take a hot bath and notice that there is water outside your body, while inside your body you are about 75 percent water. You could take your blood pressure and marvel that a fluid is circulating within your body. Notice what thirst is and develop a taste for simple, pure water. This practice is endless, because we have so many senses with which to see, smell, taste, touch, and hear the elements. We are not only built out of the elements, but we are also designed to love them. The particular sensory aspects of the elements we are attracted to are as unique to us as our voices and eyes.

Para is the Universal Soul, and in practicing this yukti, you are asking Her to take you into her kitchen and let you see how bodies and planets are whipped up out of nothing, following the Cookbook of Creation.

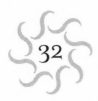

32

स्वतन्त्र

SVATANTRA

Svatantra: Independence, self-will, freedom, one's own system or school, one's own army, free, uncontrolled, full grown. *Tantra:* A loom. Metaphorically, a framework or network of interconnected threads. A system. From the root *tan:* to extend, spread, be diffused (as light) over, shine, extend towards, reach to, to stretch (a cord).

Practice

With an external practice such as asana, you can imitate someone else. You can watch the teacher do a pose and follow along. With the internal aspects of yoga, such as meditation, there is no way to imitate anyone else. We can't see what someone is doing if they are sitting there with their eyes closed. Meditation is internal yoga, just you and infinity. What actually happens inside you is unique to you. So with meditation, you need to begin with *svatantra,* freedom and independence, or else you will not end up there. You have to feel your way and follow your inner call right from the beginning.

In meditation, whenever you sense restriction, be alert to the possibility that the technique you are practicing does not suit your essence. Perhaps you are imprisoning yourself in the name of discipline. Your longing for freedom is one of the most powerful forces in your being. Yoga emerges from this longing. When you feel like quitting a specific practice or discipline, it is not failure. That system may have worked to get you through a certain phase of your life. But you have outgrown it and are now being called to a deeper discipline, one more in accord with your true nature. Your yoga is evolving into a new form, which may be unknown to you for a while.

When you graduate from a school, celebrate. The Vijnana Bhairava Tantra makes it clear that when you integrate one particular yukti and are ready to move on, another is calling you. Give yourself time to explore the practice that suits your life now and helps you to thrive in your inner and outer worlds.

33

भुवन

BHUVANA

Bhuvana: A being, living creature, man, mankind. The world, earth. All three worlds—earth, hell, and heaven, or earth, psychic, and spiritual. Place of being, abode, residence. A house. Causing to exist.

Practice

This practice is a path of wonder, in which we allow our loving attention to engage with the inquiry, how did the universe—all these people, planets, and stars—get here? What course is the universe following? *Adhva* is "road, way, orbit, journey, distance, time, method, the zodiac," suggesting you consider the revolution of planets around stars, the revolution of galaxies around their cores, and the nature of space and time.

Wonder invites attention toward the subtle, the world beyond the world. This verse uses the phrase *sthula-suksma,* "gross to subtle." Attend first to the obvious level and then allow awareness to be called into layer after subtle layer of this magical dance until you dissolve into infinity. Follow each perception from *sthula,* the massive, dense level, to the *suksma* level, the atomic. Then go beyond into *para,* that which is beyond—the infinite mystery out of which we have emerged.

Don't be surprised if your mind dissolves in awe after fifteen seconds. The mind is fast. Your natural speed might be such that once you begin to consider the multiple levels of this dancing universe, your mind might go silent in wonder within a few seconds. In a minute, you might cycle from contemplating the whole universe, to silent awe, and back again several times.

34

समन्त

SAMANTA

Samanta: Having the ends together, contiguous, neighboring, adjacent, being on every side, universal, whole, entire, all, on all sides, around.

Practice

In the course of a day, in our ordinary awareness, we forget the grandeur of the cosmos as we focus on the local. At any moment we can remember the immensity we are part of. In this practice we are invited to inhabit that simple truth: the universe is extending in all directions. Your body is the center, and above, below, to all sides, the majestic play of space and energy stretches out forever.

You may already sense infinity all around you and be slightly terrified by the vastness. This terror (*jagadbhaya*, "terror of the universe") is natural and is one of the doorways into ecstasy (*dvara*, "door, gate, passage, opening, way, means, means of entering ecstasy"). You may be able to tolerate it for only a few breaths at a time. It is a very odd sensation to be standing in your garden or on a mountain and experience the earth beneath you as translucent, a little grain of sand floating in a boundless ocean. If you had the resources, you could build a room in which the floors, walls, and ceiling are monitors showing movies of vast reaches of interstellar space with star systems and constellations, worlds upon worlds.

One of the skills involved in this practice is developing spherical awareness. Before and after meditation, stand and look in every direction. Extend your arms and move them as far in every direction as they can go. Now close your eyes and continue, sensing the nature of space all around you. In this way you gradually develop global, multidirectional awareness. As you get used to this, add multisensory awareness, in which you see, hear, and feel in all directions. When you meditate with spherical awareness, great brilliance arises.

If you want to develop a verbal mantra to go with this meditation, it could be something like this: *In all directions, relatedness. In all directions, intimacy. In all directions, belonging.*

If you enjoy spiritual language, you could formulate a thought such as, *The endless divine mystery is extending around me in all directions* or *On every side of me is infinite God consciousness.* Modify the phrase to be something meaningful to you. *Samanta* is a beautiful mantra to go with this meditation and sums up all of the above.

Another word in this sutra is *maha,* "great, strong, abundant, a feast, a festival, the festival of spring." One of the side effects of this practice is that the world begins to seem like a festival. So take someone to lunch. Make dinner for a group of friends. If you are alone on retreat, feed the birds.

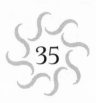

35

विचिन्त्

VICINT

Vicint: To perceive, discern, observe, to think of, reflect upon, ponder, consider, regard, mind, care for. To find out, devise, investigate. To fancy, imagine.

Practice

Breathe with all the meanings of this word *vicint* for a few minutes to open the space for your meditation. Perceive, discern, observe, reflect, consider, regard, care for, find out, devise, investigate, imagine. Here is a whole set of nuances to attention that are as distinct as different asanas.

Each term used in the definition suggests a different style of attention, a particular craft-skill in your internal yoga. In any given moment, the quality of attention life asks of you may change—from discerning to pondering, from considering to caring for, from investigating to fancying, from reflecting to imagining. Each of these is actually a very different posture or asana for tending to your inner and outer world.

An overall skill of meditation is allowing each surprising moment of your experience to invoke just the right quality of engagement. You may find yourself flowing from tending with adoration to studying carefully, then going off into flights of fancy—all in the space of a minute. This supple motion of awareness is how you let the process of meditating be so interesting that you become absorbed. The text uses the word *laya*, "absorbed, dissolved, sport, diversion, merriness, delight in anything."

दृष्टि

DṚṢṬI

Drishti: Seeing, viewing, beholding (also with the mental eye). Sight, the faculty of seeing. The mind's eye. Wisdom, intelligence. Regard, consideration. View, notion. Theory, doctrine, system. Eye, look, glance. The pupil of the eye. Aspect of stars.

Practice

Whenever you have time and the inclination, throw your awareness into empty spaces, into any container—a pot, a room, or a huge meeting hall, any interesting space with sides or walls. If you want to go on an outer expedition, visit all kinds of spaces and sacred places, temples, and cathedrals.

Be prepared to catch what happens in the twinkling of an eye. Notice what happens in an instant. There is a momentary dissolution, a quiet dissolving into space, then in the next moment you come back to yourself.

People who work with spaces as their craft are natural yogis in their own way and often are happy to share their perceptions. Go talk to potters; learn how they see the inside of pots. Talk to architects and walk around a room with them; they shape matter to make space. Find whoever designed a temple and listen to them talk about the space. Interview an acoustic engineer who designs auditoriums. Seeing is beholding.

37

वृत्

VRT

Vrt: Surrounding, enclosing, obstructing. A troop of followers. To turn, turn round, revolve, roll (also applied to the rolling down of tears). To move or go on, get along. To pass away the time. To be intent on, attend to. To have illicit intercourse with. To cause to turn or revolve, whirl, wave, hurl.

Practice

The definitions of *vrt* make my head spin. *Vrt* is the root of *vrtti,* a term often used in yoga to indicate whirlpools, mental vortexes. *Vrtti* has additional meanings pertaining to addition and occupation, working, practice, business, livelihood, and wages. *Vrtti* is also defined as the final rhythm of a verse, a commentary, comment, gloss, explanation (especially of a sutra).

The sutra suggests you go to a place *(desa)* where there are no trees, no hills, no walls, and with open eyes, gaze at nothing. Behold that wide-open space. Throw your attention into that spaciousness. As your mind dissolves in emptiness, your addictions, preoccupations, mental whirlpools—the vortexes *(vrtti)*—will gradually diminish. No matter how many times the *vrttis* intrude, return again and again to the simple beauty of bareness.

This practice is especially valuable when you are besieged by repetitive thoughts or worries, by old thinking that creates suffering. You can take a mental vacation and visualize a wide-open, boundaryless space. Sometimes there is nothing like actually going to such a place and spending a week just letting your mind empty itself out.

प्रकाश

PRAKĀŚA

Prakasha: Visible, shining, bright. Clear, manifest, open, public. Pronouncing a name out loud. Expanded. Universally noted, famous, celebrated for. Renowned throughout. Openly, publicly, before the eyes of all. Clearness, brightness, splendor, luster, light. Elucidation, explanation. Appearance, display. Manifestation, expansion, diffusion. Publicity, fame, renown, glory. Sunshine, open spot or air. The gloss on the upper part of a (horse's) body. The messengers of Vishnu. Laughter.

Practice

Prakasha makes me laugh. When the space between any two perceptions, thoughts, or objects starts shining forth, it is kind of a joke. One moment, space is just there, hiding out in the open, "No one can see me." Then, with the magic of attention, the space in between becomes bright with interaction.

The mantra (tool of thought) in this practice is the space between any two somethings—two breaths, two clouds, two mountains, two trees, two boxers in the ring, two teams on the field. In lovemaking, it is the space between two bodies, between two breasts. In a conversation, it is the space between two people.

At first, the middle space may feel like nothing. But as your awareness shifts levels toward the subtle, the space between begins to seem like the most dynamic thing happening, a magnetic field. When you get this, the invisible somehow becomes illumined and richly textured, and this is such a wonderful surprise that you may burst out laughing.

39

निरुद्ध

NIRUDDHA

Niruddha: Held back, withheld, held fast, stopped, shut, closed, confined, restrained, checked, kept off, removed, suppressed. Covered, veiled.

Practice

Focusing is easy when you are in love. When we are devoted to someone, we focus on them naturally and close ourselves off *(niruddha)* to other affections. For this practice, select something you are so interested in that you can pay attention to it forever—something you love so much you are willing to give up everything else to be with it *(tyakta,* "left, abandoned"). Immersed in this love, witness the blossoming of deep meditation, *bhavana.* Keep cultivating your interest; become more and more intimate with this one person, animal, object, art, or skill.

A universe of skills is required if we are to stay in love. *Niruddha* itself requires a light touch; restraint easily becomes suppression, and suddenly love feels like bondage. Yet not having enough restraint can endanger your primary relationship; a great love may light you up so much that you feel you can love the whole human race. Love wants to spill over, gush. But you can't share your love physically with everyone because there isn't enough time or space or condoms. We have to explore and find the right kind of restraint for each moment, each day. This skill set is ever changing, applying the exact nuance of holding and freedom appropriate in each heartbeat.

Niruddha is saying, "Be loyal to your love. Keep on going deeper with this *one*." That one baby, cat, dog, horse, woman, painting, piece of music, or garden contains the essence of the cosmos. One of the great gifts of meditation, where meditation and love intersect, is that meditation is an act of paying attention. As our attention grows stronger and deeper, we become more capable of staying interested in one person. They are new and surprising in every moment.

When we bond with another person, with an animal, with family or a team, it is as if there are invisible strings connecting us with them. Each string is a nerve connection, a living current of prana. Whenever we are working with strings, we are in the realm of tantra, in its sense of weaving together the strings of life into a fabric. Cherish these connections. The sacred function of *niruddha* is not to block out the world, but to free you to attend to love.

40

देह

DEHA

Deha: The body. (From the root *dih,* to plaster, mold, fashion.) Form, shape, mass, bulk (as of a cloud). Person, individual. Appearance, manifestation, having the appearance of.

Practice

Meditate simultaneously on the universe and your body *(deha)* as being pure consciousness.

Deha suggests appearance. We look as if we are solid and made out of matter, yet we know from science that matter is made of energy and is almost entirely space. Somehow our bodies are fashioned out of energy and space. In this meditation, you accept something deeper— that the matter of your body and the entire universe are made not just of energy and space, but on a deeper level, of pure consciousness.

When you dive into this meditation, you are not a generic person taking a snapshot of generic space. Each camera and each lens takes a somewhat different picture. Each photographer has a different eye. Each of the bus-sized telescopes orbiting the earth reveals a different aspect of the immense cosmos we inhabit. You have a somewhat different set of life experiences than anyone else who has ever lived, and when you meditate upon your body and the whole universe as being made of consciousness, there will be nuances you perceive that may not have been known before. Even if your form is only as lasting as a cloud, well, so too is a galaxy just a cloud of stars.

41

वायु

VĀYU

Vayu: Wind, air (as one of the five elements); breathing, breath. A mystical name of the letter *ya.* In medicine, the windy humor. In yoga, refers to *prana, apana, samana, udana, vyana.* In astronomy, the name of the fourth *muhurta* (a moment, forty-eight minutes, the thirtieth part of a day). The god of the wind, said to have sprung from the breath of *purusa;* he is said to move in a shining car drawn by a pair of red or purple horses or by several teams consisting of ninety-nine or a hundred or even a thousand horses; he is often made to occupy the same chariot with Indra and, in conjunction with him, honored with the first draught of the *soma* libation. *Vayu* is rarely connected with the *maruts,* although he is said to have begotten them from the rivers of heaven. Desirous, covetous, greedy, desirable, desired by the appetite.

Practice

It is impossible to be appreciative enough of breathing. In the definitions above, each word and image points to something exciting and magical. A thousand red or purple horses pulling a shining car—what an image for the dynamic power of breath and the blood vessels that meet the air as we breathe in. The greatest skill you could bring to breathing is being in awe and wonder. Some time, you might want to take a year and track all the metaphors associated with *vayu;* make your own imagery, so that when you think or say the word, you perceive a rich mandala of meaning.

Vayu also means "desired by the appetite," and this meaning points to life itself as driving our practice. Life's hunger for prana, for air, is what gives power to this practice.

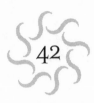

42

आनन्द

ĀNANDA

Ananda: Happiness, joy, enjoyment, sensual pleasure, the thing wished for, the end of the drama.

Practice

There is a universe of practices encoded in the thirty-two syllables of this sutra. Notice that *ananda* is used twice, to emphasize that sensual pleasure and happiness are essential. Here are a couple of mantras you can play with as a way in:

> *Sva ananda bharitam:* "I am nourished and filled with the
>   bliss of my soul."
> *Sva amritam:* "I am suffused with the nectar-essence of life."

The verse also uses the word *amrta (amrita):* "Not dead. Immortal. Imperishable. Beautiful, beloved. An immortal. A god. Name of Shiva. The plant *Phaseolus trilobus.* The nectar (conferring immortality, produced at the churning of the ocean), ambrosia. Nectar-like food. An antidote against poison. Medicament in general. The residue of a sacrifice. Anything sweet. A pear. A ray of light. Name of a meter."

You could begin meditating with the *amrita* that permeates your body—*sva amrita*—and as you shift levels, you accept that the entire universe is filled with your joy and your essence. Or you could meditate on the cosmos and your body simultaneously as being filled with your *ananda* and *amrita.*

Bliss is a necessary foundation for yoga practice. Without it, the electricity of the life-force can grate on your nerves. Bliss is nourishing, and it suffuses, lubricates, and coats the nerves with the deep pleasure of existence. When you find bliss, notice and welcome it.

Do not let any voices tell you that feeling pure joy is not a serious meditation practice. Bask in pleasure, shamelessly.

Amrita is also "an antidote against poison, a medicine." If you have ever gotten involved in service, working in the harsh, broken places in the world, you may need to get away and bathe in your own *ananda* and *amrita* for sustained periods to counteract any poison you have been exposed to. *Amrita* and *ananda* nourish and heal every cell of the body and sustain the heart as we live in the world.

43

कुह्

KUH

Kuh: To surprise or astonish or cheat by trickery or jugglery.

Practice

Life is full of surprises, and one of the sacred functions of meditation is preparing us to be poised and ready to laugh, especially when the joke is on us.

During meditation, welcome surprise, however it shows up—in thoughts, shifts of mood, or changes in your state of consciousness. Welcome the sense that you have no idea what is going to happen next in your practice. You could be feeling bubbly and energized and suddenly fall asleep. You might think you are sleepy and sit to meditate, and somehow you instantly feel energized. Before a meditation session, you might think you are in a dull and stupid place, and yet when you close your eyes, suddenly you are full of sunshine inside, and you feel wonderful. Accept that you have no idea which item of your to-do list will demand your attention. Your brain has eighty billion neurons, and they are all talking to each other. Your body has tens of thousands of miles of nerves and blood vessels, and they want a chance to commune with each other. When you welcome surprise, you are more likely to perceive the magic show that is our every living moment.

And who knows? The universe, they say, popped out of nothingness. That is what magicians are telling us as they pull rabbits out of hats. We love being astonished. Joy rises in us when we accept the surprising nature of reality.

Say you are at an outdoor wedding, where everyone is dressed up, the women have done their hair, and suddenly a rainstorm blows in and drenches everyone. That is one of nature's tricks. There is nothing to do but laugh. Welcome the laughter as a gift of the divine.

44

स्रोतस्

SROTAS

Srotas: The current or bed of a river, a stream, torrent. Water. Rush, violent motion or onset of. The course or current of nutriment in the body, channel or course for conveying food. An aperture in the human or animal body (said to be nine in men and eleven in women). The spout of a jar, an organ of sense. Lineage, pedigree.

Practice

Prana is breath, life, vitality; *shakti* is power, energy, skill. This is a meditation on the power of life flowing everywhere in the body and through the channels of perception. When you understand that *pranashakti* is singing to you through all your senses, you will be filled with transcendental happiness.

Srotas is "current"—currents of *pranashakti* or life power flowing through the body and streams of sensuous perception. The stream can be quiet or rushing and violent. The focus here is on quiet perception. Learn to be alert for these tiny sensations of the *pranashakti*, as subtle as an ant walking on your skin, flowing through your senses.

Srotas is also the flow of sensory nutrition; the sensual data flowing into your awareness is nourishing. If you don't know how to receive nutrition from simple sensuous experiences such as listening to music, working in a garden, watching a baby sleep, or looking at art, go find people who do and spend time with them. There are people everywhere in the world, on every block, in every occupation, who know this secret. They have nothing to do with yoga or meditation; they don't really need to, because they already know, inherently, how to practice this sutra.

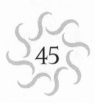

45

युज्

YUJ

Yuj: To yoke or join or fasten or harness (horses or a chariot). To make ready, prepare, arrange, set to work, use, employ, apply. To equip (an army). To put arrows on a bowstring. To fix in, insert, inject (semen). To turn or direct or fix or concentrate (the mind, thoughts) upon. To recollect, recall. To join one's self to. To be united in marriage. In astronomy, to come into conjunction with. To encompass, embrace. Exciting, an exciter. Being in couples or pairs.

Practice

Yuj is the root of both *yoga* and *yukti* and has a similar semantic range. *Yuj* refers to all kinds of joining, including sex. In the embrace of exciting sex, we can feel like we are made out of happiness. We are in union with a flow of brilliant inner energy, and we are sharing it. We want to cherish every moment, to the last drop.

In this meditation, you enter the fire of desire and prolong the experience of lust. As you join with your lover, throw your awareness *(ksipet)* right into the middle of sexual arousal, into the incredible joy, power, and fire of desire.

Making love is the highest form of yoga—and the most demanding. You are called to bring every molecule of awareness and skill to each moment and be ready for anything. You need to attend simultaneously to the energies of your own body and of your lover's. You have to be aware of every nerve that tingles in your body and in your lover's and to sense what is needed—what embrace and quality of touch to give.

The first word of the sutra, *vahni,* implies that our sexuality is an elixir we are offering to the gods. The streaming ecstatic energies and sacred juices flowing in your body are here to assist in your enlightenment. All of the practices of tantra yoga may come to you spontaneously, in the fire and ecstasy of desire, to help you go further into divine awareness. Your body may turn into a pure hum of vibration, the essence of mantras. You may taste the nectar of life. The electricity flowing along your spine and skin may shoot upward into heaven and downward into the earth. You may feel as if you are dancing, immersed in music, or dissolved into space.

46

संगम

SAMGAMA

Samgama: Coming together. Meeting, union, intercourse. Connection or contact with. Sexual union. Confluence; the confluence of two rivers or of a river and the ocean (such confluences are always held sacred). Conjunction of planets. Harmony. Adaptation. Point of intersection. United.

Practice

In this yukti, the moment of orgasm is the gateway to cosmic awareness. When we come together in orgasm, the rivers of shakti flow into each other.

There is a series of perceptions to enjoy and embrace along the way. First honor the shakti, the divine power manifesting in you and your lover. The desire for sex is a gift of the divine. Then honor the coming together of two shaktis—the shakti of your passion and the shakti of your lover. You are flowing toward each other. You yearn to gush. Then honor the sensations of orgasm, which flood every cell and nerve of your body, as a manifestation of the essential happiness of your own soul. The verse invites you to know, "This flash of joy is my essential reality."

Use all the skills of yoga you have developed in your daily practice to cherish each moment of lovemaking. When you find the meditation practice that truly suits your individual nature, it will enhance your ability to be present with this intensity.

Every other sutra prepares us for lovemaking and gives the body a chance to be ready to give and receive love. *Pranashakti* flows through our senses like a river of energy and tunes them for life, enlightenment, and sex. Orgasm is a magnificent moment, and every nerve has to be ready, willing, and able to partake of the mystery.

47

लेहन

LEHANA

Lehana: The act of licking, tasting, or lapping with the tongue.

Practice

We can bathe in the experience of lovemaking again and again, even if we are not with our lover. Welcome the memory of kissing, licking, lapping, touching, and being touched, and in meditation allow your consciousness to open up to the universe embracing you.

Love changes us. Its touch goes deep inside and remains in our cellular memory. The delight is supposed to be lasting. If you have ever been in love or want to be, you can let your heart and soul be filled with the juiciness of this love as if it were happening right now.

During meditation, recall the experience of making love and let it energize all your nerves. Sexual arousal is a form of *pranashakti* flowing through your body, nourishing you and rejuvenating your will to live. This is an important practice on the path of intimacy. We learn so much from love. The sense memory of any moment of love can be a gateway into a deeply nourishing meditation.

Simple moments of embrace change the cells of our bodies. Your daily meditation practice should keep you tuned for sex, vacations, work, and play. When you think of lovemaking and savor the feeling, your nerves tingle. This will happen spontaneously, and it will come and go. Even a second of that tingle feeds life-giving prana through the nerves. You could be lying in the sun, walking in the wind, feeling the contact of nature on your skin, and be reminded of your lover's caress. Although lovemaking memories are particularly nourishing, many kinds of memories feed us. *Bharatsmṛteḥ* is "nourished, full." *Smr* is "to remember, recollect." Notice that within the word *remember* is *member,* which in Sanskrit is *anga*. Re-membering is itself a form of yoga—connecting, linking together.

There is a joke within the word *samplavaḥ,* which means "flowing together, meeting and swelling of waters, flood, deluge, noise, tumult (especially of battle), submersion by water, destruction, *ruin.*" One day when I was working on this text, a friend called and said, "I'm *ruined.* I have the perfect job, perfect apartment, perfect yoga class, the perfect circle of friends. My life is as good as can be if you are a single woman living alone at age thirty-five. But I met a man that I love, and now I have to throw all that away and change everything so that I can be with him."

48

बान्धव

BĀNDHAVA

Bandhava: A kinsman, relation (especially a maternal relation), friend.

Practice

When you are meditating and think of someone, a friend or family member, savor the nature of the bond between you. If you love the person, there is joy in that bond. You can meditate on that *ananda.* It is a path to the soul.

Bandhava refers to bonding, and resonates with *bandha:* "connection or intercourse with; putting together, uniting; a mode of sexual union—there are said to be sixteen, eighteen, thirty-six, or even eighty-four modes; constructing, building a bridge; bridging over (the sea); directing the mind or eyes; conceiving, cherishing, feeling; arrangement of musical sounds, composition; a border, framework, enclosure, receptacle; a sinew, tendon."

Bandha is a realm of yoga techniques that involve "containing" the vital energies or prana of the body. Thus, the word suggests that any attachment, any of your relationships, if approached with skillful awareness, is a yoga. *Bandha* is building a bridge over the sea, making a connection between two hearts. Our relationships are pathways to enlightenment.

When we are bonded with other people, it is as if there are strings connecting our hearts to theirs, and these strings vibrate as they stretch. A bond of relationship is a "tendon" and also "an arrangement of musical sounds." There is a music to each of our bonds.

Bonding is an experience we all know, a very human moment. The teaching suggests we dive deeper into the joy of relatedness, of bonding, and cherish it with the total power of our attention. Take this rising bliss, this *anandam udgatam,* as a gift of the divine, meditate on it, and merge with it.

Ananda is a dimension of the divine—a vast oceanic experience, an ocean of delight. Even though we, as souls, are incarnate, we are also in oneness with the bliss of eternal consciousness, *sat-chit-ananda.* When we see someone we love, a gateway to this divine bliss opens up. Each separation and reunion with a loved one reminds us of the union of body and soul. One of the meanings of *yoga* is "union," and therefore a reunion teaches us something about yoga.

Make a practice of meditating on this joy. Each person you love or have loved is a doorway to the divine. When you think of them, it is as if you are thinking a mantra, a name of God. When you unite with them, even by cherishing their memory in your heart, you are practicing a kind of *bhakti,* love yoga. Dogs are masters of this *dharana.* When dogs see someone they love, they don't hold back. They levitate with bliss; it rises in them, and they leap. Lately, part of my practice has been to meditate on the uninhibited joy dogs express. Teachers are everywhere in our environment and in the connections we have with all other living beings. Who are your teachers on the path of love?

49

रस

RASA

Rasa: Juice, best or finest part of anything, essence, liquor, elixir, potion, nectar, semen, taste, flavor, love, affection, desire, charm, pleasure, delight, the taste or character of a work.

Practice

I love the word *rasa*. What a range of succulent meanings! You can meditate with *rasa,* which means physical tastes and also the juiciness of life in general. *Rasa* is a state of cherishing life in which you are open to the outer world and its ever-changing play, and open to your inner world and the ever-changing play of your subjective responses. *Rasa* emerges any time you are savoring your life experience, witnessing your own emotions as if you are watching a play or movie.

Juice yourself up. If you are practicing meditation, develop and cherish your appreciation for the great tastes in life. If you are attentive, a sip of pure water is delicious. You might find yourself craving sunlight, water, the air you find in a forest, the smell of garlic, the taste of apricots or ripe fruit, chocolate with sea salt, a sip of wine or high-quality juice. These desires may be telling you of an element you need for your health—your physical, emotional, or spiritual wellbeing. Yoga refines instincts; you need to listen to them. As your body awakens, so will desires; explore them as appropriate for your situation.

Meditators often practice on an empty stomach, before breakfast and dinner, when the body is getting ready to eat. Hunger arises, and you reject it. It rises again, and you dissolve it. Over time, this may result in your body becoming unenthusiastic about food and uninterested in digesting it. Your metabolism may slow down, and your digestion gets weak. Many practitioners experience diminishing vitality and health as a result. But if you cherish desires and let your body eagerly look forward to eating, you will tend to have better digestion and better instincts about what to eat and how much.

Seek out the most yummy smells and tastes available to you. Relish them. In meditation, when desire for a taste or smell arises, welcome it and meditate on it. Whenever you are eating or drinking something delicious, give an extra minute to savoring. That extra sixty seconds can be quietly life changing.

50

आरूढ

ĀRŪḌHA

Arudha: Mounted, ascended, bestridden (as a horse). Risen. Raised up, elevated on high. Undertaken. Reached, brought to (often used in compounds, such as *indriyarudha,* meaning "brought under the cognizance of the senses, perceived"). The mounting, arising. Leaping upon, covering.

Practice

The inner motion of meditation is presented here as an enthusiastic, life-embracing activity like jumping on a horse—"Let's ride!" This sutra is saying, "If you want to practice yoga, mount up! Jump onto your greatest joy and go."

Asvada is "eating with relish, also (metaphorically) tasting, flavor, enjoying." Any sensual pleasure is a gateway into meditation. The practice here is to savor the banquet of the senses, especially music, which is a joy like nothing else in the world. Mount the joy as it arises in you, and ride it into oneness with the soul.

Yoga extends the reach of our senses. When we utilize this extended reach, we fine-tune our abilities to metabolize prana, the energy of life. This sutra is inviting us to attend to the feast of the senses that is everyday life and to use the skills we practice in yoga to ascend and transcend with the joy.

51

स्वरूप

SVARŪPA

Svarupa: One's own form or shape. Your own condition, character, nature. Your own peculiar character. Wise, learned.

Practice

This verse begins with *yatra yatra,* "wherever, whithersoever." Wherever your mind finds satisfaction, there is your meditation practice. Then we see the amazing word *svarupa,* "your own peculiar nature." A reading of this verse would be, "Wherever your mind wanders, there you can experience the absolute bliss of your peculiar nature."

If you talk to people about their secret joy, that thing they love so much they live for it, there is an infinite range of peculiar activities. Rejuvenating old cars. Fly-fishing. Bathing naked in mountain streams. Training dogs. Gardening. Painting mandalas. Golf. Surfing. It doesn't matter what you love. What matters is that you love it and you choose it freely.

Svarupa is the shape of your soul. In all these practices, in everything you do in meditation, follow the shape of your own soul. Practice in a way that feels to you like your favorite hobby or indulgence—that natural way you would putter in the garden if you love gardening, wander around a city if you are a traveler, curry the horse if you are a horse person, play your instrument if you are a musician—and you are just alone, exploring.

Para ananda svarupa is "the transcendental joy of your unique character." This suggests that you get to the universal through the personal. No matter how wounded, wacky, or wonderful you think you are, celebrate your individuality.

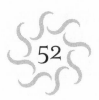

52

निद्रा

NIDRĀ

Nidra: To fall asleep, sleep, slumber. sleep, slumber, sleepiness, sloth. The budding state of a flower. A mystic name of the letter *bh.*

Practice

Sleep is an important part of meditation, and you should always welcome the impulse to fall into sleep. Take good care of yourself and tuck yourself in.

Nidra is sometimes *yoganidra:* "meditation-sleep," a state of half meditation, half sleep.

We all fall asleep for a few seconds or minutes here and there in meditation, and it's wonderful. Be prepared—have blankets and pillows at hand, so that you can luxuriate in the sleep if it happens. If you have been meditating for a while, you also might find yourself called to take naps at certain times, and many yogis find that these naps are deeper than meditation. You don't just fall asleep—you fall into magic, into the arms of the Goddess.

Meditating is a courtship. You are romancing the intrinsic divinity of life, dating *pranashakti.* There comes a time when the Goddess embraces you and takes you into her realm. What is falling asleep? It is pure surrender.

Your daily meditation practice tunes your nerves and cleans up the pathways of perception. Day by day, if you honor each impulse that arises, you attend to all the unfinished business in your mind and heal your nerves. Then you are ready. Because you are tuned to your body, you can feel the call for a nap, like a cat. And you fall into something: sometimes instead of inner darkness, it's inner light. This is *para devi prakasate* (*para,* "beyond, transcendental"; Devi, the Goddess; *prakasha,* "visible, shining, manifestation, laughter"). The

Universal Soul in the form of the Goddess, who is more ancient than time and younger than springtime, who is concerned for you, has come from beyond eternity to care for you, to fill you with her shining energy, and light you up with her laughter.

53

तेजस्

TEJAS

Tejas: Aura, glow, ray, brilliance, radiance, light, fire, luster. Spiritual power. Ardor. Splendor.

Practice

This is the sunbathing sutra, a meditation on *tejas,* radiance. Attention is invited to delight in the brilliance of *surya,* the sun. Begin with the image of *surya akasha,* the sun's luminosity permeating all of space. After a while, you will dissolve into the light. As you come back from dissolution, lightly consider the thought, *sva atma rupa,* "this is my essence." Don't be surprised if you laugh in delight. The sutra ends with a form of the word *prakasha,* "splendor, luster, expansion, and laughter."

Never do any practice unless you love it. Only meditate on the sun if you adore it. Love activates your instincts, the ones you need to be successful in this yukti and to protect yourself appropriately. *Tejas* has other meanings, including, "the bright appearance of the human body in health and beauty; fiery energy, ardor, vital power, essence; semen virile; the brain; gold." It is not just the fire of the sun that is the meditation topic here; it is the life-giving, vitalizing effect of being outdoors in the sun, the sense of being sun-kissed, filled with essence, and a sweet, subtle sexuality.

Whenever you are meditating on the relationship of your body with an element, be aware of dosage: how much of this is healthy for you in this present form, and what amount is too much? Do not look directly at the sun, ever. The light is so intense that it can damage your eyes. So you can meditate on the sun in your imagination. You could also meditate on the radiance of a light bulb, candle, or wood fire.

54

खेचर

KHECARA

Khecara: Moving in the air, flying. A bird. Any aerial being (as a messenger of the gods). A particular mudra or position of the fingers. An earring or a cylinder of wood passed through the lobe of the ear.

Practice

Sometimes the life-force in us just wants to break out and be wildly free, as if we were flying, breathing flame on people, or able to put on such a scary face that everyone would leave us alone. Children do this as the mood strikes them, and in yoga this movement has a name—*mudra*, meaning "that which gives joy."

The text lists a series of mudras, both wild and peaceful poses. Strike a pose. Feel free to throw yourself down into the corpse pose, as carefree as a skeleton on Halloween. Make a face as if you were angry or absolutely astonished, eyes wide open in awe. Sometimes in meditation practice, such gestures will spontaneously arise and carry you. There is a sense of supreme satisfaction as you fly beyond your ordinary constrictions.

Meditation is powered by our life energy, which wants to break free. And when it does, *pranashakti* is both peaceful *and* wild. We need to bust out some new moves. This often happens to people after a couple of years of sitting meditation; their bodies just get tired of sitting, and that is it—sitting is over. From now on, let's dance.

If we have come to yoga for healing, we may have needed our practice to be a cast or cage so that the bone in a broken wing can set. Now it is time to stretch our wings and fly again, so our practice needs to change. We feel an inner urge to abandon the cage of the practice that got us this far. This is not a failure of yoga; it is the success.

55

निराश्रय

NIRĀŚRAYA

Nirasraya: Having or offering no prop or stay. Supportless. Shelterless. Alone. Lying open.

Practice

There is a time to take shelter in props, and there is a time to be out in the open. When you have been doing something in sequence, after many repetitions you may find you can glide over some steps very lightly and touch down on others. This is one of the implications of *nirasraya.* You can set aside or skip over the prop of your technique.

Part of the delight of watching athletes is seeing the way they flow through their events, almost levitating. This same type of flow also develops in meditation—*antar yoga,* the inner flow of your technique. After you have gone through the steps of your practice many times and you know them by heart, go ahead and allow yourself a kind of carelessness, an easy freedom. Fly through the sequence and skip parts if you want. There comes a time to just lean into the practice as if you are skiing. At this point, you leave behind your sense of sequence and lose your addiction to support.

The mind moves at the speed of thought, and you can perceive many thoughts in one second. Sometimes your mind will delight in doing something in a few seconds that used to take half an hour or all day.

The opposite is also true: sometimes you may want to slow down a process. Human beings invent meditation techniques almost continuously, the very ones described in the Vijnana Bhairava Tantra. These come and go so quickly, in just five or ten seconds, that you may not even notice you've engaged in them. The inner teacher, the wisdom of life, has offered you a bit of instruction, an attitude adjustment, a moment of rejuvenation. When you recognize a sutra and relate to it, you have probably already practiced it spontaneously—*nirasraya,* "without props"—many times. One day you may sense the need to map out a series of steps, feel the nuances, and practice them individually. You may practice this way for minutes or months, until it becomes time to leave the technique behind and return to *nirasraya.*

56

व्योमन्

VYOMAN

Vyoman: Heaven, sky, atmosphere, air, space, ether (as an element), wind or air (of the body), a temple sacred to the sun. The tenth astrological mansion. Preservation, welfare.

Practice

This yukti is an appreciation of space. One way to explore space is to stand or sit and form your arms into a circle and become aware of enclosed space. Just notice what is there; be curious. Let space be itself, infinite, as you embrace it. Embrace the nothing.

Imagine you are encircling the whole universe. What quality of awareness do you bring to this embrace? What texture of creativity, love, and welcoming do you want to give?

Now shift perspective. Be the universe enclosing you with love, welcoming the birth of something new.

57

निपत्

NIPAT

Nipat: To fly down, settle down, descend on, alight. To rush upon, attack, assail. To fall down, upon, or into. To throw one's self at a person's feet. To fall into ruin or decay, be lost. To enter, be inserted, get a place. To direct (the eyes) toward.

Practice

This is a meditation on the experience of being ravished, transfixed, and overwhelmed by something you see in the physical world. You see someone so magnificent that immediately you have the impulse to throw yourself at his feet. You see a baby crawling along, and you are overcome with adoration, falling to your knees beside her and making cooing sounds.

Awe occurs spontaneously; be ready to go with it. See a marvelous work of art, the ravishing gorgeousness of nature. There is skill in being so open that we can be slain by beauty. We throw ourselves at the feet of that manifestation. The yukti here is aesthetic rapture; we transcend on the *rasa* of amazement.

58

जिह्व

JIHVA

Jihva: The tongue. The tongue or tongues of *agni,* various forms of flame. Three flames are named in the Rig Veda. In astrology, the twenty-eighth yoga.

Practice

This sutra refers to a whole world of practices having to do with the tongue in its role as a doorway into the subtle body. We are invited to attend to the tongue as an altar that receives the food that fuels the fire of life. The physical tongue accepts the offerings placed on it. It cherishes the food, relishes it, welcomes it into the temple of the body, where it soon becomes warmth and energy. The subtle tongue, the tongue made of prana, receives the energy in the food and transmutes this directly into vitality.

Agni, a central concept in this yoga, means "fire, sacrificial fire (of three kinds, *garhapatya, ahavaniya,* and *daksina*), the god of fire, the fire of the stomach, digestive faculty, gastric fluid."

Explore your tongue in all its senses—taste, temperature, touch, and movement. The tongue can perceive many tastes, textures, and temperatures.

If you enjoy drinking, pour two glasses of high-proof alcohol, such as brandy. Set one on fire and watch it burn. Then sip the other. Realize that food and drink really are fuel for fire. You are a slow-burning flame.

In lovemaking, when you are aroused and feel like kissing someone, explore the relationship of your tongue and your clitoris or penis. Explore the movement of the tip of the tongue. Explore the connection that runs down through the *madhya,* the middle of your being; this connection is a dancing flame through your whole core.

This meditation leads to a remarkable feeling of peace *(shanti)* as you accept the essential reality of flame.

59

क्षण

KṢAṆA

Ksana: Any instantaneous point of time, instant, twinkling of an eye, moment. A leisure moment, vacant time, leisure. A fit or suitable moment, opportunity. A festival. The center, middle.

Practice

This is an afternoon-nap-type of practice, or *shavasana,* in which you lie down and give in to gravity so completely that it feels like you are suspended in space. At first you feel the earth, the floor, or your mat or bed beneath you, then that feeling dissolves, and you are simply floating.

This sensation can happen in an instant, and it is to be cherished. There is a shift of perception inside this paradox. You lie down and give in to gravity, let your weight drop, and the instant you surrender into the weight, you become light. In the twinkling of an eye, the sensation shifts to a feeling of boundlessness. When the moment is right, something liberating can happen, effortlessly. It feels so good it must be a sin. This moment of leisure becomes an inner festival, a celebration.

60

चल

CALA

Cala: Moving, trembling, shaking, loose.

Practice

This sutra is about *dancing*. Shaking your booty is a sacred activity. The yukti here is to spaciously embrace *divya augha,* the flood of divine sensations aroused by dancing. *Divya* is "to long for heaven; divine, heavenly, celestial; supernatural, wonderful, magical; charming, beautiful, agreeable; the divine world or anything divine." *Augha* means "a flood, a stream."

Everyone who has danced knows that when you're dancing, you are flooded by celestial sensations. *Calana* is also "shaking, wagging (the tail), making loose." Rock out! What makes you want to wag your tail, throw off all restraint? Put on music that makes you want to move.

Another area of exploration, which you may already know and celebrate, has to do with the rocking sensations of riding horses or any sport in which your pelvis is being rocked. Snowboarding, skiing, and certain styles of surfing involve a lot of hip swaying. The rocking creates undulation through your spine, waves of energy rippling everywhere, and you can ride these waves into the union of your body and the divine.

61

आकाश

ĀKĀŚA

Akasha: A free or open space, vacuity. The ether, sky, or atmosphere. In philosophy, the subtle and ethereal fluid (supposed to fill and pervade the universe and to be the peculiar vehicle of life and of sound). Brahma (as identical with ether).

Practice

Lie on your back, gaze upward at the sky, and become one with the mystery. Children do this and it's fun. Whether beginners or advanced, meditators need to bathe in space. There is nothing like it, no substitute for this type of gazing. Something of the *atman,* the nature of the soul, becomes clear. If for some reason you are stuck in your cubicle at work, you can cultivate the feeling of spaciousness by imagining the sky at night. Look at the imagery astronomers produce. But if you can, go to any outdoor space that's available. Build up an appetite to indulge yourself in space.

In this yukti, you dissolve into space, transcend with space, merge with it, become it. Meeting yourself in this way can be somewhat terrifying (*bhairava* is "the property of exciting terror"). At the same time, it is a relief to let go of the constriction of being an individual.

62

लीन

LĪNA

Lina: Clung or pressed closely together, attached or devoted to, merged in, sticking. Lying or resting on, staying in, lurking, hiding. Dissolved, absorbed in, disappeared, vanished.

Practice

There is so much teaching in this one word. If we take the definition as a teacher, we hear that on the path to becoming *absorbed* in meditation, we might *cling* to the object of attention, such as the sky *(viyat).* We feel *devoted* to it. In the next heartbeat we are *resting* in it, *hiding* in it and being safe. Then we *disappear* into it—we *vanish.* These are subtle internal postures of attention, and each may arise, stay for a while, then dissolve into the next quality.

Devoting, resting, clinging—your own sequence will be unique to you, may take only a few seconds, and may vary from moment to moment. On another day you might close your eyes and go straight to *absorption*—immediately you are absorbed in the infinite sky. Yet another day you simply feel a little bit *restful.* That's it. Welcome all these nuances and let them shift and change into each other continually.

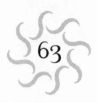

63

तमस्

TAMAS

Tamas: Darkness, gloom, the darkness of hell or a particular division of hell, the obscuration of the sun or moon in eclipses, mental darkness, ignorance, illusion, error, one of the three qualities or constituents of everything in creation.

Practice

Run a loop in your mind: dreaming, deep sleep, awakening, dreaming, sleeping, awakening. Think of what you do in twenty-four hours, the states of consciousness you roll through. Meditate on the rhythm, the flow from one state to the other. Over and over, this whole wacky cycle rolls on and on. The yukti here is to meditate on the succession of these states of consciousness and thus become your true body—eternal consciousness, *bhairava.*

The idea of a yoga practice is that we awaken, orient ourselves toward a greater source of nourishment and inspiration, and then go to work. As a gift of practice, something shines through, a kind of luminosity permeating the world. Here you are, flowing through day and night, exertion and rejuvenation. Whether you are working, resting, or sleeping, the uncreated light wants to shine through and dispel the gloom.

Work is a way of engaging with the world. Work is also love and what you give to others. Your to-do list might feel like hell some days, but the light of consciousness wants to illuminate your work as well as your meditation practice.

64

कृष्ण

KṚṢṆA

Krishna: Black, dark blue. Wicked, evil. The dark half of the lunar month, from full to new moon. The fourth or kali yuga. A crow, an avatar of Vishnu. Blackness. Iron, lead. The black part of the eye. The black spots in the moon. A kind of demon or spirit of darkness.

Practice

Picture this: You are alone in a strange forest or desert at midnight, in the dark of the moon, in a storm, and it is pouring rain. With your eyes open, you can see nothing. You hear only the sound of the rain. There may be a flash flood. There is an uncomfortable pounding sense that something you can't see is going to come racing out of the blackness and clobber you. The yukti here is to use the terribleness of darkness as a gateway into the mystery of the soul. Meditate on this terror, and something mysterious happens. You become one with the blackness. This yukti tells you to take your worst fear and merge with it.

You may have your own equivalent of this scenario. Or perhaps the experience is purely internal: you awaken at two in the morning, in your own bed, filled with an eerie loneliness. When we face a terror, the vibrancy of it becomes part of our consciousness, and we are not the same.

As part of preparing to translate the Bhairava Tantra, I lived outdoors on retreat in Hawaii for a year. For months I camped out in an area of black lava, miles from anyone, a few feet back from the ocean. When it rained, I would sleep in my Jeep because I had no tent. It was uncomfortable, so sometimes at night in the storms, I would stand outside in the warm rain in the middle of the night. I came to love being immersed in pitch black— black lava, black sky—and the howling wind, the swirling roar of the storm, and the crashing surf.

Notice this sutra has *bhairava* again—the terror of facing the unknown. It is strangely liberating to go through the fear to the other side, which is indescribable. Beyond and inside the wildness of nature, there is intense friendliness.

65

प्रसार

PRASĀRA

Prasara: Spreading or stretching out, extension. A trader's shop. Opening (the mouth). Going forward, advance, progress, free course, coming forth, rising, appearing, diffusion. Range (of the eye). Boldness, courage. A fight, war. An iron arrow. Speed. Affectionate solicitation. In music, a kind of dance.

Practice

This is a meditation on darkness. In your mind's eye, see darkness spreading, diffusing *(prasara)* everywhere, into infinity. Embrace the blackness and become one with the body of infinite I-AM consciousness.

Darkness is a mystery, both terrifying and blissful. I tend to be somewhat afraid of this practice, even though it is the very first meditation I did as part of the scientific research on meditation in 1968. I usually feel a kind of shudder, like when jumping into a cold pool or ocean, when I meditate on darkness. There is a set of strange sensations until I get used to it, and then it is such a relief.

There was a season in 1972 when, over a period of months, I sensed darkness coming from the back of my brain, spreading forward and threatening to engulf me. It was a creepy, background sensation, as if black tar was taking over my brain. This happened so slowly that I was only subliminally aware of it. I instinctively recoiled from it and thought I was depressed. Finally, one morning it got intense enough that I consciously noticed it while meditating, and I gave in.

Once I relaxed into it, the darkness quickly spread throughout my brain, body, and the space in front of me. It was restful. I turned into inky blackness, and it was sort of refreshing, like slipping into a warm bath of pure blackness. It changed my cells and that was that. I had been clinging to the light—apparently, the light side of the yin-yang dynamic—and now I was letting the opposites dance in me in their own way. Even though I typically arise at four in the morning and do yoga and meditation in the darkness, loving the resonant silence, I have to return to this yukti again and again.

66

इन्द्रिय

INDRIYA

Indriya: Fit for or belonging to or agreeable to Indra, the god of the senses; a companion of Indra. Power, force, the quality that belongs especially to the mighty Indra. An exhibition of power, a powerful act. Bodily power, power of the senses. Virile power. Semen virile. Faculty of sense, sense, organ of sense. The number five as a symbol of the five senses (in addition to the five organs of perception—eye, ear, nose, tongue, and skin).

Practice

In yoga, the senses—seeing, hearing, smelling, tasting, touching—are the *indriyas,* "the companions of Indra," who is the king of the gods. The senses are delightful to the divine. The senses are the entourage of God, always entertaining.

In the literature of yoga, Indra is a party animal with an insatiable appetite for *soma,* the alcoholic and psychedelic drink that is the nectar of life. If we take this metaphorically (always a good idea with Sanskrit), it means that the senses permeating our bodies are to be celebrated as divine. Yoga practices play with the senses and extend their range. *Tantra* is "extend, stretch, weave together." We use the senses to weave together flesh and spirit, this moment and eternity.

Cherish your senses as gifts of the divine. Breathe with each sense for a few seconds. You could think the name of each sense and inwardly cherish it, welcome its music, then welcome its continual flow of information about the outer and inner world. Add the senses of movement and balance, essential to everyone and especially yogis. "Now I am awake to touch . . . vision . . . hearing . . . smell . . . taste . . . touch . . . balance . . . movement." Over time, you will notice a delicious enhancement of your ability to notice your world, both inside and out. This is a simple practice of being grateful for every sense, and it will enrich your daily experience no end.

When one sense is affected, they all are affected. If you close one room of the party, the guests congregate in the other rooms. When you close your eyes, your inner eyes open; you can become more aware of your skin sensations and your sense of hearing. People do this spontaneously; they close their eyes and sigh when receiving a massage or when listening to music.

ज्ञान

JÑĀNA

Jnana: Knowing, becoming acquainted with. Knowledge, the higher knowledge (derived from meditation on the one Universal Spirit). Knowledge about anything cognizant. Conscience. Engaging in.

Practice

This is the *aha* sutra—a sudden glimpse beyond the ordinary. We are astonished, and in moments of discovery, insight, and revelation, the whole body comes alive. The eyebrows rise. The mouth opens, and we may gasp, "Ah!" It is the sudden sensation of being flooded with knowledge, *jnana.* That gasp of "Ah!" or "Aha!" is a natural mantra.

If you have had this experience, then you can invoke it intentionally in meditation; you can use the feeling and the *ah* as a focus.

There is a universe of techniques here. One loving approach is to use *jna augha* (pronounced *jnaana aughah*) as a mantra. *Jna* is "to know, remember, recognize." *Augha* is "stream, flood." So the meaning of the mantra is, "streams of divine knowledge flowing through me."

68

वर्ण

VARNA

Varna: A covering, cloak, mantle. A cover, lid. Outward appearance, exterior. Luster, beauty. Color, tint, dye, pigment (for painting or writing). Character, nature, quality. A letter, sound, vowel, syllable, word. A musical sound or note, also applied to the voice of animals. The order or arrangement of a song or poem.

Practice

The yukti here is to be alert for a sound that emerges from the interface of spirit and matter, the infinite and the individual. It is the primordial song of soul entering the body, almost an animal sound. The sound emerges from the lovemaking of body and soul.

You can't speak this sound; you can't think it. In meditation, when you are at the level where soul and body are loving each other, you may hear it.

In moments of intense, intimate lovemaking, in the surrender and letting go, you may hear a sound emerge spontaneously from the throat of your beloved. This is the closest we can come to the self-existent mantra of creation. In meditation, welcome this profound surrender and cherish its sound resonating within you, whenever you come into its presence. Let your consciousness merge with that sound, and be touched by the primal creative power of life.

अनावृत

ANĀVṚTA

Anavrta: Uncovered, undressed. Unenclosed, open. Unlimited, free.

Practice

The yukti here is meditating on the body as having the form of unlimited space stretching in all directions. You are naked before infinity, unlimited and free. As you fall into freedom, you realize your true body is *chitih shakti*—the divine energy and power manifesting as your individual consciousness.

You can enter the yukti playfully and imaginatively: "This body is made out of heaven, out of the infinite sky stretching away in all directions."

Along with the freedom resulting from this practice, there is a sense of being undressed. You know you are in the midst of this practice if suddenly, even with all your clothes on, you feel naked. Some people feel this way naturally, and it's a problem for them. If you feel too transparent, invent a series of hand motions—like what you see orchestra conductors doing. Make up your own motions of activating a force field around your body, a subtle boundary made out of vibrating space. With your hands, paint a beautiful sphere of shimmering energy around you at a comfortable distance. Do a few minutes of motion in this way, and then go for a walk and notice how you feel.

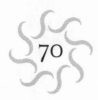

70

विभिद्

VIBHID

Vibhid: To split or break in two, to break in pieces, to cleave asunder, to cause to split, to divide, to separate, to open, to pierce, to sting, to loosen, to untie, to break, to infringe, to violate, to scatter, to disperse, to dispel, to destroy, to alter, to change (the mind). To be split or broken, to be burst asunder, to be changed or altered. To alienate, to estrange.

Practice

Any moment of wounding immediately produces a healing response from life. Whenever you experience pain or violation in any form, use the terror as a gateway. Stop and feel the intensity. Let it wake you up. Unite with pure, shining universal consciousness, and begin to heal.

We are many-bodied beings, with bodies corporeal, emotional, mental, and celestial. We have a physical body, *anna maya kosha.* We have an emotional body—to coin a phrase, *vibhava maya kosha,* or "body of emotional drama." *Mano maya kosha* is the mental body, and *ananda maya kosha* is the body of bliss. When we get injured on one level, it can throw us through a door in space-time into the next dimension. Meditation helps us to develop the ability to quickly, almost instantaneously, relax into a pain sensation.

The verse also uses the word *suci:* "The sharp point or tip of anything or any pointed object. A kind of military array in which the sharpest, most active soldiers are placed in front. An index, table of contents to a book. In astronomy, the earth's disc in computing eclipses (or the corrected diameter of the earth). Gesticulation, dramatic action. A kind of sex (coitus)."

When the sharp point of pain pierces us, a table of contents to our suffering gets written in our bodies. As we heal, the healing process encodes wisdom into our cells and writes a song of healing into our flesh. When our reality gets punctured, this spontaneous mantra rises in us: *ouuuuch*. It's a particle of OM, calling out to life: "Help me, I'm hurt here." When we are hurt, physically or emotionally, we can call out to the forces of life. OM is the primal song of creation joyously expanding, and *ouch* is the beginning of reconnecting with the joy.

71

चित्त

CITTA

Citta: Noticed. Aimed at, longed for. Appeared, visible. Attending, observing. Thinking, reflecting, imagining, thought. Intention, aim, wish. The heart, mind. Memory. Intelligence, reason. In astrology, the ninth mansion.

Practice

In meditation, gently consider this:

> There is no mind.
> There is no intellect.
> There is no ego.
> I am pure consciousness.
> I am pure Being.

Sometimes meditating on these words just once is liberating. Let the light of this passage shine inside for a day, then go out and live. Do not force the recognition of this truth; let it come to you gently.

This sutra is part of a sequence of yuktis about being startled out of your ordinary perception and opened to the Beyond.

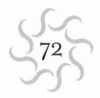

माया

MĀYĀ

Maya: Measuring. Creating illusions. Art, wisdom, extraordinary or supernatural power (only in the earlier language). Illusion, unreality, deception, fraud, trick, sorcery, witchcraft, magic. An unreal or illusory image, phantom, apparition. Duplicity. Compassion, sympathy. The name of the mother of Gautama Buddha. An alternate name of Lakshmi.

Practice

This is a declaration of independence meditation: "Let the world turn; let the illusions spin. Let everyone else believe the scripts they are playing out. Party on, all you people."

Maya refers to the gorgeousness of the universe and all art, poetry, and magic. *Maya* is the power of a performer to embody a character and enchant us, the power of a storyteller to weave the threads of the characters and dialogues together into an absorbing tale.

Maya is beguiling. The universe is supposed to be so beautiful that we are endlessly enchanted and drawn into scenario after scenario. We are supposed to fall in and forget everything else for two hours, as we would with any good movie. That's why we buy a ticket. *Maya* is also *vimohin*—"perplexing, bewildering." Somehow we love this aspect of the drama.

This being Sanskrit, there are always jokes embedded in the statement. In the context of all the other sutras, this one is saying, "You all can believe in the reality of *maya,* but I am standing here on the firm ground of absolutely *nothing.* I will just stand here in midair for a while and enjoy the show."

इच्छा

ICCHĀ

Iccha: Wish, desire, inclination. In math, a question or problem. In grammar, the desiderative form.

Practice

This yukti is something you can do anytime you perceive the rise of a desire: spot the initial flash or sparkle of the desire as it begins to rise. Usually this requires great attentiveness, so at first you may only notice it during clear meditations.

You have a choice: you can absorb the energy of the desire and dissolve it, you can modify it, or you can use the desire itself as a means of transcendence, following it back into the source of all desire.

The English word *desire* is said to be from the Latin *de sidere,* "from the stars." Desire is from the heavens, and to follow your desire is to follow your star. You have a dozen or more desire-stars to follow, your own constellation. These include friendship, exercise, food, sex, play, and power. Desires often come as a sequence—you want to eat good food, in a great place, while feeling love and laughing with your friends.

The technique here is to savor the energy of desire and use it as you would a mantra, a focus for meditation. Desires flow, like an electric current; let that flow of juice nurture and energize you. Imbibe the sparkle, dissolve, transcend with that desire, and be fulfilled.

भाव

BHĀVA

Bhava: Becoming, being, existing, turning or transition into. State, condition, true condition, reality, manner of being, temperament, any state of mind or body, way of thinking or feeling, sentiment, intention, love, affection, attachment. The seat of the feelings or affections, heart, soul, mind. Wanton sport, dalliance.

Practice

If we allow the definition of *bhava* to teach us, we hear an unending stream of inspiration: "As you engage with any of these practices, be loving and affectionate toward who you are. The intention is to turn into yourself, become yourself. As you connect with your heart and soul, let there be wanton sport and dalliance—play, fun and games, friskiness, recreation, and relaxation."

The future case of *bhava* is *bhavet,* which is used thirty times in the Vijnana Bhairava Tantra, always as the last word of a verse, representing a possibility, a hoped-for state, a potential: "It could become." Becoming is mysterious.

Bhava, in turn, is based on *bhu:* "To become, be, arise, come into being, exist, be found, live, stay, abide, happen, occur. To cherish, foster, animate, enliven, refresh, encourage, promote, further. To addict or devote oneself to, practice. To manifest, exhibit, show. Becoming, being, existing, springing, arising. The place of being, space, world, or universe. The earth, ground. Soil. Floor. Pavement. A spot or piece of ground."

If we listen to the teaching of *bhu,* we hear: "Meditate in a way that fosters and enlivens you. Let your practice encourage you to become who you really are. Investigate your addictions; find out what secret is hidden there—what you are really craving—and convert it to a practice. Become devoted to your practice. Cherish your relationship with this spot of ground, the floor, the soil, the pavement, this world, space and the universe."

There is so much meaning in *bhava, bhavet,* and *bhu;* each word in each definition suggests a skill, a *vijnana* (understanding, recognizing, intelligence, skill, proficiency, art). The greatest skill may be to cherish your own being as an expression of the mystery of being and becoming and your place in the divine play.

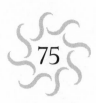

75

अर्थ

ARTHA

Artha: Aim, purpose. Cause, motive, reason. Advantage, use, utility. Generally named with *kama* and *dharma,* used in wishing well to another. Thing, object (said of the membrum virile). Object of the senses. Substance, wealth, property, opulence, money. In astrology, name of the second mansion, the mansion of wealth.

Practice

The current of desire flowing through us at all times is acknowledged in the word *artha*.

In the background of yoga philosophy is a life-embracing concept, the four *purusharthas* or aims of human life:

Kama—sensual pleasure; also desire, longing, sexual love
Artha—wealth
Dharma—duty
Moksha—emancipation, liberation; release from worldly
    existence; setting free

Yoga practice is to serve all of the *purusharthas,* helping us to function better in order to achieve all our desires and fulfill our obligations. When you are flowing through all the *purusharthas* in your own way, there is the feeling of living the life you were designed for.

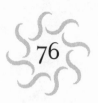

76

निराधार

NIRĀDHĀRA

Niradhara: Without receptacle or support.

Practice

When your head becomes cluttered with knowledge, you need a housecleaning. Anything that is not supported by your own direct living experience, toss it out. Maybe it is time to just throw out everything you used to think you know, and start fresh.

There is always something daunting and unsettling when your previous model of reality falls apart. At the same time, the freedom is exhilarating, and the spaciousness makes room for something new.

तन्मय

TANMAYA

Tanmaya: Made up of that, absorbed in or identical with that.

Practice

We all arise from the same source, whatever that is. The laws of nature are identical in my body and those bodies over there.

Humans have an instinct to commune with the universe and with all the other creatures in creation. In this meditation, you follow that instinct and develop a kind of kinship with everything that is in a body—be it a bug, a person, and even a planet. If something has a body, it is a relative of yours.

You can explore this yukti as a walking meditation. Each time you see any living being—a bird flying by, an ant on the ground, a tree, another human being—consider the mantra, "The same consciousness pervades my body and every body." Look at photos of the earth, the other planets, the stars, and do the same.

This is one of those little perceptions that you might touch on but think is insignificant. Or you might assume such perceptions belong only to advanced yogis. But these experiences can happen to anyone and are a gift of grace.

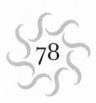

78

काम

KĀMA

Kama: Wish, desire, longing, love, affection. Object of desire, love, or pleasure. Enjoyment. Sexual love or sensuality. Love or desire personified, the god of love. A stake in gambling. A species of mango tree. A kind of temple.

Practice

Love is a temple. Whenever you enter here, bring your ready wit to witness the play of the elements and savor the light show.

Cherish the passions that electrify you while you are meditating. Welcome *kama* in all its forms—desire, lust, longing, adoration, and the sense of taking a risk, of gambling with your life. What arises when there is an obstacle to love? Anger, *krodha*—we are aflame with anger, the desire to burn through all obstacles. We get perplexed, *lobha*. And then we swoon, *moha*. Then perhaps we start laughing, *mada* (hilarity, rapture). Uh-oh, *matsarya,* envy and jealousy! Each of the passions sends signals through your whole body and makes your chakras spin with a different hum. Your body may flow through a sequence of passions every few seconds while you are meditating. This is healthy.

If you have an interesting daily life, part of your meditation time will be spent reviewing and replaying any emotions that got stuck in your chakras or were not finished. Attention always wants to finish what was unfinished. This is why it is so beneficial to welcome all energies that arise in meditation. All those thoughts, sensations, and emotions are just information. You are feeling them because awareness is sorting through the various forms of prana.

The average adult reads text at 250 to 300 words a minute, or four or five words per second. We can understand a friend chatting away at several words per second, and we can recognize facial expressions in a flash. We can read our own emotions that quickly, as the energies play through our nerves and senses. When you witness the flow of your passions during meditation, your practice will be as riveting as your favorite soap operas, reality TV, novels, and movies, because your practice is your adventure, your drama, your divine play of life.

79

इन्द्रजाल

INDRAJĀLA

Indrajala: The net of Indra. A weapon employed by Arjuna. Sham, illusion, delusion, magic, sorcery. To juggle. The art of magic.

Practice

This whole universe is magic, a vast arena of illusions put on for your entertainment. Matter and light are fountaining out of nothing. Whirling flames fill the sky. It is all a kind of juggling. The world we see is art, the most wonderful creation; creativity is overflowing everywhere. Everything is moving, revolving—every particle of existence is on the potter's wheel. When we meditate on this knowledge, joy arises spontaneously.

Look up at the sky. Then look at astronomy images of the same stars. Modern science, particularly physics, astronomy, and astrophysics, has outdone stage magicians in revealing the universe as a magic show. Huge telescopes are orbiting the earth, gathering light from thousands, millions, and billions of light-years away. The images are beautiful beyond description and reveal outer space to be a great work of art.

Awaken to your inner world as magic. Our senses receive the energies streaming in from the world and arrange them onto the canvas of our perception. As you meditate, consider all thoughts, emotions, and sensuous impressions as your personal form of magic show.

80

दुःख

DUHKHA

Duḥkha: Uneasy, uncomfortable, unpleasant, difficult. Uneasiness, pain, sorrow, trouble.

Practice

During meditation your mind will be drawn toward whatever pain and sorrow is going on in your body and your life. In any given moment you might feel an ache, which then turns into an irritated sensation, a pang, sting, or soreness. How do we deal with our world of trouble? There are thousands of different strategies for handling uncomfortable sensations, but the simplest one is to allow your attention to be called to the pain and give it space.

The word *duhkha* is literally "bad space" (*dur* is "bad or difficult," and *kha* is "space"). *Kha* is also an axle hole, so *duhkha* is the image of a wheel out of balance, or rough going. (*Su* is the opposite of *dur*, "good," so *sukha* is "good space," or the wheel that is rolling swiftly and easily.)

Kha suggests that we get interested in space itself and from there learn about how to balance the wheels of life. In yoga there is the concept that life energies spin like wheels; *chakra* means "wheel, a potter's wheel, a whirlpool." Your chakras are wheels of energy in motion, each one representing an area of instinct and expression. During meditation you will feel, with a kind of microscopic perception, tiny ways they are out of balance.

Our chakras can hurt from giving too much and not receiving enough, and also from receiving too much and not giving enough. We ache to give the best in us, and we long to be in a flow with our outer and inner world. If you pay attention to an ache, it will try its best to teach you everything, speaking its language of sensation. The quality of attention required to hear it is spacious embracing and tenderness.

If you have a full life—a lover, a job, kids, pets, and projects—you will feel many kinds of pain during meditation. This pain is not to be avoided. It's a signal, not noise. You are a craftswoman or craftsman, tending to your potter's wheel. What feels like pain may be feedback that your work-in-progress is out of balance. The potter puts her hand just so, and balance is restored.

81

मनस्

MANAS

Manas: Mind (in its widest sense as applied to all the mental powers), intellect, intelligence, understanding, perception, sense, conscience, will. The internal organ or *antah-karana* of perception and cognition, the faculty or instrument through which thoughts enter or by which objects of sense affect the soul. Sometimes joined with *hrd* or *hrdaya,* the heart. The spirit or spiritual principle, the breath or living soul that escapes from the body at death. Thought, imagination, excogitation, invention, reflection, opinion, intention, inclination, affection, desire, mood, temper, spirit.

Practice

Your mind is not what you think. It is vast and a source of awe. If you get interested in *manas,* the yogic concept of "mind," give yourself a chance to delight in how rich the word truly is.

As a meditation, let your attention rest on each word of the definition for one breath: mind, intellect, intelligence, understanding, perception, sense, conscience, will, imagination, invention, opinion, intention, affection, desire, mood, temper, heart, spirit, breath, living soul.

82

घट

GHAṬA

Ghata: Intently occupied or busy with. A jar, pitcher, jug, large earthen water jar, watering pot. A peculiar form of a temple. An elephant's frontal sinus. A border. Suspending the breath as a religious exercise.

Practice

Ghata has a series of jokes in its definition, suggesting that jars are busy and maybe even practicing their own form of pranayama. The yukti here is playful and childlike. Take something simple and ordinary, such as a watering pot or pitcher, and imagine that it has a personality. Imbue it with knowledge *(vijnana)* and desire *(iccha).* Maybe the pitcher even remembers the earth it was formed from and knows a thing or two about transformation.

Animated movies are created by people who have this kind of whimsical perception. Cartoonists think that their bicycle gets cold and lonely if they leave it on the porch at night. Notice in yourself whenever you do this in your own world. Do you talk to your plants or your car? A computer is a kind of jar, a container for billions of tiny bits; do you think that your computer has its own personality? This is animism, the sense that everything is alive and adorable.

When we look at the world in this way, it is as if we receive a transmission of secret knowledge from each little object in the world.

सम्बन्ध

SAMBANDHA

Sambandha: Binding or joining together. Close connection, union, or association. Conjunction, inherence, connection with or relation to. Personal connection (by marriage), relationship, fellowship, friendship, intimacy with. A friend, ally. A collection, volume, book. Prosperity, success. Fitness, propriety.

Practice

To the extent that your heart is open, in meditation you will find yourself tending to the texture of each relationship in your life. You will feel your heartstrings stretching and may even hear them vibrating. On the path of love, we use yoga to prepare ourselves to be alert and awake to this magnificent mystery—that there are other people in the world and we love them. Technically speaking, we enter cosmic consciousness by meditating on the texture of bonding, *sambandha.*

We all have many relationships—with friends, family, coworkers, teammates, lovers. Each requires its own precise way of holding, its own rules for what an embrace is. Each bond, each connection, each relationship in our life requires the best we can bring, and each moment of contact is surprising.

Every kind of relationship is a kind of embrace, whether you are physically touching or holding someone in your heart. Each person you meet says, "Show me some love," offering you an opportunity to reveal the love inside you. The feeling is exquisite, with its own texture and magic. You create when you relate. When you listen to someone and really see them, more is going on than you may know—a sacred, powerful exchange between "you" and the "other."

84

स्वशरीर

SVAŚARĪRA

Svasarira: One's own body or person.

Practice

Compassion is a natural human emotion: *com,* "together," and *pati,* "to suffer." When we see our friend hurt her hand, we feel the injury and say, "Ouch!" In this meditation, you take your natural empathy and multiply it with the power of sustained attention.

A lifetime of practices is here. One gateway in is to marvel at individuality, the way each of us, with our own *svasarira,* is an expression of the All, and yet so utterly unique.

Awareness of the fragility of life intensifies this appreciation. *Sarira* means "support or supporter, that which is easily destroyed or dissolved, the body, bodily frame, solid parts of the body (the bones), any solid body, one's body, one's own person, bodily strength" and suggests that even the solid parts of the body are easily destroyed. So cherish this temporary embodiment, for soon enough we will all be gone and onto our next adventure, if there is one. Do not abandon your body before it is time. Embrace your body and use it to extend awareness into the mystery of incarnation.

विकल्प

VIKALPA

Vikalpa: Alternation, alternative, option. Variation, combination, variety, diversity, manifoldness. Contrivance, art. Difference of perception, distinction, indecision, irresolution, doubt, hesitation. Admission, statement. False notion, fancy, imagination. Calculation, mental occupation, thinking. Antithesis of opposites.

Practice

This is a wild technique! Let your mind wander anywhere it will, but don't let it rest when it tries to stop. Keep it moving. In this way, you do not allow all your mental occupations and preoccupations, *vikalpas,* a chance to spin their hypnotic web. Whenever your mind goes to a pair of opposites, "I like this and I don't like that," don't give any respect to the distinction. Move on before the opinion even has a chance to shape itself. When you deny your mind anything to hang onto, there is an opportunity to wake up to the true nature of mind, which is beyond all its creations and contrivances.

व्यापक

VYĀPAKA

Vyapaka: Pervading, diffusive, comprehensive, omnipresent, widely spreading or extending, spreading everywhere. In law, comprehending all the points of an argument, pervading the whole plea.

Practice

In this meditation, first you attend to the vastness of infinity, then you attend to your own "I-am-ness" as part of and one with infinity. Release your awareness to refresh itself in the vastness of the universe, then consider the mystery of your own existence as an inseparable part of everything.

For some, this is a spontaneous realization. It is also a prayer and a set of stunning statements for meditation. Here are some phrases you might want to explore:

Present everywhere is knowledge of the universal spirit.
Pervading everything is the power of spirit.
Comprehending all is the supreme consciousness.

The Sanskrit here is so beautiful. Whisper this mantra, if you feel attracted to it, and rest in the delight of freedom: *Sarva jnah. Sarva kartaa. Vyaapakah Paramishvarah.*

Sarva is "every, everything, all together, in all parts, everywhere." *Jna* is "knowing, familiar with, intelligent." *Sarva karta* is "the maker of all." *Vyapakah* is "omnipresent." *Paramishvara* is "far, distant, remote in space, beyond, extreme, ancient, past, future, next, name of the Supreme or Absolute Being, the Universal Soul."

87

विश्व

VIŚVA

Visva: All, every, every one. Whole, entire, universal. All-pervading or all-containing, omnipresent. The faculty that perceives individuality.

Practice

At some point in a love relationship, you may find it appropriate to say, "You are mine, and I am yours." Here is a wild thought: Creation is your primary relationship. In this sutra, you are invited to talk to your Beloved, the universe, in an intimate and tender way: "I am yours, and you are mine. I am at one with you."

Visva is the faculty of perceiving individuality, so you are invited to meditate on the relationship of individuality and infinity. Your mantra here is the texture of that relationship:

I am at home in the rivers and tides and all currents
    of Creation.
I am at one with Bhairava, the consciousness that
    permeates everywhere.
Everything everywhere is singing, "I AM—love me."

You could use lines such as this as a prayer of the heart.

If you are more of a scientist than a lover, you can stay in wonder and use the mystery of individuality as the focus. The fact that anything exists at all is still a great mystery. No one knows why the Big Bang occurred.

88

क्षोभ

KṢOBHA

Kshobha: Shaking, trembling, agitation, disturbance, tossing, emotion. In drama, an emotion that is the cause of harsh speeches or reproaches. A strong current of water.

Practice

The technique here is to work yourself to the point of exhaustion, then throw yourself down to the ground. Surrender to gravity. Meditate on the trembling of fatigue and be born again. The mantra and the gateway is *kshobha shakti.*

There is a yoga of tiredness, thank God. And we are all good at it. Everyone I know is running themselves ragged. Being exhausted by honest work is good preparation for the *samadhi* of rejuvenation. One of the meanings of *tantra* is "extending ourselves, stretching our capacity for attention and exertion." There is a sweet science to wearing ourselves out just the right amount. This sutra focuses on the practice of wearing yourself out physically, and then, with the attentiveness of a yogi, entering shaking exhaustion and finding therein a gateway into shakti, the vibratory nature of the life-force.

Kshobha is a "strong current of water," and there is a current of OM inside the trembling. We all know the magic that happens when we lie down and surrender to fatigue: it is bliss, and you earned it. In this yukti, use the power of your yoga-enhanced attention to meditate on *kshobha shakti* and enter bliss.

89

अशक्त

AŚAKTA

Aśakta: Unable, incompetent, powerless. This is the opposite of shakti, which is "power, powerful, mighty."

Practice

Powerlessness is a gateway. There are days when reality unravels before your eyes. You are disrupted, torn down, stripped of what you believe. Your foundation is shaken. When this happens, enter the powerlessness and use it as a focus for meditation.

Anytime you feel incompetent and ignorant, let your mind dissolve into that unknowing helplessness. You are already in the disturbance, so you may as well go all the way in with full attention. You now realize you know nothing, so become curious and melt into wonder. The forms of power you have known are gone. Now you can rebuild and learn entirely new ways of dancing with shakti.

Meditators know that when they are relaxed and at ease, the memory of painful times comes to awareness to be healed. Welcome these shocking and embarrassing memories when they come because they are teachers. If you learn from your own history, you don't need to repeat it.

Note: The phrase "unmind your mind," used in the sutra, comes from Lakshman Joo, one of the great teachers of this text, a master from Kashmir who wrote many books on Shaivism.

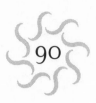

90

सम्प्रदाय

SAMPRADĀYA

Sampradaya: Tradition, sect, doctrine transmitted from one teacher to another.

Practice

Transmissions of wisdom can come quite suddenly. You might be out walking, notice a dog glancing at you, and see fifty thousand years of love and companionship in a second. You might witness the birth of a child, and you start seeing not just that particular baby being born, but also all beings everywhere being born. Standing alone at night in the wilderness, under the star field, you might see not just that particular night sky, but also beyond—stars emerging, planets coalescing. You might look at one particular thing, and suddenly the soul is detached from matter; the specific form you are seeing dissolves, and somehow you are seeing through that form into eternity. In these moments, you receive the transmission, and you feel a sense of inner freedom and happiness. We can receive these transmissions anywhere, at any time.

Sit in open spaces, with your eyes open, gazing. Receive light, color, movement, shapes, as if you were newly born to this world.

91

सनातन

SANĀTANA

Sanatana: Eternal, perpetual, permanent, everlasting, ancient, primeval.

Practice

There is a song, an eternal hum, permeating all of creation. Your body is part of the universe, so it is vibrating also. At certain times in yoga practice, sports, and intense moments of living, you may become attuned to the hum of creation and be able to meditate on the sound of your own life-force resonating in the body.

The senses are designed to notice changes, not something that is steady. We don't hear what is always there. So here is a trick, a yukti: Close your ears, with your fingers or earplugs. Introduce some contraction into the lower *dvaras* or doors of the body, the muscles around the perineum, anus, and urinary passage. If you know *mula bandha* or *ashwini mudra,* this is a time to practice them. Explore what happens when you introduce pulsation—rhythmic contracting and releasing. Singers use techniques such as this to attune to their own note and amplify the resonance of their voice.

Now simply listen. Be open to whatever you are hearing. Let the vibration of your own life-force teach you about itself. There may be a quiet sound, like a stream flowing—the current of life. You might sense it as silence, as radiance, as a vibration that is not a sound, but just a feeling or a hum. Welcome the unexpected song. The primordial chord that began resonating before you were born, *sanatana,* sustains you continually and is always here. This is home. You already know this sound; simply return to rest in the Unstuck Chord.

You may not need to actually plug your ears each time. Your attention may go inside naturally as soon as you invite the internal sound.

This practice can happen spontaneously in lovemaking. As the charge of energy builds and builds, the muscles at the base of the pelvis contract rhythmically, and you may find yourself in the palace of the Creator, listening to the hum of life. Again we see how in yoga we cheerfully accept every part of the body, every nerve center, and every tube or opening in the body as invaluable for enlightenment.

92

चित्तलय

CITTALAYA

Citta: Noticed, aimed at, longed for, appeared, visible, attending, observing, thinking, reflecting, imagining, thought, intention, wish, aim, the heart, mind, memory, intelligence, reason. In astrology, the ninth mansion. *Laya:* The act of clinging to, to become attached to someone, to disappear, be dissolved or absorbed. Lying down. Melting, dissolution. Rest, repose. Sport, diversion, merriness. Delight in anything. An embrace. The union of song, dance, and instrumental music. A pause. A swoon.

Practice

In meditation, we court the experience of mind dissolving into nothingness. It's restful, and when we come back to ourselves, it's an embrace, a party, the union of song, dance, and instrumental music—a Bollywood musical!

Dissolving can be intense and scary. Adventures in the outer world can prepare us for the swoon of *cittalaya.* Looking into depths, such as wells and canyons, can give us a chance to practice relaxing into the fear of falling. Roller coaster rides are intense and exhilarating. In some sports, you give in to the drop. In snowboarding, skiing, surfing, base jumping, and parachuting, you fall into the gravity well and steer.

Outdoor explorers and athletes encounter meditative states in the course of their daring adventures. They glow as if they were on a meditation retreat, but they can't tell you why. They are encountering *cittalaya* in an informal way. It happens so instantaneously that they wouldn't be so bold as to say they are meditating, but their minds are dissolved in delight.

If you are fortunate, you have come across some phenomenon that makes you feel as if the ground beneath your feet were opening up—a moment of intense love, a great musical or theatrical performance, the divine streaming through someone, a magnificent act. You are encountering something so brilliant that all your thoughts fall away.

93

अवस्था

AVASTHĀ

Avastha: To go down into, to reach down to; to go away from; to take one's stand; to stay, abide, stop at any place; to abide in a state or condition; to remain or continue (doing anything). To be found, exist, be present. To fall to, fall into the possession of. To enter, be absorbed in. To penetrate, as sound. To be settled or fixed or chosen. To cause to stand or stop (as a carriage or an army). Appearance (in a court of justice). Stability, consistence. State, condition, situation (five are distinguished in dramas). The female organs of generation.

Practice

This is a God-consciousness technique. People often think of meditation as stilling the mind and stopping the flow of thought. This sutra invites you to consider the opposite.

Avastha, reach down into your deepest being. Take a stand in divine consciousness. See the whole world from inside this state. Perceive everything as the functioning of the divine, the Mysterious All-Pervading One. If you don't like religious terminology, you can use the Mystery of Whatever Set the Laws of Nature in Motion.

The sutra begins with *yatra yatra,* "wherever your mind wanders, in the outside objective world or your inner secret world," and *tatra tatra,* "there is the gracious, friendly, benevolent universal consciousness." The skill here is to find a way to rest in the knowledge that "wherever your mind moves, you are moving with the One Infinite Life."

Minds wander—that's what they do. Hearts are always looking for love. The heart, by design, longs to be in the rhythm of giving and receiving. Life is flow and motion. Both mind and heart want to connect with the essence of life, and *yoga* means "connection." Attention is dynamic by nature, always on a quest. In this practice, the yoga is in the wandering and searching. We are called to honor all this questing as *yatra,* a pilgrimage.

94

भरिता

BHARITA

Bharita: Nourished, full.

Practice

We need food of many kinds. There is the food we eat with our mouths. There is also food for thought, food for the soul, and nourishment for our hungry hearts. There is something nourishing about good music—it is a kind of food. And there is a nourishing quality to simple sensuality, like walking in nature, with the sun shining on your skin and the wind ticking the hairs on your arms. Certain people are nourishing to be around.

We are invited here to let our meditation practice be nourishing in all these ways.

The technique is to receive all sensuous perceptions as a gift of the cosmic intelligence that is everywhere. In meditation, accept everything coming in through your channels of perception as being an emanation from infinity, and let your soul be suffused with nourishing fullness.

In meditation, pay attention to your senses and follow each one from the level on which you receive it through the channels of sensuous delight, into the soul. *Bharita,* the sense of being nourished, is accessible to you though every sensual perception. All of your senses are pathways for the divine nature of life to talk to you, sing to you, touch you, feed you, delight you, entertain you.

Start from wherever you are, and as the soul, welcome each and every sight, sound, touch, smell, and taste as a manifestation of that which is everywhere, the All-Pervading Lord. This practice may take many years, as you learn to transcend through smell, taste, touch, vision, and hearing, and other senses, such as balance and motion.

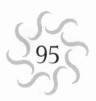

95

कुतूहल

KUTŪHALA

Kutuhala: Curiosity, interest in any extra-ordinary matter. Inclination, desire for. Eagerness, impetuosity. What excites curiosity. Anything interesting, fun. Surprising, wonderful. Excellent, celebrated.

Practice

This is the "there are no atheists in foxholes" sutra. The images are intense: when fleeing from battle, running so fast that your brain melts; when seized by terror, dread, dismay, or burning heartache; when totally confused; when hiding from danger in a hole in the ground, a forest, or a cave; when keeping a terrifying secret; when starving, ravenously hungry. You can wake up to the Great Spirit in the midst of any of these shocking experiences—which are about as unmeditative and unyogic as you can imagine. The throbbing intensity of your need carries you across the invisible threshold into the presence of the One Self-Existent Spirit.

Thankfully, you can wake up in the wonderful, to *kutuhala*— "eagerness, impetuosity; anything fun and surprising." The "extraordinary matter" might be a surprising reversal that gives an underdog sports team the win. A roar of enthusiasm goes up from eighty thousand voices. You can even wake up with a sudden sneeze—*kshut!*

Meditation is surprising. There is no predicting what you will experience from one moment to the next, and this is a good thing. You'd think that if you have a busy life, your mind will be noisy during meditation, and if you have a year off, an extended vacation, your mind will be quiet. But it does not work out that way. Sometimes the exhaustion of raising kids, running a business, having a love life, makes you so perfectly tired that meditation is just bliss. And if you took a year off to sit on a hill, your brain might be busy day and night processing your past experiences. There is just no telling. All you can do is prepare your body for meditation and then accept what arises. And the best preparation for meditation is to live your authentic life, do your work, follow your passions, explore who you are, and give everything you can give to each moment.

If you have survived traumatic experiences, you will have flashbacks during meditation. When these flashes of memory occur, welcome them. They will come anyway, and if you set the table, you take charge of the interaction. Each time you access terror or dread, you have the opportunity to soothe it a bit and massage some of that fear out of your system. You may need to learn a variety of meditation practices, such as those described in this text, to create enough inner safety to meet yourself on the level of terror and trauma.

It is a great challenge to develop life-affirming experiences that are as incandescently powerful as the traumatic ones. This sutra reminds you, "You were witness to something shocking, and you survived."

96

स्मर

SMARA

Smara: Remembering, recollecting. Memory, remembrance. Recollection. A loving recollection love, especially sexual love. Kama-deva, the god of love.

Practice

This is the time-travel sutra. During meditation, a memory may grab you and carry you away. One moment you are here and the next you are *there,* in that time and place, seeing and feeling what you saw and felt then. By the mystery of memory, your *here* has been teleported to *there.*

You might be remembering a wonderful lover or longing for a land that was once home. Perhaps you are thinking of noble actions you have witnessed. You might find yourself recalling meetings with inspiring people, fantastic conversations, or moments of *shaktipat,* when you received a transmission of something great. If you met Jesus, you are supposed to remember this communion forever and eternally be in its embrace.

Technically speaking, you are using a cherished memory, *smara,* as a meditation object, in the same way you would breath, a mantra, or the chakras. As your mind and heart engage with that memory, you enter heightened awareness. You savor the *rasa*—the deliciousness and aesthetic relish—of a specific moment. Intense positive emotions—inspiration, gratitude, pride in accomplishment—are worthy of being cultivated in this way.

An odd twist in this particular memory technique is that you allow self-abandonment. *Tyaj* is "abandon, leave a place," and *tyajet svasaririam* is "abandoning your body." When we are really in love, there can be a sense of hanging suspended. We love the other person so much that love elevates us to the point that we don't really care about our body. Artists, musicians, dancers, and mothers can be this way about their bodies. If it is safe, go ahead and let yourself be carried away like this in meditation. Leave your present body behind. Leave your mind behind. Just be there in that time and space, reliving and recollecting. Here is a mystery: after a while, you may find you are floating free between worlds, flooded by divine consciousness.

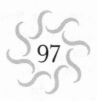

97

शून्यालय

ŚŪNYĀLAYA

Shunyalaya: An empty or deserted house—"abode of the void."

Practice

Attention has rhythms and cycles. We focus on our tasks for a while, perhaps a couple of hours; we are on a roll. Then at some point, we realize we have been absent or daydreaming. One of the meanings of *shunya* is "absentminded." You can utilize your naturally occurring absentminded states as a meditation.

As with many of the yuktis, this meditation may occur spontaneously or it may be cultivated. *Vinyasya* here means simply "to be put or placed upon." Place your attention somewhere—just gaze at something. Then gradually, softly, allow your attention to turn within. This is something attention does by itself; you will be completely focused on something, and then without noticing it, your attention dissolves. You probably think you have spaced out, and you are right. This spaciousness is a gateway.

When you come across someone who is absorbed in this way, don't interrupt them. Stand twenty feet away or so and let them finish their reverie. After a while—usually not more than twenty minutes—they will notice you.

If you have a healthy daily meditation practice, you will space out much less during the day, because you are giving your attention time and space to refresh itself in spaciousness. The *laya* of *shunyalaya* is "delightful, refreshing." You had a vacation, and now you are back.

If meditation is *making* you spaced out, then modify your practice. Do more physical activity, meditate for a shorter period, engage your passions, and make sure you are well nourished. Find a sport you love that requires you to pay close attention and keep your eye on the ball. It takes many years to integrate *shunyalaya.*

A certain amount of meditation-induced drunkenness is normal. When you discover that everything is made out of space, you can feel like Gene Kelly in "Singin' in the Rain." You don't care that it is raining or that everyone else is hurrying to work and scowling. Life is so wonderful that you just want to gaze at that baby in the carriage. After a while, you learn to hide your drunkenness without suppressing it, to keep calm and carry on.

98

भक्ति

BHAKTI

Bhakti: Distribution, partition, separation. A division, portion, share. Division by streaks or lines. A row, series, succession, order. That which belongs to or is contained in anything else, an attribute. Attachment, devotion, fondness for, devotion to. Trust, homage, worship, piety, faith or love or devotion to (as a religious principle or means of salvation, together with *karman,* "works," and *jnana,* "spiritual knowledge").

Practice

During meditation you will find yourself thinking of the people you love. You will be attending to the texture—the tantra—of your relationships and feeling what is there. This is your heart vibrating and pulsing with your connection. You can transcend on *bhakti,* on love and devotion.

When you love someone, you carry them inside you and will think of them all the time, including during pranayama, *shavasana,* and meditation, even if you try not to. You can't help but be bothered by your love. Your awareness is sneaking off to practice bhakti yoga and will do so no matter what style of class you are in, no matter what you call your meditation system. In the bhakti yoga stories, otherwise honorable and diligent women (the *gopis*) are always getting up in the middle of the night and slipping away to worship Krishna down by the river. In daily life, attention steals moments of *bhakti* here and there to muse about your lover, baby, cat, dog, or creative project. Part of love is worrying about people, praying for them, attempting to find words to say what you feel. All of this is welcome in meditation.

Loving any one being, one person, expresses your devotion to your local part of the infinite universe. This is a tangible thing you can do, an act of power and creativity. The everyday practice here is to know that no matter who or what you love, this love is yoga in its most fundamental form: linking, connecting, valuing the other, honoring the relationship. There are many kinds of love, many textures of relationship, and each moves and challenges us in a different way. There is erotic love and all those wild energies of sexual devotion. There is friendship, parental love, family love, unconditional love. Every form of love is sacred; every relationship, temporary as it may be, teaches us about eternity. Bhakti yoga says that you can be in an erotic, passionate relationship with God; you can be friends and equals with God; you can even feel parental and protective of God. All rivers flow to the ocean.

99

वस्तु

VASTU

Vastu: Becoming light, dawning, morning. The seat or place of any really existing or abiding substance or essence, thing, object. In philosophy, the real (opposed to that which does not really exist, the unreal). The right thing, a valuable or worthy object. Goods, wealth, property. The thing in question, matter, affair, circumstance. Subject, subject matter, contents, theme (of a speech), plot (of a drama or poem). In music, a kind of composition. Natural disposition, essential property. The pith or substance of anything.

Practice

When you focus on something that engages your entire interest, the rest of the universe disappears. This is wonderfully peaceful.

Find something so compelling that you want to engage with it to the exclusion of everything else—at least for a while. Getting lost in something is a natural experience. Little kids do this when playing. Children of all ages can get totally absorbed in books. Teenagers get fully focused in games, sports, video games, music. *Vastu* has vast meaning—wealth, property, the plot of a drama, music, a poem. The only thing that matters is that your *vatsu* is engaging, that it calls you completely.

Yogis and meditators need to make sure they have and indulge in benevolent obsessions, whether it is a music group, romance novels, movies, games, Mardi Gras, or comic book conventions. It is healing to have your whole intellect and intuition, all your mental powers, absorbed in your area of interest, whether it is fly-fishing or martial arts. For some people, it may be gambling or shopping. Everything else in the universe drops away, and you are free. All your troubles are forgotten. Your whole being is appeased, tranquil. You are walking on air.

100

शुद्धि

ŚUDDHI

Shuddhi: Cleansing, purification. Purity, holiness, freedom from defilement, a purificatory rite. Setting free or securing (from any danger), rendering secure. Justification, exculpation, innocence (established by ordeal or trial), acquittal. In arithmetic, leaving no remainder. One of the shaktis of Vishnu.

Practice

Following the rules, eating right, doing yoga, and meditating, you get healthier and healthier. Then one day you notice you are starting to be disgusted by everything. The world seems impure, people are impure, and food is impure. This is a dangerous side effect of practice. If you start disliking your body and being disgusted by contact with others, you can lose your primary relationships or develop eating disorders.

If you are attracted to this sutra today, it may be time to leave behind the mental preoccupations with purity and impurity and the overly obsessive thinking yogis are prone to. *Vikalpa* has many meanings, including "false notion, imagination, calculation, mental occupation." *Nirvikalpa* is "without *vikalpa*." After a certain point in practice, you cannot afford to let other people's rules rule you.

IOI

सामान्य

SĀMĀNYA

Samanya: Equal, alike, similar. Shared by others, joint, common to. Whole, entire, universal, general, generic, not specific. Common, commonplace, vulgar, ordinary, insignificant, low. Equality, similarity, identity. Equilibrium, normal state or condition. Universality, totality, generality, general or fundamental notion, common or generic property. Public affairs or business. In rhetoric, the connection of different objects by common properties. Jointly, in general, in common.

Practice

Notice that ordinary people are full of the wisdom of life. Or you could say, "The reality of cosmic awareness is everywhere, in everyone."

A mantric phrase from this sutra you may enjoy is *sarva bhairavo bhava*—"Everywhere the infinite consciousness is becoming." *Sarva:* "everywhere, at all times, in every case." *Bhairava:* "the Terrific One, the primordial awareness." *Bhava:* "becoming, existing, manner of being, temperament, passion, emotion, love." *Sarva bhairavo bhava.*

When I first started meditating, I happened upon this perception unknowingly, and it was like stepping into another world that looked just like this one, only magical. It seemed to me that ordinary people were walking around in God consciousness. They were already in on the secret. They just got up in the morning, fed the dogs, and went to work. After my meditation teacher training, I felt that I was the one with elite knowledge. Over time, I came down off my throne, which was painful.

Regular people, who don't practice yoga or meditation, are sensible. They don't try to get their dogs to become vegetarians. Those of us who are constantly meddling with our organs of perception, dialing in new energies, are always losing our common sense. As the range of our senses increases, we are ecstatic, delighted, and expansive. We think we have discovered the secret of life, until eventually we realize that all kinds of people are already there. Dancers at the ballet know more about movement and stillness than we do. Mountaineers know more about mental silence than we do. Singers know more about breath than we ever will. Fishermen know more about patience than we do. The mother with three kids who gets everyone to school on time knows more about grace under fire than we do. If you are a yoga teacher, you may realize someday that your students know more about *shavasana* than you do. The reality of God is common to all. It is not specific to you at all. This is a cheerful, humbling perception.

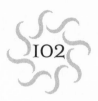

102

सम

SAMA

Sama: Any, every. Even, smooth, flat, plain, level, parallel. Same, equal, similar, like, equivalent, like to or identical or homogenous with. Always the same, constant.

Practice

This sutra points to a daring level of equanimity requiring you to differentiate yourself from the collective trance. At one level this sutra is a heads up—a notice saying that a time may come when it is appropriate for you to rise above and beyond the opinions of others. Your inner work will have led you here. Listen to the song of life within you, make your choices, go your way, and leave behind the whole struggle to be hip and to avoid being uncool.

The Sanskrit here sounds like the plot of a daytime soap opera: *mana* means "opinion, arrogance, indignation excited by jealousy (especially in women), sulking; a blockhead, an agent, a barbarian." When you are established in inner equanimity, it's all the same *(sama)* to you, whether the players like you or not.

Keep in mind that everyone will still have their opinions, and may feel indignant about your aloofness and superiority. They may sense that you are not obeying the herd, and they may be envious. Envy is the desire to have what the other has, so some part of them wants this freedom. Bless them on their path.

This sutra is a hint to keep favoring the inner happiness that percolates up from your deepest *bhava* ("becoming, being, existing, turning or transition into") during meditation. Allow joy, pleasure, delight, and ease to keep on permeating your being, and let the soap opera continue on its own, without you. Let the other characters in the soap opera continue on their own without you; they will be fine.

103

ब्रह्मन्

BRAHMAN

Brahman: The one self-existent spirit, the Absolute.

Practice

While you are meditating, images and sensations of what you like and dislike will arise, calling your attention, inviting you to mix it up somehow. Instead of taking sides, explore the texture of the middle spaces, all the nuances of energy and emotion. *Brahma,* the one self-existing spirit, witnesses all qualities and is not bound by them.

Set everyone free. Set yourself free from your previous dislikes and likes. Let your brain reboot. Start fresh from this moment. Everyone and everything are part of *brahman,* the Absolute. Everything you have ever perceived is an intrinsic part of how you arrived here, in this moment. You do not need to be bound by the coloring, *raga,* that you put on things in the past. That was then. This is now. Deliver yourself from the trap of believing all those evaluations. *Mukta* is "let loose, set free, delivered, emancipated." Let all those prisoners out of jail.

Get intimate with the continuum of infinite variability between the extremes. There is wide-open space here in the middle, a spaciousness embracing all human emotion. Dislike or passion, these are notes on the keyboard; know and appreciate all octaves. You are not just one set of notes; you are the player of notes, and you are the Great Silence from which the notes emerge.

A caution: this practice gives you the power to make yourself into a completely bland person with no *raga,* no passion, whatsoever. It is like becoming tasteless white bread, distilled water—no salt, no spice, no taste, no minerals. This is a gateway to depression and emotional malnutrition. Your healthy adaptation to life depends on having a rich life of passion appropriate to your unique character, your age, and your life path. Are you on the path of renunciation or the path of intimacy? Celibates need to dissolve passion. If you are married, dissolving passion will just destroy your marriage.

During this meditation, your passions will tend to melt into peace. During your everyday life, stay close to your preferences and encourage your likes and dislikes.

बोध

BODHA

Bodha: Knowing, understanding, waking, becoming or being awake, opening of a blossom, blooming. Taking effect (of spells). Exciting (a perfume). Perception, apprehension, thought, knowledge, understanding, intelligence, consciousness. Awakening, arousing. Making known, informing, instructing.

Practice

This is an invitation to appreciate the knowing that is beyond objects. Consciousness wakes up and blossoms, *bodha,* into intimacy with that which cannot be grasped. This is a stage of transcending that usually flashes by in a fraction of a second, as everything you think you know dissolves into space, *shunya.* Even if this awareness lasts a flicker of time, it is still valid and, over time, will continue to blossom. Take a breath and inhale its perfume.

Notice what happens when you come up to the edge of your understanding, the limits of perception. Get to know what it is like to fall off the edge of the world into emptiness, no-thing-ness. Some phases of meditation are very much like training in any sport; the coach has you do exercises to refine your skill and reduce effort. In this sutra, the tendency to grasp, to try to grab hold of knowledge, is replaced with spaciousness. Gently, gently, you let the body and mind get used to how wonderful it is to know nothing.

The last word of this verse is *bodhasambhava,* a beautiful mantra to use as a reminder. *Bodha,* "blossoming, awakening, arousing." *Sambhava,* "together, coming together, union, intercourse, sexual intercourse, acquaintance, intimacy." *Bodha sambhava:* to come into intimacy with pure consciousness.

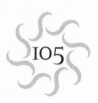

105

समावेश

SAMĀVEŚA

Samavesa: To enter together or at once, meeting, penetration, absorption into. Co-existence.

Practice

This is a fancy version of what kids do for fun—lying on their backs in the grass and looking up at the cloud-filled daytime sky or star-filled night. Gaze at the all-pervading spaciousness and with your awareness enter *samavesa,* the vastness.

Place your mind in outer space, *bahya akasha.* Reach out and touch the stars with your awareness. Then enter the vastness of the cosmos and know it as your home. This is not just a metaphor. This is a physical reality—your molecules came from space, from the exhalation of a primordial sun.

Bahya akasha is a beautiful sound you could use to propel your mind into outer space. *Bahya,* "being outside, outer, exterior, strange, foreign." *Akasha,* "a free or open space, a vacuum; the sky or atmosphere; the subtle and ethereal fluid supposed to fill and pervade the universe and to be the peculiar vehicle of life and of sound." Become that vehicle, flying through the space you behold.

106

तरङ्ग

TARAṄGA

Taranga: "Across-goer," a wave, billow, a section of a literary work that contains in its name a word like *sea* or *river;* a jumping motion, gallop. Cloth, clothes. To move like a billow, to wave about, to move restlessly to and fro.

Practice

This is a completely wacky practice: wherever the mind moves, in that moment, move on. Don't let the mind rest anywhere. Keep it jumping, keep it skipping over the top of the waves.

This sounds just like what we do anyway when we are distracted. In *Four Quartets,* T. S. Eliot used the phrase "distracted from distraction by distraction." Some days it seems like most of us are running around this way.

The Sanskrit is cute: *yatra yatra manas yati. Yatra yatra* means "wherever, whithersoever." *Manas* is mind in its widest sense—intellect, intelligence, understanding, sense, the spiritual principle, the breath or living soul, thought, imagination, desire, mood. *Yati* is "goes." You could use *yatra yatra* as a kind of fly swatter to keep the mind moving.

Each thought is a wave. One of the skills of surfing is to know how to dive under the waves so you don't get caught in the churn. In this meditation, you keep your mind skipping along the surface, free of any one wave, then you let it dive of its own accord. It's a rebound effect. You take the mind's natural motion, amplify it to exhaustion, and then let it rest in the depths, motionless and still (*nistaranga,* from *nis,* "out, forth, free from").

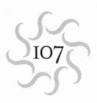

107

भया

BHAYA

Bhaya: Fear, alarm, dread, apprehension. Fear of or for. Terror, dismay, danger, peril, distress. Danger from.

Practice

When fear rises during meditation, welcome it, feel into it. Enter the vibratory world of sensations underneath that emotion.

Many of our thoughts during meditation have their origin in what we are afraid will happen. Most of the uncomfortable emotions and sensations you feel during meditation have some connection with fear, anxiety, or nervousness. This is not to be denied. Loving opens us up to loss. If we go for it in any arena and follow our passions, we put ourselves at risk. We can learn to make fear our friend.

The name of this text is the Vijnana *Bhairava* Tantra. *Bhairava* has many, many meanings, including "terrific"—the aspect of universal consciousness that accepts our terror as prayer and opens the door to revelation. Contemplating infinity can lead to terror and ecstasy at the same time. Meeting the soul is terrifying.

Therefore, terror is not shameful; it is to be embraced. Terror can be subtle, as in the recognition that life is short and you have to get on with what you are here to do and experience. The alarm goes off and propels us to wake up and seek God. Every human emotion, every impulse, is an opportunity to awaken to the immediacy of life.

Several meditations are suggested here. One could be to meditate with the phrase *bhaya sarvam,* "everyone is afraid." (*Bhaya,* "fear, alarm, dread, dismay." *Sarva,* "all, whole, entire, everyone.") Suns are probably afraid when the time comes for them to die. Who knows?

Another meditation is to use *bhairava* as a mantra, and be aware of the vast range of meanings such as, "God is here, inside my fear" and "The universe is indeed vast and terrifying, and yet permeated by a friendly consciousness. I am intimate with that One."

The trembling we feel in terror is a vibration in our bodies. Every cell is buzzing. Listen to this sound rising up from the depths of your being.

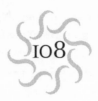

108

अहम्

AHAM

Aham: I.

Practice

Aham is the source of all mantras and can be heard in a variety of delightful ways—for example, as *aha* followed by *mmm.* It can also be heard as *ah* followed by *ha* and then *mmm.*

Ah! Ha! Mmmmm.

Aha! Mmmmmm.

Aaaaahhhh haaaaaaaa mmmmmmm.

These are sounds we make all the time, because we like to. We say "Ah!" in surprise, "Ha!" in laughter, and "Mmm!" in pleasure. We say "Aha!" when we have sudden insight, and we can say "Mmm, thank you, universe, for existing."

Whenever you explore your relationship to mantra as sound, use your own personal principle of onomatopoeia—the feeling that the sound is itself the meaning. You can tell what mantras are good for you by how they feel.

Aham points to the mystery of consciousness, that there is a witness to creation. *Aham* is a form of *pranava,* the primordial shout of exuberance that set the universe in motion, and is similar to OM or *Aum,* but more personal.

Sit or lie down somewhere safe and engage with the mantra *aham,* either in Sanskrit or as the English, "I am." A couple of times a minute, quietly whisper *aham* with your inner voice, subvocally, and notice what happens. Pay attention to the spaces before and after the mantra. You can ask *aham* to repeat itself within your awareness, so you can lean back and simply listen. Delicately pulsate with the sound. Do not feel you need to fill the silences; rather, allow the sound to evoke silence, to remind you of the way silence is humming with peaceful aliveness. Over time, learn to embrace *aham* with spaciousness and to tolerate the sense of individual identity existing against a background of infinity.

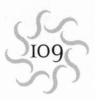

109

नित्य

NITYA

Nitya: Innate, native, one's own. Continual, perpetual, eternal. Constantly dwelling or engaged in, intent upon, devoted to, used to. The sea, the ocean. Constant and indispensable rite or act.

Practice

Eternity is your native state. You have choice about how you want to dwell here. You can be devoted to any quality that inspires you and engage with it continually.

This sutra invites you to inhabit your native state by immersing yourself in a mantra of your own. Ask yourself, "What quality would I love to be permeated by?" Notice what arises. Come up with one, two, or three qualities. Give them names, and use those words as a mantra. This meditation can become your constant companion.

Any quality you are craving—peace, love, harmony, joy, order, freedom, communion, creativity—is a good mantra to use. Your desire for that quality is itself a form of prayer and a shakti, an impulse of power from the depths of your being. The words to use are different for each of us, and they change over time as we evolve.

Shabda is "sound, noise, voice, tone, note; a word, speech, language; the right word, correct expression; the sacred syllable OM." When you name something you love, it becomes a mantra for you. The right word for you is an articulation of your yes to life and your version of OM in this moment.

Ask the spiritual energy you feel in the mantra to repeat itself in your heart as you move through your day. Your body will grow to love this feeling of being your own portable sanctuary. Everywhere you go you will feel at home. You are a native of eternity.

110

अतत्त्व

ATATTVA

Atattva: Non-essence.

Practice

In Sanskrit, when you add a short *a* before a word, it negates the word's meaning. For example, *yoga* means "connection, union," so *ayoga* means "separation, disjunction, separation from a lover." *Tattva* has a range of meanings, including "essence; true or real state, truth, reality; the essence or substance of anything." Therefore, *atattva* means non-essence.

Say you have learned the three flows of shakti, the nine states of the soul, and all thirty-six *tattvas* of Kashmir Shaivism. Now you realize it is all a joke—that all this knowledge has no substance, no base in reality. It's *atattva*.

You have stepped behind the curtain and are witnessing the magician at play. Indra is the god of the senses, and Indra's network of the senses is how we perceive anything at all. Our bodies are permeated with an internet of miraculously functioning nerves and senses, and the brain takes many millions of bits of information every second and creates the world we perceive. This is grand magic.

Consider that the act of perceiving is a kind of lovemaking with the elements of light, sound, vibration, gravity, and the chemistry involved in smell and taste. The sutra uses the word *vraj,* "to go, walk, wander, to go to have sexual intercourse with." There is a subtle erotic sense of being tickled and teased by the great magician.

III

आत्मन्

ĀTMAN

Atman: To breathe. To move. To blow. The soul, principle of life and sensation. The individual soul, self, abstract individual. Essence, nature, character, peculiarity. The person or whole body considered as one and opposed to the separate members of the body. The understanding, intellect, mind. The highest personal principle of life, *brahma.* Firmness. The sun. Fire.

Practice

Contemplate your essence, your individual and peculiar self, every sensation you have ever felt, your entire sense of life, your personality, everything you understand—the wholeness of who you are. Breathe with this awareness. Adore the miracle of this tiny spark of fire existing in the midst of infinity. You are a small sun, shining forth against a backdrop of vastness.

Now contemplate infinite spaciousness and emptiness, *shunya.* The emptiness of space is so accommodating that it makes room for hundreds of billions of galaxies, each with hundreds of billions of stars, and is not crowded at all. Thus, the universe easily makes room for you, your atman, to be here and breathe and witness infinity.

What is a sun but radiance? Why can we see stars a billion light years away? Because of the utter clarity of *shunya,* emptiness, the space that allows everything to exist. Outer space is so clear that there are particles or waves of light touching the earth's atmosphere right now that originated in the ecstasy of ancient suns, which no longer exist. The clarity of space allowed those little photons to travel across the universe and make it here, bringing their message, "I was once part of a sun. Now I give my light to you."

Only atman knows these things from the inside. Only the soul knows the soul. The questing mind goes silent in awe of infinity.

112

प्रतिबिम्ब

PRATIBIMBA

Pratibimba: The disc of the sun or moon reflected (in water). A reflection, reflected image, mirrored form. A resemblance or counterpart of real forms, a picture, image, shadow.

Practice

For the Great Self, there is neither bondage nor liberation. *Na me bandha, na moksha me:* "Not for me bondage; neither am I liberated. I was never lost in the first place."

Bhairava, the One Who is Enjoying Everything Everywhere, is saying, "The sun reflects off the water. If the angle shifts and you do not see the reflection, does that mean the sun has gone away? You have the power to form conceptions, to make mental models of the world. If you make a model that says you are separate from Me, does that mean I have gone somewhere? When your *buddhi,* your power of forming conceptions, forms the idea that you are separate, isolated and lonely, you become terrified. The universe then seems like a dangerous place."

The concepts of bondage and liberation are scary (*bhita:* "frightened, alarmed, terrified, timid, afraid of or imperiled by, anxious about"). Terror is part of the path. The name *Bhairava* itself means "frightful, terrible, horrible, formidable." When you become scared, use that as energy for your awakening.

Know that your essence is not trapped in this body. You are not bound by the space-time continuum. The soul, that which you seek, is not trapped in matter.

Engaging with the Sutras

There are many ways to explore the Radiance Sutras and develop a meditation practice with them. One way is just to show up and dive in. Read them once in a while and let them influence your *pranashakti,* your life force, in the background. Another way is to develop a relationship with one of the sutras and spend time with it on a regular basis. You can ask your inner wisdom to lead you to the right sutra and teach you the most useful way to play with it.

Here are a few more hints for cultivating a healthy and life-affirming meditation practice with the sutras.

Respect the power of your love. Answer the call of the sutras you love. It is powerful to spend even one minute being in the presence of what you adore.

Make yourself at home. One of the great gifts of meditation is learning how to be at home in yourself and in the world. As you come in and explore your relationship with these practices, be welcoming and nonjudgmental toward yourself.

Open embrace is the style of attention called for in most of these 112 practices. This is the opposite of concentration. The posture is that of opening your arms wide to the universe and to your inner world.

Be playful. The word *lila* (pronounced *leela*) is Sanskrit for play and amusement—and the sense that the universe has been manifested as an act of play by the divine. As you engage with these tantric techniques, give yourself permission to be at play, so that you can find your individual path in meditation.

Be gradual. Allow yourself to gradually become familiar with a sutra. Notice where in your body you respond to the images and sensations that the text evokes. When you practice, delight in the gentle progression from the outer level of experience to the interior, intimate levels. This may take only a few seconds, but it's gradual. The text uses the word *sanais,* "quietly, softly, gently, gradually."

Ride your rhythms. When you practice with these sutras, there will always be flow and fluctuations in the *pranashakti,* the vibrant energy of your body-mind system. Your experience will change second by second, and many sensations, emotions, mental pictures, remembered conversations, dreamlike thoughts, desires, and energy sensations will come and go. The waveless state usually lasts only a second or two. Welcome it all, then return to your focus in an effortless way. Yogis often go through an entire mythic journey in a few minutes—Hearing the Call to Adventure, Refusal of the Call, Crossing the First Threshold, the Road of Trials, Meeting the Mentor, Seizing the Elixir, Resurrection, and the Return to the Ordinary World. Meditative experience is often intense.

Ask questions of life. Practicing tantra does not mean imposing techniques upon yourself. An attitude of wonder and inquiry is one of the greatest skills you can develop. Cherish your questions, and then be alert so that you can see, feel, and listen to life's responses.

Be succinct. In exploring what you love in a certain sutra, feel into what is the most wonderful word or phrase for you today. When you say or think those one or two words, the whole sutra will be there, vibrating. There are times when shorter is better. You can select an English or a Sanskrit word or phrase, welcome it into your awareness, and cherish it.

Learn by heart. When you find a sutra, a line, or a phrase that resonates with you, memorize it. Learn it by heart. In this way, you can close your eyes and let it roll through your awareness. Remembering is *smara,* loving recollection.

Learn what effortlessness is. When you allow your attention to be called to something you love, the flow is natural. Effortlessness is a great skill and emerges spontaneously from operating in accord with your essence, your *prakriti* (your essential nature). Effort comes in only when you try to block out thoughts, sensations, or emotions.

Find what works for you. There is no one prescription for a meditation practice. Some people are able to practice the sutras' techniques on the fly, as they move through life. They can enter and exit meditative states within seconds, almost invisibly. I love to meditate for half an hour in the morning and again late in the afternoon. Other people make time for meditation every couple of days or on weekends. The main thing is to explore, test what works, and don't make yourself feel bad for not fitting into an imagined ideal.

Don't do too much. Get used to enjoying yourself. Begin with a minute or two of practice. Over days, learn to stay in the practice for a few minutes longer. Twenty minutes of meditative rest is very powerful. Spend a year or two getting used to the effects of meditating for twenty or twenty-five minutes in the morning and evening before going longer. This is just a guideline, though; if you are teaching yoga or doing healing work, you may find that you need to meditate more, to keep your energy field shimmering.

Honor the no. Not all of these practices are for everybody. The Vijnana Bhairava Tantra is a mini encyclopedia of yoga meditation techniques. Some will call you to come in and play. Some will be scary. Others will just not feel like *you*, so feel free to simply ignore them. Saying no creates a container, a boundary, leading to the possibility of a profound yes at some other time. A healthy relationship includes the freedom to say, "No, not right now."

The skills of meditation are the skills of loving anyone or anything. Meditation is not a separate set of skills apart from living and loving people, places, and things. In your inner life, learn to hold yourself as skillfully as a cook holds a spatula, a cellist holds a cello, a singer holds a note, a mother holds a baby—think of how lightly and yet firmly, how stable and yet responsive the holding is in each situation. The holding changes continually in response to the changing situation. The skills of meditation are like this in a subtle way: you are holding and releasing thoughts, emotions, sensations, and perceptions.

Allow yourself to rest in the truth of your being. When you are attending to a sutra that speaks to you, there will be waves of exhilaration and restfulness—the power of outward expression of your truth and the power of resting in your being. Both will evolve over time. As you learn to rest in your essence, a special, almost magical kind of meditative rest will develop. This aspect of the physiology of meditation has been researched extensively at Harvard Medical School and other universities over the past forty years. Meditative rest is a type of rest deeper than deep sleep.

Meditation is not making the mind quiet. It is tolerating all the noise without resistance and discovering the silent depths. Meditation is not sitting still. It is enjoying your motion on all levels, including the subtle levels, where stillness and exquisite motion seem to be one and the same.

Honor your individuality, for it is a great mystery. Everybody has a different style of engaging the forces of life as they flow through the *nadis* (energy arteries), chakras (rotating wheels of energy), and muscles. The song Bhairava and Devi are singing to each other is one of intimacy with energy. These practices lead to an intensified relationship with the life pulsating within and around us. Cherish the differences between you and others, for intimacy is based on an appreciation of differences as well as commonality.

Be tender toward your wounds and all that you feel is flawed, broken, or defective in yourself. As the sutras say, these wounds are gateways to infinity. Allow the life-giving prana to circulate freely in your being and body and to heal the places you are ashamed of, the places that ache.

Check in with your inner child. Take time to daydream about your childhood quiet times, your forts and secret places, those times when you spoke to the sky and earth, for in these times and places, you were natural and untamed.

Take naps. If you have been playing with the sutras for a while, you may find that your naps become sublime and feel like meditation. These catnaps can create a feeling of being drenched in rejuvenation and healing. Many of us have a sleep deficit, and the more you pay that off, the more you can enter deep states of meditation.

Use all your senses. You have a dozen senses, maybe more—vision, hearing, smell, taste, touch, plus senses of joint position, balance, motion, stretching, lung inflation, blood pressure, hunger (blood sugar), thirst (hydration), and perhaps magnetoception (the ability to sense magnetic fields). Each sense is a way of being in contact with the vibrating, pulsating field within which we are dancing. Learn all your senses, practice using them, engage with them in pranayama (breathwork), asana (movement), *dharana* (holding a thought), and *dhyana* (appreciation), and daily life. Become intimate with the full range of each sense and delight in the nuances and combinations.

Get elemental. Space, fire, air, earth, water, are the general *tattvas,* or elements. The Vijnana Bhairava Tantra invites you to develop your own playful and informal relationship with each element, as it pulsates in the *outer* world and *within* you. Learn to be intimate with each element with each of your senses—the *sight* of water flowing, the *sound* of waves, the *smell* of the air near rivers and oceans, the *taste* of anything you drink, the *touch* of the shower water all over your skin. Find your favorite experiences and continually cultivate and expand your list.

Be instinctive. Learn also to relate to each element with each of your instincts, of which you have many: homing, exploring, trail-making, resting, nesting, feeding, bathing, forming communities, pair bonding, mating, playing, self-expression, protection, and others. So you can, for example, *rest* with fire, as in luxuriating in the presence of a candle or fireplace. You can be *fed* by fire, in the form of the heat that cooks your food. You can *bathe* in fire, in the form of sunbathing or just exposing your skin to the sun. You can experience an erotic relationship with sunlight when hiking or doing outdoor sports. Everything you do in the outer world to enrich your sensuous perception of the elements will also enrich your inner world when you are practicing meditation.

Welcome infinite variety. A healthy meditation practice involves welcoming the free flow of all elements, with all your senses engaged, and all of the instincts free to give their gift. The combinations and permutations are as vast as the stars in the sky, and in this way, each moment of meditation is novel, startling, and fascinating. You enter a lively peace born of embracing life in its fullness, and your body, your perception, and your spiritual practice will be continually refreshed. Let each of your senses delight in each of the elements, in every instinctive tone; this is a healthy practice.

Welcome your emotions. To the degree that you open your heart to life, you will feel flooded by emotions of all kinds. Each emotion is a world of energy flows and sensations throughout the body. Some of the major moods described in the yoga literature include laughter *(hasya)*, erotic love or lust *(rati)*, sorrow *(soka)*, anger *(krodha)*, enthusiasm *(utsaha)*, fear or terror *(bhaya)*, disgust *(jugupsa)*, and astonishment *(vismaya)*. We can see these emotions as a color wheel, a mandala; each one has its place and its gift to give to the vibrancy of life. It is not necessarily a good meditation if you are sitting there feeling peaceful the whole time. A good meditation means you get what you need to thrive in your life.

Cherish nuance. Blue light oscillates at around six hundred trillion times a second; red light, only four hundred trillion times a second. Green light is in between, in the five hundred trillion range. Yet we can easily perceive the difference; our senses have evolved to notice and utilize the various frequencies, all these tiny wiggling energies. We also sense nuances of emotion. We sense the subtle differences between worry, regret, discouragement, envy, weariness, depression, anxiety, grief, shame, agitation, despair, impatience, and indignation. We distinguish between lust, love, adoration, and admiration. Some nuances are fleeting, lasting a fraction of a second; others demand your attention for a long time.

Noticing emotion may involve detecting many processes within the body and around the body. We are simultaneously gauging our hormonal and muscular situation, along with assessing what is going on in our outer world. We interpret all this information and attempt to shape prana, our natural energies, to respond to the life situation. Be inviting, accepting, and friendly toward your moods in all their varieties. Each is a form of the life force, prana, as it flows.

Welcome emotional release. An intimate relationship with *pranashakti,* the energies of life, is like any relationship—you laugh and you cry. Therefore, welcome thoughts and emotional release as an intrinsic part of the process. Crying and laughing may not seem meditative, but they are cleansing, nourishing, and rejuvenating, and signs of a healthy meditation. The heart and the chakras (the instinctive centers of the body, such as the sexual area, solar plexus, heart, throat, and head) get to reboot themselves, start afresh. Chronic muscular tension blocks the flow of prana and emotion in the body, and as you let go of that tension, you may find you have a backlog of emotions to tend to. Get good at this tending. If it's all too wild, work with a mentor who is adept at dealing with emotion.

Savor your emotional experience. When we attend to the flow of emotion with the skills of yoga, there is the possibility of transmutation. The raw experience of life becomes refined. Erotic energies lead to a lovemaking between body and soul. Angry energies turn to the element of fire. Sorrow leads to compassion. Humor leads to levity, a light heart. Even the most base emotions, when we engage with them as yogis, can turn to gold. We extract the essence, the juice, or *rasa,* of experience, and bliss, *ananda,* emerges. Attending to the energy flows in the body is similar to witnessing a movie, play, or dance performance: you are witnessing the play of life as you. As you cherish your experience in this way, you can spend more time in wonder, awe, and peacefulness.

Write your own sutras. Give yourself the opportunity to speak and write from inside your own current of perception. There is a flavor, a style, of sensing the energies of life that is unique to you, and your world needs it.

Don't put your enlightenment outside of you—not in India, in the past, in the future, in gurus or experts. Honor the revelations that come from your own direct living experience.

Note the difference between the path of denial and the path of intimacy. In the past, yoga was the domain of males who practiced a particular asana toward life—*sannyasana,* "throwing down, laying aside, giving up, resignation, renunciation of worldly concerns." Those who practice this posture toward life are called *sannyasin,* or renouncers, and they generally take vows of celibacy, poverty, and obedience to their superiors in the tradition. The ideal is to be poor and homeless and yet free within, as well as free to practice yoga and meditation all day. This is the ancient path, and it was profound; the energy that would otherwise go into raising children and running a business goes into practicing and preserving the knowledge of meditation. Historically, almost all meditation texts were composed by male renouncers, and so the language system and techniques were shaped for their lifestyle of detachment and denial. All of us who practice meditation today owe these renouncers a debt of gratitude. They kept the faith.

In the modern Western world, yoga is practiced mostly by women and men who live in the world and have families and jobs. This is the path of intimacy, and in many ways it is the opposite of renouncing. Those on the path of intimacy work *with* attachment, desire, and responsibility, honoring and embracing each aspect of life, as time, energy, and ethics permit; their yoga evolves though love, work, play, and honoring the bonds of friendship and family. Instead of taking vows of celibacy, poverty, and obedience, those on the path of intimacy experience sexual relationships, work to generate wealth, and explore the play of independence and cooperation with others.

Always practice in accord with your inner nature, whether you are on the path of denial or the path of intimacy.

Give up altogether on judging your experience. During meditation, your brain and body are running maintenance programs. There is a lot of healing going on. Often you will be hurting and feeling your exhaustion. If you were an athlete getting a massage, you wouldn't say, "It was a bad massage because the therapist was rubbing my sore muscles."

Make peace with thoughts. If you are going to meditate, make peace with the flow of thought. The brain is always making connections, whether you are meditating or not. Hundreds of thoughts come and go every hour; this is what brains do. When you close your eyes and pay attention, you may become vividly aware of the intricate lightshow that manufactures all we see, hear, feel, think, and sense. If you are not willing to make peace with thoughts, then do something else for your development. Get into dance or sports. Take singing lessons. Learn an instrument.

Don't enforce a speed limit. You don't have to write yourself speeding tickets. Eyes and brains work fairly rapidly: third-grade students generally read two-to-three words per second, and college students average over seven words per second. When you are meditating, you might have seven perceptions per second. Not a problem. People often talk about meditation as slowing down. Consider the opposite: appreciating how fast attention moves. Even though your awareness might be vibrating rapidly, your body and your breathing will often slow down if you are doing one of the sitting or lying down meditations. A speeding mind and slow body can happen simultaneously.

Welcome your wildness. There a meme in children's cartoons in which someone opens a door, discovers a monster roaring "RAAAARRRGH!" and then slams the door and shudders. This shows up in adult movies also: the characters are in a quiet room and walk outside into a tornado of human activity. When some people close their eyes to meditate, they immediately sense wildness and feel out of control. This is not a failure to meditate; it is a glimpse of the astounding reality that is always here.

Cultivate the opposite. If you are in love with one side of a polarity—outside-inside, dancing-stillness, visual-tactile, passion-serenity, wildness-peacefulness, freedom-discipline, independence-communion—begin to inquire into the joy of the opposite, which will arise anyway. Yoga flows between the polarities—breathe out then breathe in, turn toward the left then turn toward the right, bend forward then bend back. Train yourself to think in terms of the balance between opposites and the continuum of energies flowing between the poles. Tolerating the play of opposites is called *tapas* in yoga and valued because this builds strength.

Look at art, listen to music, read poetry, and dance. The arts, including the expressive arts, speak of the sacred, each one in its own way. Art educates the senses and creates community, sharing revelations with others around the world throughout time. Whenever possible, attend live events, openings, and performances, for artists of all kinds are yogis in the sense of being utterly devoted to bringing forth onto the earth the revelation of truth and beauty. Artists seek to articulate, each in their own medium, the resonance of *pranashakti* in our times, the unfolding revelation. Be in the presence of artists—musicians, singers, dancers, painters. Know that the attention you bring is a blessing to them, as you appreciate their work from a deep place within.

Develop expression commensurate with your communion. Learn to express yourself from inside your ecstatic energy flows and sacred spaces; otherwise, the energies you awaken will just ache. Expression takes the form of movement of all kinds, including dance, sports, and speaking from inside the current of your passion. *Mudra* is soul-infused movement, and *mantra* is evocative speech.

Get coaching on your meditative practices. For example, I'm a meditation coach, and I enjoy working with people in person, on the phone, and by email. When you work one-on-one with a coach, you and your coach can honor your individual experience.

Be open to teachers. The best teacher for you on any given day may be the one who embodies the quality you are craving the most, and they may teach in ways other than words. A massage therapist, vocal coach, wilderness guide, or an instructor of dance, art, yoga, breathing, surfing, or martial arts may be your inspiration.

Stay in touch. There are lovers of life around every corner. Find others who share the same enthusiasm as you. (One way is to sign up for my mailing list; see my website to do so.)

Come to workshops with us at yoga and retreat centers worldwide. Don't think, "Oh, everyone is more advanced than me," or "I don't have the right yoga pants to wear." You are always welcome. Take our online courses or download audio programs to stay tuned in to the community of others exploring The Radiance Sutras.

POSTLUDE

THE LAB

One day in 1968, when I was a freshman at the University of California, I signed up to participate in a brain-wave biofeedback study. Learning to control your brain waves by looking at flashing lights sounded interesting. Also they paid more than I was making mowing the greens at a nearby golf course. Due to the flip of a coin, I was selected to be a control subject in the study, meaning that I received no instructions whatever; I was just hooked up with electroencephalogram (EEG) wires stuck all over my head and left in total darkness and total silence, in a soundproofed room in the physiology lab, for two to three hours at a time, every day for several weeks.

At the time, I had never heard of meditation. Not knowing what else to do, I simply paid attention to what was going on. Gradually my senses opened up in ways that I had no words to describe. My sense of self melted into the dark. I merged with blackness and infinity and entered a world of spacious peace. Space itself seemed to be made out of harmony.

Walking out of the lab each afternoon, I felt refreshed and wonderful. It was as if my entire previous life had taken place in a mild sleep state, and now I was fully alert. It was as if I had never seen the world before, and everything alive seemed to glow, especially the trees. I began to appreciate every detail of light, every touch of air, every sound, with extraordinary clarity. Light itself seemed soluble, an elixir I was drinking in through my eyes and the pores of my skin.

I would have been astonished, but the intensity was balanced by a magnificent serenity. I was drenched in moving peacefulness. The perceptions seemed natural—this is the way the world has always been—but I had been too oblivious to notice.

I was delighted. The feeling was similar to the peaceful joy of surfing, but more intense and steady. I felt like myself, but this was a self I had never spent time in before. I was very much in my body, aware of the current of life flowing through me, and at the same time I could feel an extended sense of touch reaching out in all directions. I was in love with existence.

The experiment continued for weeks. I enjoyed going to the lab each afternoon and sitting there in the dark for hours, then walking out into the light and discovering a new world. I got used to living in this free and open state in which I just breezed through tasks that previously had been chores.

I noticed that even taking calculus tests was easy; my mind was lucid, and I could remember a formula that I had glanced at the night before, then derive its applications right there during the test.

The heightened sensing and superb functioning lasted for a month or so after the experiment was over. It was a continuous and self-maintaining state. Then it started to fade away, and I missed it.

The physiology lab seemed like an interesting place, and I needed a job, so I started to work there. At a meeting one afternoon, a female graduate student read from the Vijnana Bhairava Tantra, just a few lines of the conversation between Shakti and Shiva. Her words vibrated in the air with brilliance. After the meeting was over, I asked her about it. She handed me the book, a paperback copy of *Zen Flesh, Zen Bones* by Paul Reps. It was open to a page:

> Radiant one, this experience may dawn between two
> breaths. After breath comes in (down) and just before
> turning up (out)—*the beneficence.*

> As the breath turns from down to up, and again as
> breath curves from up to down—through both these
> turns, *realize.*

Or, whenever inbreath and outbreath fuse, at this instant
touch the energyless energy-filled *center.*

As I read that, a quiet happiness filled my being. This description
felt intimate and familiar, an echo of my experience in the lab. An
electric current lit me up from the inside out, everywhere in my body.
In one instant, everything changed. I was standing there in the lab,
but the world was full of new possibilities, because the words in the
book spoke to the heart of what happened during those hours in the
dark room and afterwards. I immediately jumped into my car and
drove to the nearest bookstore to buy the book. Standing there in the
bookstore, I read:

> Wandering in the ineffable beauty of Kashmir, above
> Srinagar I come upon the hermitage of Lakshmanjoo.
> It overlooks green rice fields, the garden, of Shalimar . . .
> Water streams down from a mountaintop. Here
> Lakshmanjoo—tall, full bodied, shining—welcomes
> me. He shares with me this ancient teaching from the
> Vigyan Bhairava and Sochanda Tantra, . . . and from
> it Lakshmanjoo has made the beginning of an English
> version. It presents 112 ways to open the invisible door
> of consciousness.

Hmm, I thought, so there is a teacher by the name of Lakshman Joo
who lives this teaching, and he says there are many doors to consciousness and each one can be practiced.

In this way, my first taste of the revelations the Vijnana Bhairava
Tantra came from sitting in silence and darkness, with no knowledge
of meditation. The next came through the written word, the sense of
being electrified by the current of power behind the words of Lakshman Joo and Paul Reps. It was obvious to me that they were writing
from inside the same pulsating current of life force that I was being
introduced to.

My experience in the lab taught me that meditative attention
occurs spontaneously. From the Bhairava Tantra I learned that there
are many pathways into meditation. Learn to shift your attention
slightly, and you will find them, and you will find the ones that are

svanurupa, suited to your character ("natural, innate, well suited"). The life force flowing through the body invents techniques as needed—just tune in. These two insights, of the instinctive natural-ness of meditation and the tremendous variety of approaches, have been guiding and inspiring me ever since.

In 1969, as part of various research projects at the university, I started teaching meditation. When people would come for instruc-tion, I asked them to tell me about their natural "meditative" kinds of experiences: "When have you felt peaceful, glad to be alive?" I found that as they spoke, they would enter the meditative states they were talking about. After an hour or ninety minutes of listening in this way, I would ask them to browse through the Vijnana Bhairava section of *Zen Flesh, Zen Bones* and show me which of the practices they recognized as being natural to them, or which they just were interested in. Whichever one they selected, we would work together to develop that into a daily practice for them.

In 1970, I was trained as a teacher of Transcendental Meditation (TM) by Maharishi Mahesh Yoga. TM utilizes several of the practices in the Bhairava Tantra and is an elegant system. After completing the teacher training, I immediately went on to three months of advanced training. At Maharishi's suggestion, I spent twenty-eight days in total darkness, from full moon to full moon. From before dawn to early eve-ning, I would flow through asana, pranayama, and meditation, over and over. During that time, I found that my body was also flowing through the 112 practices of the Vijnana Bhairava Tantra. Each of the practices would arise as needed then fade into the background. After a week or so in the dark, there were moments and days of pure terror, in which I was face to face with what felt like ultimate destruction.

When you become silent in meditation, you are, whether you know it or not, inviting all the noise in your soul to come to the sur-face to be resolved and turned into harmony. If you have any traumas, they invite themselves to come to awareness and be healed. If there is anything to have flashbacks about, they come, because this is the best possible situation for them to flash back and forth and reoccur until their healing purpose has been fulfilled. This happens whether you want it to or not. I did not want it to, but I wanted to be healed and integrated, feel at home in the world, and be free of the profound loneliness aching in my soul.

Out of the silence arose a flood of memories, a continuous stream of the storehouse of impressions. I relived my entire life over and over, backward and forward, with particular focus on everything painful. Attention would zoom in on a moment of pain or agony, amplify it, then zoom out to embrace the solar system and this blessed little ocean-covered rock we are on. Then again, awareness would focus in, like a microscope, on another painful memory encoded in my muscles or senses. I viewed it from inside, then all around, then backward, then forward, amplifying, amplifying, intensifying beyond all limits of endurance, until I finally let go and let the pain have its way with me, which felt like dying. This process was merciless and thorough—no molecule went untouched. The pain became elemental, like a blowtorch, intolerable, heating up the atoms of my being. At other times I felt like a lump of coal being crushed by the earth for an eternity, but there was no sense of slowly being turned into a diamond.

For the first two weeks, I wanted to run screaming out of the room. Maharishi had instructed me to just "feel de body," stay with the sensations, so that's what I did. The pain got worse and worse until it was the only thing in the universe. Finally, out of desperation, I relaxed into being the space that embraces this solar system. Within this sphere, the earth is just a grain of sand, held lovingly in the orbit of the sun. This went on over and over, relentlessly, until every trauma was healed, every harm forgiven, every agony erased.

I noticed that my body was meeting each impossible demand with one of the brilliant methods of the Vijnana Bhairava Tantra. Each blast of flame, sensation of being crushed, encounter with terror, or feeling of being ripped apart molecule by molecule required a specific skill and demanded to be met with one of the meditations described in the text. We all have survival instincts that come to us when we desperately need them. I felt that for my survival, I needed to stay in that room. When faced with each intolerable energy, I would let go into a skill, a way of welcoming the energy so that it was transmuted into something else. I had just a hint of technique, but it was just enough to allow me to stay and face everything steadily.

There came a moment, a breath, in which there was nothing left to fear, nothing anywhere in my being I had not faced. I waited for something else to arise and looked around in the inner universe with an attitude of welcoming, of "bring it on." But nothing came. There was nothing but a vacuum, an incredible, vibrating nothingness.

I took another breath.

And mind dissolved into empty space. Heart dissolved into a spaciousness that was somehow very friendly. Then I simply dissolved into vast darkness—the space embracing the solar system, with a teeny dot in the center, shining steadily.

I stayed in the room for another week, just savoring what had happened, resting in a quiet, self-sustaining, steady ecstasy as I flowed through asana, pranayama, meditation, pranayama, asana, pranayama, meditation, over and over again.

One day, some inner prompting told me it was time to emerge. I arose around 4 a.m. as usual, did asanas, and meditated. Then I walked outside and found myself in the presence of the full moon, which was extremely bright to my dark-adapted eyes. The moon was on its way to setting behind the mountains. I turned my back to it and looked out over the Mediterranean and the stars glowing above the water. I felt a deep, intimate communion with everything. After a while the horizon started to glow, and I watched and waited. When the sun rose over the sea, there was glory in the sky. When I took a breath, there was an elixir of new life in that salty air coming off the ocean. With that breath, the thought came to me from somewhere, "Now I can live." I was a changed person. I was simpler. At the same time, an ancient witness within had emerged, someone who had seen millions of sunrises and delighted in every single one.

Later that day I walked down the beach to where Maharishi was staying. I told him that I had a strong feeling that "If I could stay in the room for three years, I would become enlightened." It was such a deep yearning in my heart, in my entire being.

Maharishi chuckled, then looked at me with those fathomless eyes and said, "Go and teach, hmm?" My head dropped. He said, tenderly, "Go and teach, and come back. More advanced trainings." That was it.

Then a spiritual flashbulb went off inside, flooding my entire being in an instant.

"Thank you, Maharishi," I said. I was at peace, happy.

I knew—it was obvious—that Maharishi himself would rather be in a cave somewhere, or on a mountainside in the Himalayas, meditating, breathing the pure air, cherishing the silence. But there was a call he could not refuse: to go to the West and teach meditation. His heart had led him to be here.

When I returned to California, I moved to Laguna Beach and spent my days surfing, teaching meditation, and going to college at University of California, Irvine, in that order. For the next five years, until 1976, I exuberantly taught TM in Southern California, primarily in Orange County and Los Angeles. I taught at UC Irvine, in various businesses, in six different high schools, and in people's homes.

During this time I was a subject in physiological research on meditation underway at UC Irvine Medical School and the University of Southern California. These studies were not fun. There were no deluxe soundproofed rooms. But I felt that I owed the meditation research community a great debt. So when a scientist would call and very politely request my participation in a study, I would almost always say yes. The location was often a physiology lab with hundreds of rats in cages along the wall, smelling of rat food, rat droppings, and ether. Here I would sit and meditate while doctors stuck needles in my veins to take blood samples and measure changes in serum cortisol or blood flow to the brain. Other times the study was intended to measure oxygen consumption or galvanic skin response or brain waves.

Having participated in the research was a great asset for teaching in the universities. When I would be lecturing and showing slides of the scientific research on meditation, professors and doctoral students would challenge the data. I could gracefully field their questions and say, "I don't know," when appropriate, and this led to an easy rapport. After a few years, a group of professors started suggesting I get a PhD, because it seemed like a natural next step for me.

I entered a PhD program in the Social Sciences Department at UC Irvine, where I studied meditators' subjective experiences and the language they use to describe these experiences. The cognitive sciences and semantic anthropology had developed wonderful tools to reveal people's inner maps of the world. I created a technique for interviewing meditators in which I would sit with them for up to two hours and listen, occasionally asking leading questions.

I interviewed meditators of all kinds, including athletes, soldiers, hunters, dancers, atheists, Zen practitioners, Buddhists, Christians, stay-at-home mothers, and rebel, do-it-yourself meditators. These were people who usually would not, in the course of things, ever talk in depth of their meditative experience. In hundreds of sessions, I invited them to enter peaceful and ecstatic states, of whatever kind they had access to, and then speak from inside the experience.

Since then, as I have been teaching (and practicing) the yogas of the Bhairava Tantra, I've spent quite a few thousand hours sitting with people in the silence as they meditate and then listening to them talk about their experience.

LISTENING TO PRANASHAKTI

Engaging with the methods of the Bhairava Tantra for forty-plus years has opened up my senses so that I can see the energy shimmering around someone who is in the process of a spiritual awakening, listen to the song of their life-force flowing, and feel the current of their individual integrity. I have learned from this that the radiance, the spiritual power of that awakening, is their real teacher. My task as a meditation guide is to help them recognize the awakening, cooperate with it, and find the appropriate meditation practice to support it.

People who are interested in meditation are often on the verge—or in the midst—of intense revelations that they do not have the skills to fully accept or the language to express. In fact, it is this awakening-in-progress that calls people to come learn about meditation. This is what teaching meditation is about. I coach people in how to accept and roll with the yoga practice that is happening spontaneously.

Awakenings do not come uninvited, in my experience. We just forget that we've invoked them. At some point the day or year before, we asked life to lead us onto a better path, and then things shifted around in the background to make that possible. The methods, the *yuktis,* that Bhairava sings to Devi are ways that evolution gets our attention.

In my teaching, I always listen to people as much as time allows. What students say is actually more interesting than what teachers say, because in their fumbling for language, they are right on the edge of the abyss—in the uncertainty bordering on ecstasy that this text sings of. It's an unusual exploration in language, and I love it.

If you listen with silent attention and just let people speak from the heart about what they love, after a while, perhaps an hour or so, they'll tend to close their eyes and slip into meditation spontaneously. When they emerge, if you can get them to speak, what they say is drenched in vibrant peace and sounds similar to one of the practices in the Bhairava Tantra. It is as if one of the sutras is on the tip of their tongue. When someone is being called to meditate, there is often something in the 112 methods that is already vibrating in their nerves, and this is their natural technique.

When people are in ecstatic meditative states and you can get them to say something, they tend to generate simple succinct language, usually just a couple of vibrant words. "I breathe in, and I feel that life is giving me a fresh beginning," a young woman said after her first meditation session. Another woman opened her eyes and spoke from inside a vibrating silence: "I feel at home—at home in existence." That was all she said, simple and stunning. A woman who had been doing yoga for several months and was just discovering meditation said, "I feel as if I am drinking in peace through every pore of my skin." A young man looked around the room and with a mischievous sparkle in his eye said, "Everything is glowing, as if lit from within."

Two seemingly opposite qualities come together: a lively sense of pulsation and a peaceful silence. When the person I am meditating with enters this fusion, they glow with life. When I ask them to speak, to make words from within such a pulsating silence, it feels like a joke, but people usually manage a phrase or two. I call this listening to *pranashakti*—listening to the spirit becoming flesh, listening to the song being sung at the intersection of the life force with the body.

When I write down the phrases people say, there is a condensed meaning suggestive of poetry. We could say that their speech has a mantric quality; it is speech that is evocative of the inner world. The thought-impulse seems to rise up out of a field of silence, become a sensation in the body, shape itself into a few words, and then, after the words are spoken, the silence becomes louder than ever. In Radiance Sutras workshops and one-to-one sessions, people speak this way naturally, because that is what they are experiencing. The language is always surprising and fresh as it emerges from the encounter of awareness with the subtle energies flowing through the body.

TRANSLATION AS RAPTURE

One day in 1987, after I'd finished writing my doctoral dissertation, a quiet thought came to me: I should start working on a version of the Vijnana Bhairava Tantra. The words and phrases I use in *The Radiance Sutras* are inspired and informed by years of listening to how people speak when they are in contact with the soul, giving voice to *pranashakti*. They are also the result of an ongoing dance with the living, impish language that is Sanskrit.

Much of the work was done in the hours before dawn, starting at four in the morning or earlier. I find that it is the freshest time for this type of writing. There is a vitality in the air, a wave of pure fresh energy sweeping across the earth in advance of sunrise. Writers and meditators can ride this energy.

This early morning rush has a name in Sanskrit—*brahmamuhurta,* "the time of Brahma." I have also heard it called *navaswan.* In Vedic timekeeping, this time is said to start about two hours before dawn and last for forty-eight minutes. The Sikhs also have a term to describe this time: *amrit vela,* "the ambrosial period." They feel it is an auspicious time for spiritual practice.

If you are rested and ready for it, ready to sit and enjoy the pre-dawn quiet, *brahmamuhurta* is a treat. One moment, it is "the still of the night." Then something changes—there is a zing in the air, and the darkness is lively.

When I am in a sutra-writing cycle, I often go to bed by nine or so and get up at three or four in the morning to take advantage of *brahmamuhurta.* I pick a sutra, or it selects me, and I walk around inside it, chant it and dance with it for an hour or two, in Sanskrit and English (if I have gotten any English yet).

I first approach the text as mantra—I listen for the meaning encoded in the sequence of syllables, as one would listen to music. When you chant Sanskrit, after a while, it picks you up and carries you. When this happens, it is as if the sutra is whispering itself in the silence, pulsating and undulating. This is what I pray for. I know that if I just stay there, suspended between the worlds, trusting the silence, eventually I will get a fresh flow of words in English that conveys some of the juiciness of the original mantric speech.

The Sanskrit of the text is incredibly succinct. Each of the 112 central verses describes a yoga technique (called a *dharana* or *yukti*) in six to twelve words, depending on how long the compounds are, using about three dozen Devanagari letters. At the speed of a professional chanter, each verse can be said in twelve seconds. They get their point across in twelve seconds! This brevity is a feat of engineering. The composers packed many bits of information into each syllable.

My preferred speed is very slow by comparison; I usually take about thirty seconds to say a verse. I like to linger with each sound and notice its effect on my nerves and the way the sequence of syllables activates or redirects the flow of prana in my body. Sanskrit has a tendency to keep on vibrating even when the verbal and subvocal repetition ceases. Over the years, I spent an hour or more with each word and a day, week, or month with each verse. The text is only a couple of thousand words, in 162 verses, so this is a doable task and great fun.

After immersing myself in the mantric quality of the text, I shift to the semantic level, and to that I add usage—the way the word is used in the tantric tradition.

The Language of Enchantment

Sanskrit is a language of enchantment, and chanting it takes you to an inner world we all share, a living, worldwide web woven from prana, the life force. Your body is the access portal. Touch a word with your awareness, and it begins to pulsate and shimmer, then tell you tales of its origin. Be alert, though—any word may allure you into a magic realm. The pulsation of consciousness is stirred as layers of meaning resonate in your heart and scintillating imagery lights up your inner vision. Suddenly, you are inside the awareness field of the sages and *rishis* of the Vedic tradition.

This is not a world of the past. It is a subtle level of the present—a friendly world, warm and musical. When you enter it, you feel as if you have happened upon some cheerful and gabby oldster storytellers sitting around a fire, eager for an audience, for fresh ears to regale with their tales. Once they let you in, you can't say, "Oh, I have to go. The phone is ringing." You have to stay until they finish the story, which may take several hours or days—or in my case, years.

This is Indra's net, the primordial consciousness net. Instead of taking you to every random thought anyone ever posted on some website, it takes you to the best thinking and feeling of the meditators and *rishis* throughout time. Their code is *samskrita,* an "artificial or constructed" language, intentionally devised to safeguard their real-izations, the secrets they discovered in their caves and in the cave of the heart. It's the music of the heart. They invite you in: "Come sit by our fire, and we will tell you the truth. Your world needs this. Become a water-bearer, a conveyer of this wisdom."

Your body is the computer, your inner vision the screen, and you access it by meditating on the words. Each sound, word, and phrase resonates in the physical body, the emotional body, and through-out the subtle levels of your being. The internet being accessed is the vibrating field of intelligence permeating the space in which we breathe and think. Instead of using electricity, it uses the life force, the energy of breath.

Assembling the Mosaic

In order to attune myself to the richness of what Shakti and Shiva are singing to each other, I build a semantic web for each word of the text. This is a technique, borrowed from cognitive anthropology, for building a mosaic, or a mandala, of the meaning of a word.

The verses are made up of a dozen or fewer words each. I give every word of each sutra its own group of cards. Up to twenty-five cards represent the way the word is defined in the Monier-Williams *Sanskrit-English Dictionary.*[1] Another cluster of cards indicates how the term is used in the Vedas, Upanishads, Bhagavad Gita, and vari-ous texts of Kashmir Shaivism. The cards are spread out on the floor, and I walk around in them for a few hours or days, until I feel that the richness of the word is vibrating in my body. Then I lay out the cards for all dozen of the words in a particular sutra, and see what I've got. That is the mandala of the sutra. This detailed look at the individual words leads me into a deeper sense of what other workers in the field understand about the techniques being discussed.

Then I start to pray for English words and word sequences that resonate with the intention behind the Sanskrit. I may pace around among these cards for a week, just wondering and listening to the mantric quality of the Sanskrit and the corresponding English.

You can't sit still to do this type of writing. You have to walk, dance, stand, feel the earth beneath you, and open your arms wide to embrace the universe. You have to risk falling in love with the practices and be willing to be transformed by that love. Each time you approach a sutra, you have to approach it anew. Let the tantra sing to you and make your whole body vibrate with its song.

After looking at the pattern of cards on the floor for a while, a current of revelation begins to flow—sometimes immediately, other times after a few days or weeks. Sometimes I have to beg for mercy. "Come on, reveal yourself. I am hanging in suspense here. It's four in the morning, and I have been showing up here for a month."

There are places where the Sanskrit is cryptic, as if to guard its secrets, and the scholarly translations have only hinted at the deeper meanings or spoken in technical language resembling computer code. In other places, the text is actually not obscure; it just assumes that you are sitting on a hillside in Kashmir with all the time in the world to ask your questions.

Keep in mind that all of the meditation methods presented in the Vijnana Bhairava Tantra are practical and very human—experiences of feeling at one with life, the kinds of things lovers and children know.

Multiple Levels of Meaning and Sound

Sanskrit is gloriously polysemous (*poly*, "many," plus *sema*, "sign"). Because there are multiple layers of information in each Sanskrit word and each layer evokes realms of wonder and awe, the Vijnana Bhairava Tantra reverberates with clues to multiple layers of experience. Everywhere in this text, the Sanskrit lexicon is used with superb skill to indicate nuances of meditative experience.

For example, verse 39 (sutra 16) describes a mantra practice. Bhairava uses the word *pluta,* defined in the Monier-Williams *Sanskrit-English Dictionary* as "floating, swimming in, bathed, over-flowing, submerged, filled with, flooded." This is a remarkably sensuous description of the experience of meditating with a mantra—especially as attention shifts from verbal pronunciation to subvocal speech and then to the energy impulse of the sound as it dissolves into oceanic silence. If you interview mantra yoga practitioners and ask them what they experience as they melt into silence, you'll get these sorts of descriptions. Those who know how to meditate deeply with sound often say, spontaneously, "I feel flooded by the mantra, floating with it, bathed in the sound." The usual translation of *pluta* is simply "protracted."

When working on my latest version of the sutras, I prefer to use as much of the full semantic range of each word as I can fit onto the page without cluttering up the flow. If you ever wonder where a metaphor in a particular sutra came from, just look in the Sanskrit-English dictionary and follow the trail.

The language of the sutras is coded as densely as if you said in English, "B. B. King, Clapton, Hendrix, Paige." That is eight syllables evoking a style, a set list, a series of legendary, era-defining performances by these adept guitar players, and the awakening that the music evoked in the listeners. Or think of these eight syllables: *Bach, Beethoven, Wagner, Mozart.* Just these few words evoke worlds of revelatory beauty.

Each thirty-two-syllable verse of the Vijnana Bhairava Tantra is a message sent to the future: "Here is the greatest thing I have ever learned. I have encoded it so there is not one extra syllable, one extraneous thought. It's as perfect, polished, purified, consecrated—as *samskrita*—as I know how to make it. My prayer is that this message makes it through to you intact, you who will be born in a distant time and place."

The text is saying, "Here are 112 yoga practices, each described in about a dozen seconds of chanting. We call them *yuktis,* and each is a gateway into divine awareness. Cherish these as a treasure, a gift from us to you."

In addition to technical information regarding the skills of meditation, the verses convey images and jokes. The composers were irrepressible punsters. When Devi dares her lover, Bhairava, to speak the secrets of yoga, she uses the word *samshaya,* one of the meanings of which is "doubt." The primary dictionary definition of the word, however, is "lying down to rest or sleep," from *sam* ("together") and *shaya* ("lying, sleeping"). *Shaya* also means, "a bed, a couch." This is the second sentence Devi speaks, and already she is suggesting that perhaps they can lie down together and he can tell her all about it.

The language of the Vijnana Bhairava Tantra abounds in earthy humor and sexual innuendo. When Bhairava describes the yoga of kissing in sutra 47 (verse 70), the word he uses is *lehana.* Usually translated as "kissing," *lehana's* actual definition is "the act of licking, tasting, or lapping with the tongue." To lovers, *licking* is an utterly different word than *kissing.* When monks and nuns translate this word, they edit out the juiciness.

There are images everywhere in the Sanskrit, and I have attempted to use as many as possible so that you can access the visceral experience of the practice that is being described. Some translations of this tantra are so abstruse that even if you have been doing one of the practices described in a verse for years, you can't recognize it.

Rasa, used in sutra 49, has the basic sense of "juice" (of plants or fruit) and "the best or finest or prime part of anything, essence, marrow, liquor, drink, syrup, elixir, potion, nectar, semen, taste, flavor, love, affection, desire, charm, pleasure, delight." *Rasa* is also aesthetic relish—"the taste or character of a work, the feeling or sentiment prevailing in a work of art."

Nitya, used in sutra 109, is often translated as "eternal," but its full definition is more personal: "innate, native, one's own, continual, perpetual, eternal, constantly dwelling or engaged in, intent upon, devoted or used to, the sea, the ocean."

These terms, and many others, have oceanic semantic fields. I don't attempt to reduce them to a corresponding word of English in a one-to-one mapping. Rather, I set the mantra-field vibrating and listen for English that hints at the mystery.

In addition to the semantic field of each word, there is the sound of it, which is often succulent. Sanskrit is designed to be euphonic, both to the physical ears and to the internal hearing. The verses are intended to be chanted and to convey messages in rhythm. Levels of sound and silence open up, and the chant gets more and more interesting as it gets quieter and quieter. In yoga there is the concept of four levels of sound:

Vaikhari-vak, the spoken word, where there are syllables,
    words, and sentences;
Madhyama-vak, the in-between or middle sound, subvocal
    speech, the sound you hear in your mind;
Pashyanti-vak, seeing, sensing, and beholding the vibratory
    effect of the word;
Para-vak, the transcendental sound.

In between each level of sound are exquisite transitional areas, where one sound melts into the other. I ask the Sanskrit of the sutra to repeat itself like a mantra in my heart, so that I can listen with every cell of my body. I am willing to be pulsed by the fluctuations and impulses that the sounds set up in my nerve circuits and the cool flame that flows along my spine. After a while I become enchanted. Often, a soft, warm luminosity fills the room. Even though it is before dawn, the atmosphere becomes kind of rockin'.

I ride the *vak* elevator up and down, a whispered *vaikhari-vak* to *madhyama-vak* to *pashyanti-vak*. I inhabit the vibrating energy field at the level just before thoughts become words. This feels like being in a hot tub of prana, with bubbles of tingling impulses everywhere. Then I let the impulses that gave rise to the Sanskrit give me English words, which I sort of sand down a bit, like a woodworker, so they are smooth.

This is very physical work, letting the sutra hit you and then responding to it. Because the sutras are so varied, I find it's best if my posture also varies, so I flow between walking, standing, swaying, dancing, lying down, and sometimes sitting still. Each posture or asana allows me to hear different currents of revelation. In this way, I let the chord of the sutra strike me, then I seek words that articulate the experience.

In places, Sanskrit is consciously onomatopoeic: if you listen to it sensitively, something in the sound of the words and rhythm of the chanting evokes in you a feeling of what is being described. The words resonate simultaneously on all levels: physical, sensual, emotional, mental, and spiritual. In so doing, they evoke a vibrational integration or correspondence among all these levels. This multidimensionality provides endless possibilities for jokes, plays on words, and double and multiple entendres.

There is something more in Sanskrit: in certain words there is a mystery beyond onomatopoeia. An ancestral memory is invoked, echoes of ancient altars—a feeling of communion from heart to heart going back through the ages to the primordial ur-language, the first attempt to name things.

Softly I chant in Sanskrit, savoring its sound for a while, and then let it echo inside me, moving energies around in my body until I get corresponding English words. I look up the root structure of the words to track how they metamorphosed over the ages from Indo-European through Greek and Latin into modern English. I am like a hunter following a trail through a forest wet with dew, in the lively darkness before dawn, knowing that just around the hill over there I will find what I am seeking.

THE PLAY OF SANSKRIT AND ENGLISH

Sanskrit is finely crafted, designed for use in the oral tradition, in which important meditative texts and revelations are memorized, chanted, and passed on over many generations. It was built to last. Because of this sacredness, Sanskrit appears to be fixed in time, not developing, evolving, or adding new words. It is considered a liturgical language, and it is as frozen as a bug in amber. Sanskrit is the language of the ancient texts, but not the language people use to talk about their experience and their life in the present.

The population of India is more than a billion, and yet according to the 1991 census there were a total of 49,736 fluent speakers of Sanskrit—about .005 percent of the population. The 2001 census found that 14,135 listed Sanskrit as their mother tongue.[2] For decades, there have been attempts in India to revive Sanskrit and encourage students to learn it. The High Court of Madras had to rule in 1998 that Sanskrit is "not a dead language."

The English language is in many ways the opposite of Sanskrit. English is a wild, ever-changing, ever-evolving language, always in search of the next adaptation of itself, always transforming to meet the future, always redefining its words according to popular usage. English is as brilliant in its unperfectedness as Sanskrit is in its perfection.

As part of its adaptability, English is always adding new words, including words from Sanskrit, such as *pranayama* and *bhakti*. It's doing so because Sanskrit words are so useful for describing states of consciousness and yoga practice, which more and more English speakers are exploring.

A nationwide survey conducted by the United States government in 2007 found that 9.4 percent of the adult population had practiced meditation in the previous year, representing about twenty million people.[3] About the same number of people had practiced yoga in 2007. All of these meditation and yoga practitioners reach for words to describe the subtleties of their experiences and what they are feeling. As they do, they use the occasional Sanskrit word, which then becomes part of conversational English. Writers take part in these conversations and then confidently use a Sanskrit word here and there while writing for magazines, newspapers, blogs, novels, nonfiction books, songs, and movies. Then it moves to the global scale, such as the Gayatri mantra used in the movie

The Matrix and Madonna chanting *shanti* in a pop song. In this way Sanskrit words are steadily added to English vocabulary. This has been going on for at least 150 years, since Emerson and Thoreau and others began reading translations of the Upanishads and Bhagavad Gita and then talking and writing about what they love in these ancient texts. Thus, Sanskrit words like *yoga, mantra, guru, chakra, dharma, karma,* and *avatar* are now a lively part of American discourse.

The Vijnana Bhairava Tantra begins with these words: *sri devi uvacha shrutam deva maya sarvam rudra yamala sambhavam.* Five of these ten words are already in English dictionaries: *sri, devi, shruti, deva, rudra.* Others words from the text that have made it into English dictionaries are *agni, akasha, amrita, ananda, bhakti, Brahma, buddhi, dhyana, Durga, Gita, guru, Indra, indriya, kama, Krishna, Kali, maha, mahatma, manas, Marut, maya, moksha, Mitra, prana, pranava, puja, Rudra, sadhu, Shakti, Shanti, Shiva, shunya, tamas, tantra, tattva,* and *veda.*

Swami Yogakanti of the Bihar School points out that as Sanskrit words become English, various spellings and pronunciations are explored. This always happens when words migrate from one culture to another: their pronunciations change, because each language has unique sounds, and then the words are spelled differently, according to whatever system the receiving language uses. For example, the Sanskrit word for meditation, *dhyana,* became *chan* in China, and in Japan it became *zen.*

It doesn't help that English has a crazy spelling system, and words are often not written as they sound. (Linguists describe English spelling as chaotic, erratic, and irrational.) So when ancient Sanskrit words are brought into English, they are going from the most precise spelling system on earth into a raucous and wacky system, where they are misspelled and mispronounced, which is why we have so many creative variations in spelling among different English texts. Unfortunately, the semantic range is also reduced.

Something similar happened a thousand years ago, when tantric teachings were taken from India to Tibet and translated into Tibetan. In *Foundations of Tibetan Mysticism* (London: Rider and Co., 1959, 27), Lama Govinda remarks:

If the efficacy of mantras depended on their correct pronunciation, then all mantras in Tibet would have lost their meaning and power, because they are not pronounced according to the rules of Sanskrit, but according to the phonetic laws of the Tibetan language (for instance not: OṀ MANI PADME HŪṀ, but 'OṀ MAṆI Péme HŪṀ').

This means that the power and the effect of a mantra depend on the spiritual attitude, the knowledge and responsiveness of the individual. The śabda or sound of the mantra is not a physical one (though it may be accompanied by such a one) but a spiritual one. It cannot be heard by the ears but only by the heart, and it cannot be uttered by the mouth but only by the mind.

Harvey Alper notes in his encyclopedic *Understanding Mantras* (Albany: State University of New York Press, 2008, 443):

And, then, there is the knotty problem of pronunciation. Americans, after all, do not get the sound right. This is bound to be troubling. From the Vedic age to the present day, in mantras the sound is the thing. An apologist might respond, neither do Indians. The Vedic ideal notwithstanding, there is no single absolutely correct way to pronounce Sanskrit, as regional variations in pronunciation, not to mention the migration of mantras from India to Central Asia and East Asia, abundantly prove.

Shakti or *sakti, Shiva* or *siva, chakra* or *cakra*—it is anyone's guess how these words will be spelled and pronounced as they enter wider usage.
You say *Shakti,* and I say *sakti.*
You say *Shiva,* and I say *siva.*
Let's call the whole thing off.
Apologies and an offering of *soma* to appease Panini,[4] who is running up quite a tab, as we all continue this scandalous enterprise of receiving Sanskrit, finding it useful, and putting it to work in our daily lives while we explore the impact of yoga and meditative disciplines.

OTHER VERSIONS OF THE BHAIRAVA TANTRA

I am very grateful to the students, scholars and disciples who have worked to make the Vijnana Bhairava Tantra available in various translations. Many of these writers learned the teaching directly from Lakshman Joo (1907–1991), a renowned sage and scholar of Kashmir Shaivism.

As far as I can ascertain, *Zen Flesh, Zen Bones,* by Paul Reps, was first published by Doubleday in 1957 and is still in print. This was the first book on meditation I ever held in my hands, in 1968. It's how I began this whole adventure.

The entire Bhairava Tantra is condensed into one section at the end of the book, the rest of which is Zen stories. Reps, in his introduction, said that he started with an English version by Lakshman Joo and then did eleven more drafts until he got it into the form that he published as "Centering." The whole text is only sixteen pages, about eight verses per page. The English is beautiful and simple. It has a somewhat beatnik flavor to it, *dig it:* "Consider your essence as light rays rising from center to center up the vertebrae, and so rises *livingness* in you." For decades, I couldn't imagine any other way of reading the sutras.

The Paul Reps translation was used by Osho (Rajneesh) in his exuberant *Book of Secrets* (New York: St. Martin's Press, 2010), based on a series of lectures he gave. He goes on for more than thirteen hundred pages in his talks on the 112 meditations of the text.

Vijnana Bhairava: The Manual for Self-Realization, by Swami Lakshmanjoo and edited by John Hughes (Culver City, CA: Universal Shaiva Fellowship, 2007), is seven audio CDs (plus a 225-page book) of Lakshman Joo teaching the Vijnana Bhairava Tantra, chanting the Sanskrit, and then explaining the practices. This is the authoritative version of Lakshman Joo's transmission on the Bhairava Tantra. (Note: Hughes prefers to spell the author's name *Lakshmanjoo;* I prefer *Lakshman Joo.* In a debate, he would win.) Each of the verses is given in Devanagari (Sanskrit's written form), with a Romanized transliteration and pronunciation guide, plus a link to the place on the audio CDs where you can listen to Lakshman Joo chanting the verse and commenting on it.

John and Denise Hughes were trained by Maharishi Mahesh Yogi as teachers of Transcendental Meditation in India in 1969. During the training, Maharishi asked Lakshman Joo to come speak to the students. Several years later, in 1971, John and Denise returned to India to study with Lakshman Joo. John made tape recordings of Lakshman Joo's teachings and transcribed them, then went over the transcriptions with him. John and Denise have studied these teachings for decades and are custodians of Lakshman Joo's lectures.

Lilian Silburn's 1961 book *Le Vijnanabhairava Tantra: Publications de l'Institut de Civilisation Indienne* is in French. If you don't speak the language, find a French speaker, perhaps a poet, and have her read it to you. That is what I did, and it was wonderful. She spoke the text in French and then translated, on the fly, into English. Lilian's writing is imbued with a sensual flow and vibrancy. She is another of those who studied with Lakshman Joo in India. To get a feeling for her approach to this tradition, there is an English version of her *Kundalini: The Energy of the Depths,* translated by Jacques Gontier, published by State University of New York Press in 1988. Silburn's writing has an embodied feel to it, and she is not afraid to speak of arousing the vibratory energies and letting the sacred liquor flow.

Jaideva Singh is another of those who studied at the feet of Lakshman Joo. I came across his *Vijnanabhairava or Divine Consciousness: A Treasury of 112 Types of Yoga* (Delhi: Motilal Banarsidass, 1979) soon after it was published, through contacts at the Siddha Yoga organization.

The book begins with a blessing by Swami Muktananda. Jaideva Singh's writing is dense, and his translation and commentary explain some of the techniques with notes, footnotes, asides, and references to technical terms. It has a dry, scholarly, academic flavor. I have consulted it extensively over the past twenty-eight years and have worn out several copies. Fortunately it has been reprinted as *The Yoga of Delight, Wonder and Astonishment: A Translation of the Vijnana-Bhairava* (Albany: State University of New York Press, 1991). An excellent part of the SUNY edition is the ten-page foreword by Paul Muller-Ortega, in which he gives an overview of the relevance of the Vijnana Bhairava Tantra in the tradition of Kashmir Shaivism.

In 2002, Indica Books of Varanasi, India, published *Vijnana Bhairava: The Practice of Centring Awareness; Commentary by Swami Lakshman Joo.* (Yes, they spell it *centring.*) According to the introduction, "three disciples of Lakshman Joo" collaborated to put forth this version: Bettina Baumer and Sarla Kumar edited Lakshman Joo's notes, and Prabha Devi wrote a foreword. But this Sanskrit translation and commentary appears to be lifted, without giving credit, from notes and transcripts of the audio recordings by John and Denise Hughes as they interviewed Lakshman Joo. What apparently happened was that over the years, as John and Denise completed different drafts of their manuscript, they gave copies of the work in progress to Lakshman Joo, who made his *mahasamadhi* in 1991. A few years later, Prabha Devi felt inspired to reveal this treasure, this gift of the master's divine grace, to Dr. Sarla Kumar and Dr. Bettina Baumer, other students of the master. According to John Hughes, in the preface to his *Vijnana Bhairava: The Manual for Self-Realization,* the Indica edition is based on his preliminary manuscript and is "both incomplete and fraught with mistakes."

This story tells us a couple of things about the tantric tradition, besides the fact that it is a far-flung communion of passionate, individualistic people. It often happens that a disciple will do years or even a lifetime of work, then take no credit and give all honor to the guru. This is in keeping with the egolessness of disciples. There is a humility we all feel in response to the gushing wisdom behind these teachings.

One of the gracious things scholars do is point to everyone from whom they have drawn inspiration. It's called a footnote. But in the tantric tradition, by its very nature, people are off doing their own wildly idiosyncratic thing, making music, making babies, and dancing.

If you look in the backs of the translations I cite here, they do not make any mention of each other. It could be that they are working with a theory of immaculate conception. I make no such claims—I've devotedly read all the other translations of the Vijnana Bhairava Tantra cited here, dozens or hundreds of times. Their work has helped mine immeasurably. I can't thank them enough. Each one brings out and illuminates different aspects of these extremely condensed sutras.

Sri Vijnana Bhairava Tantra: The Ascent, by Swami Satyasangananda Saraswati (Yoga Munger, India: Publications Trust, Bihar School of Yoga, 2003), is a magnificent work of scholarship, and at 499 pages, it is among the most comprehensive of the translations described here. It is also very readable. The book includes a ninety-page introductory section. Each verse is given in Devanagari, followed by a transliteration with word boundaries indicated and component terms defined, thus including a full glossary for every word of each verse.

Swami Satyasangananda is female and has brought brilliant intellectual clarity and rich feeling to the text. I adore her at a distance. She was initiated into *sannyasa* in 1982 by Swami Satyananda of the Bihar School. She makes no mention of Lakshman Joo, so apparently this is a separate line of transmission of the teachings. There are some differences in the way she unfolds the descriptions of the techniques, compared to the other translators. She lives in a religious order and has taken vows (including celibacy, I imagine), and therefore she often tilts her translations in the direction of renunciation and suppressing desire, which is entirely appropriate for a renouncer. As much as it is possible for a nun from India to speak to us in the West, she has.

Daniel Odier included a short translation of the Bhairava Tantra in an appendix to his book *Yoga Spandakarika: The Sacred Texts at the Origins of Tantra* (Rochester, VT: Inner Traditions, 2005). His version has a free-flowing quality. Each verse or technique is translated in two or three sentences, and the entire appendix is only eighteen pages. He attempts to briefly describe each method and leaves terms such as *Bhairava, Bhairavi, Shakti,* and *Shiva* untranslated. Daniel is an initiate of Tibetan Buddhism, Kashmir Shaivism, and Zen. He lives in Paris and teaches in Europe and the United States.

Eric Baret is another French writer and teacher in the tradition of Kashmir Shaivism, based in Paris. One day in 1993, I was visiting Santa Fe, New Mexico. By then early drafts of *The Radiance Sutras* had been circulating around the United States and Europe, and somehow a copy came into Eric's hands. He lives in France and happened to be visiting Santa Fe at the same time. Out of the blue he called, introduced himself, and said, "I am in town. Let's get together!" Eric showed up at my door, radiating joy. Over the course of several days, he generously went over the manuscript with me line by line and gave me valuable tips and corrections. Thank you, Eric!

Mark S. G. Dyczkowski is a tantric scholar researching what he calls Kashmiri Shaivism, and his work has been a great help to me in understanding the layers of meaning in some of the words used in the Bhairava Tantra. His book *The Doctrine of Vibration* (Albany: State University Press of New York, 1987) is an example of research combining passion and intellectual clarity.

Dmitri Semenov published (in June 2010) a translation of the Vijnana Bhairava Tantra, available from the self-publishing website

Lulu (lulu.com). Dmitri writes, "The interpretation is almost never literal, but interpretive. The interpretation relies heavily on my own personal experiences." Dmitri is a Russian mathematician and a student of tantra, and he brings a refreshing tone of precision to the translation.

Each of these translations brings out different nuances of the information coded into the text. Layers of sound and meaning are playing, and you can choose to listen to one layer or the interaction of two, three, four, or more layers. In *The Tantric Body,* Gavin Flood discusses the optative mood in Tantric texts and points out that "the main verb, 'he should meditate' . . . is in the third-person singular optative, a mood which, according to the famous grammarian Panini, is used in five senses: to denote a command *(vidhi),* a summons *(nimantrana),* an invitation *(amantrana),* a respectful command *(adhista),* an enquiry *(samprasna)* or a request *(prarthana)*" (London, I. B. Tauris, 2006, 179; diacritical marks omitted). This is brilliant semantic engineering. Each of these tones is profound and has its place; the optative mood gives you options.

As Flood and Panini point out, what is often translated as "He should meditate" can be taken simultaneously as a command, summons, invitation, inquiry, and a request. In a text such as the Bhairava Tantra, the sentence "He should meditate," although semantically correct, is a bit insulting to Shakti. It is as if a group of elite males, impressed with their own importance and erudition, are proclaiming to each other how clever they are: "The *yogi* should meditate either in the heart or in the *dvadashanta*" (verse 37, corresponding to sutra 14). That is not how you enter these practices if you are in a Western body and a householder.

I find the *invitation* mood to be much friendlier (*amantrana,* "inviting, speaking to, calling to, greeting, welcome"). The Radiance Sutras is a *bhashantaram,* a rendering of the text into the vernacular. Therefore, I have structured the language to be engaging and inviting, not distancing and elitist. I have taken as the basic *mood* of discourse the sense that Bhairava is speaking to our bodies through Devi's body, through her shakti, which is our very life force; this is happening now, in the present moment, because Bhairava and Devi are always present; and these are not merely esoteric techniques being discussed, but openings or doorways into the sacred that are available to us all in the rhythm of a day. In the text, Devi is already enlightened, but she is asking to be reminded of the ways in which a being who is immersed in creation can wake up to infinity again. Bhairava is her lover, and he adoringly complies.

When I first looked at the Vijnana Bhairava Tantra in 1968, it was as if Devi handed me a ball of light and said, "Here—here are the teachings you have been looking for. Step into this reality. Live and breathe it. Share it with all who come your way and ask." Not knowing any better, that's what I did. I just accepted the ball and ran with it, never looking back.

These forty-some years have been, and continue to be, a journey of wonder and delight.

NOTES

1. Sir Monier Monier-Williams, A Sanskrit-English Dictionary, etymologically and philologically arranged, with special reference to cognate Indo-European languages. (Oxford: Clarendon Press, 1899).
2. Government of India, Ministry of Home Affairs, Office of the Registrar General and Census Commissioner, "Statement 1: Abstract of Speakers' Strength of Languages and Mother Tongues, 2001." Available online at censusindia.gov.in/ Census_Data_2001/Census_Data_Online/Language/Statement1.htm. Arvind Kala, "Hegemony of Hindi," The *Times of India* (January 6, 2007). Sujay Rao Mandavilli, "Sanskrit and Prakrit as National Link Languages: A Balanced Assessment," *Language in India* 8 (May 5, 2008).
3. P. M. Barnes, B. Bloom, and R. Nahin, CDC National Health Statistics Report #12, "Complementary and Alternative Medicine Use Among Adults and Children: United States, 2007" (December 2008).
4. Panini, often considered the greatest linguistic genius of all time, set forth the rules of Sanskrit morphology in 3,959 sutras, in a text of eight chapters called the Ashtadhyayi, thus defining classical Sanskrit. The text is the oldest existing grammar in any language, and research is still being done on the subtleties of Panini's rules, to shed light on how human language works. He is thought to have been born in Northwest India, in what is now Pakistan, and to have lived in the sixth, fifth, or fourth century BC. According to the Panchatantra, Panini was killed by a lion. Speculation ever since has been that the lion was the reincarnation of a Brahmin priest whose life was ruined when he couldn't remember one of Panini's 3,959 rules during an important recitation on *Hindu Idol.*

Resources

Private sessions. There are over a hundred major meditation techniques, and each one has dozens of variations. If you would like help finding your way and developing a daily practice that suits your nature, sessions are available in person, on the phone, or by video over the Internet. Because Lorin's work focuses on the fine structure of individuality, meditators of all traditions and levels of experience seek him out for coaching.

Online courses. We offer teleseminars on meditation, which you can attend by phoning in or listening on the web.

Audio courses. Audio recordings of Lorin's talks and guided meditations are available for download, or if you prefer, you can order recordings on CD. Visit lorinroche.com. The audio book *Meditation For Yoga Lovers* is available from soundstrue.com.

Video mini-seminars. Check out the four-minute videos of Lorin Roche exploring different topics related to developing a meditation practice.

Retreats and Workshops. Radiance Sutras workshops are held at retreat centers around the world. It is a delight to get away for a weekend or a week and immerse yourself in the freedom to explore your own innate experience and get coaching.

The Feminine Path. Lorin teaches with his wife, Camille Maurine, who is a world expert on meditation and the female path. Together they wrote *Meditation Secrets for Women,* a handbook for developing your own practice, based on your individual soul nature. Over 80 percent of yoga students in the modern West are women, and this is a significant revolution on a historic scale. To find out more, visit camillemaurine.com.

Meditation Teacher Training. There aren't enough meditation teachers in the world! Tens of millions of people want to begin meditating, if only they can find a way that works for them. Pranava Meditation Teacher Training is now being offered and is registered with Yoga Alliance as a two-hundred-hour program. Discover more at lorinroche.com.

ABOUT ACCOMPANYING MUSIC

For the past few years, musicians Dave Stringer, Denise Kaufman, Donna DeLory, Joni Allen, C. C. White, Christine Stevens, Steve Gold, Joey Lugassy, Ena Vie, Howard Lipp, Zoe Elton, Dearbhla Kelly, and others have been putting the Radiance Sutras to song. This has evolved into jam sessions, called Sutra Sessions, in which musicians and singers improvise to the Sutras. These sessions are ecstatic and amazing. We often have an open mike, and members of the audience come up and read their favorite Sutra. Join our mailing list to find out about events near you.

Dave Stringer, Donna DeLory, Joni Allen, and others have been composing and recording stunningly beautiful songs of the Radiance Sutras. For a free download of one of the Radiance Sutras put to music, visit lorinroche.com.

Acknowledgments

Much gratitude to the merry band of yoginis and yogis around the world who have blessed me, encouraged the writing, lovingly edited the text, and read it back to me, drenched in shakti.

Camille Maurine, my Shakti, wife, and creative partner, just by walking through the room illuminated many teachings in this text. Camille also spoke the verses to me many times, dancing while she edited.

Denise Kaufman created, in collaboration with Dave Stringer, the Sutra Sessions, live jam sessions with musicians improvising to the Radiance Sutras. Sean Johnson and Gwen Colman brought their New Orleans groove to the sutras. Joey Lugassy, Donna De Lory, Christine Stevens, Joni Allen, C. C. White, Craig Kohland, Steve Gold, and others have given their gift of music to the school of sutra rock.

Victor Miller, Eric Baret, Ari Davis, Ilene Segalove, Emilie Conrad, Ana Claudia Cunha, Felicia Tomasko, Micheline Berry, Tesa Silvestre, Melanie Foust, Tia Reiss, Elyse Neuhauser, Dr. Christopher Key Chapple, and Dr. David Gordon White have all contributed in wonderful ways. Dr. John Casey, of Loyola Marymount University, fine-tuned the Devanagari text and created the phonetic spelling. Thanks also to Dr. Wendy Doniger, Dr. Mark S. G. Dyczkowski, Dr. Gavin Flood, Frederick M. Smith, and Dr. Hugh Urban for their writings and valuable input.

The brilliant Shiva Rea and the wildly wonderful tribe she has called together have embraced me and enriched my understanding of Shakti immeasurably. May Devi bless their community.

About the Author

Lorin Roche, PhD, began exploring the 112 meditations of the Vijnana Bhairava Tantra in 1968, and it has been a nonstop love affair ever since. He began meditating as part of a scientific research study at the University of California and was soon assisting the research and training subjects to meditate. After advanced training as a meditation teacher in 1970, Lorin taught in think tanks, universities, military bases, high schools, hospitals, retreat centers, and private homes. He was involved in the physiological research on meditation until 1975, when he switched to studying the emotional and subjective experience of meditation. Lorin received a doctorate from the University of California at Irvine in 1987. In his research, he used the tools of cognitive anthropology to study the language of experience—the way meditators describe their inner worlds. His master's degree research investigated the hazards of meditation and the crisis points in a meditator's development; practicing the wrong technique for your personality and body type can produce harmful effects, and even the right type of meditation can challenge your system and produce evolutionary crises.

Lorin is a pioneer in developing personalized meditation practices, designing the techniques around an individual's inner nature. In addition to *The Radiance Sutras,* Lorin is the author of five books on the life-affirming path of meditation, including *Meditation Secrets for Women,* written with his wife, Camille Maurine.

Lorin's teaching celebrates individual uniqueness and aims at activating your internal guidance systems and bringing forth your instinctive knowing. In order to transmit the joyous wisdom of the Radiance Sutras, Lorin has created two related meditation systems: Pranava Meditation®, which utilizes the richness of the Sanskrit language and is oriented toward the yoga community, and Freedom Meditation®, which uses common sense terminology and focuses on inner knowing. He teaches and consults worldwide with businesses and universities to create custom meditation programs that suit their needs and cultures. For more information on private coaching, lectures, workshops, teleseminars, and meditation teacher training, visit lorinroche.com or contact him via email at lorin@lorinroche.com.

ABOUT SOUNDS TRUE

Sounds True is a multimedia publisher whose mission is to inspire and support personal transformation and spiritual awakening. Founded in 1985 and located in Boulder, Colorado, we work with many of the leading spiritual teachers, thinkers, healers, and visionary artists of our time. We strive with every title to preserve the essential "living wisdom" of the author or artist. It is our goal to create products that not only provide information to a reader or listener, but that also embody the quality of a wisdom transmission.

For those seeking genuine transformation, Sounds True is your trusted partner. At SoundsTrue.com you will find a wealth of free resources to support your journey, including exclusive weekly audio interviews, free downloads, interactive learning tools, and other special savings on all our titles.

To learn more, please visit SoundsTrue.com/bonus/free_gifts or call us toll free at 800-333-9185.

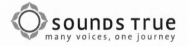

SOUNDS True
many voices, one journey

FICTION
Kapla
Kaplan, Andrew.

Dragonfire /

DRAGON
FIRE

Also by Andrew Kaplan

HOUR OF THE ASSASSINS
SCORPION

DRAGON FIRE

FIRE

ANDREW KAPLAN

WARNER BOOKS

A Warner Communications Company

Chapter headings and symbols are quoted from: *I Ching*, Sam Reifler, ed., Bantam Books, 1981 ed.

Bengali hymn quoted from: *The Religions of Man*, Huston Smith, ed., a Mentor Book, New American Library, 1961 ed.

Security regulations of Tuol Sleng prison quoted from: *National Geographic Magazine*, Vol. 161, No. 5, May 1982.

Book design: H. Roberts

A Warner Communications Company

Printed in the United States of America

First Printing: July 1987

10 9 8 7 6 5 4 3 2 1

Library of Congress Cataloging-in-Publication Data

Kaplan, Andrew.
  Dragonfire.

  I. Title.
PS3561.A545D7   1987   813'.54   86-40420
ISNB 0-446-51337-6

*To those for whom Southeast Asia
was more than a place on a map*

and

to Justin, age 3. I really like you too.

ACKNOWLEDGMENTS

This book was written in the south of France, a fact which created its own peculiar set of advantages and difficulties. My thanks are therefore due to a number of people who assisted in the early proofing and word processing of the manuscript, particularly Jake and Susan Lowe, Colette Stoltz, and the people at Fortune Systems International in Monte Carlo, especially Eva Ehojoki and Brooke "Pete" Taylor, president of Fortune Systems International. It should also be noted that without the unwavering support of my agent, June Hall, and my wife, Anne, this book would not exist.

AUTHOR'S NOTE

The symbols and sayings that begin each chapter are taken from the *I Ching,* or *Chinese Book of Changes.* The *I Ching* is almost as old as China itself. The version that has come down to us was used as an oracle by the Mandarins of the Chinese court, and it is still widely employed by fortune-tellers throughout the Far East. As such, it provides a unique window into Asian thinking.

The *Book of Changes* originally evolved from a simple Yes or No oracle based on tortoiseshell patterns, where a solid line (———) indicated Yes, or Yang (crudely translated in the West as the masculine force), and a broken line (— —) indicated No, or Yin (the opposing, or feminine, force). But the need for greater subtlety was felt early on and a second and then third line was added, to form a "trigram."

Each of these three-line trigrams (eight combinations are possible) came to represent a unique aspect of the world, such as Heaven (☰), Thunder (☳), Fire (☲), and so on. In addition, each trigram is associated with specific symbolic attributes. For example, the trigram for Marsh and Mist (☱) also represents happiness, pleasure, magic, destruction, sensuality, youngest daughters, the animal characteristics of the sheep, the color blue, autumn, the direction west, etc.

However, the *I Ching* is not so much concerned with things as they are (which the Chinese considered illusory anyway), as it is with things in the process of change; hence the name, *Book of Changes*. Each line may change from Yang to Yin or from Yin to Yang, and each trigram may combine with another to form a six-line "hexagram."

Normally, the first statement of the prophecy describes the configuration of this hexagram. For example: "The wind blows above the earth" means that the hexagram consists of the trigram for Wind on top of the trigram for Earth. The remaining statements are prophecies, which may sometimes seem obscure, but which would have been perfectly clear to a Chinese courtier. For example, the statement "The man places mats of white grass beneath objects set on the ground" is a warning to take extraordinary precautions.

There are sixty-four possible hexagrams (eight squared). The ancient Chinese believed that these sixty-four hexagrams encompassed all of human experience.

DRAGON FIRE

Because Thou lovest the Burning-ground,
I have made a Burning-ground of my heart—
That Thou, Dark One, haunter of the Burning-ground,
Mayest dance Thy eternal dance.

—A BENGALI HYMN

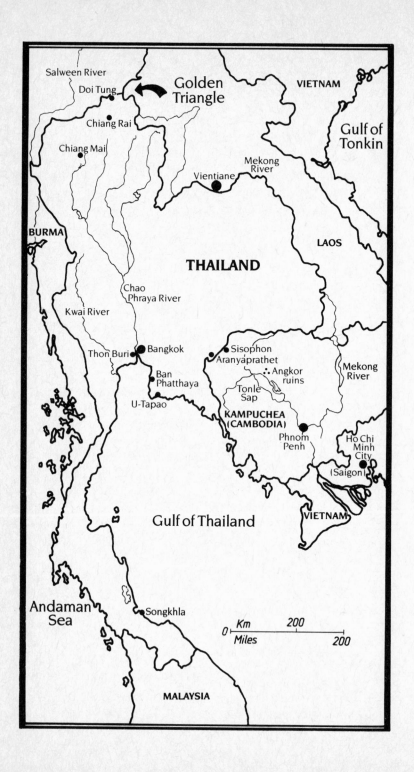

In the plain between the hills of Kulen and the giant lake called the Tônlé Sap, the ancient Khmers of Cambodia built a vast complex of temples, of which the most famous is Angkor Wat.

The temples were an attempt to create in stone a kind of map or enormous scale model of the Hindu universe, but after the Hindu deities failed to protect the city from a disastrous Cham invasion in the twelfth century, the pragmatic Khmers dedicated their new temples to Buddha.

But many of the existing temples retained their old pagan and Hindu associations.

One of these, the Phimeanakas (completed circa 1000 A.D.), is located within the Angkor Thom complex, north of the temple of Angkor Wat. The ruin is a single pyramid made of laterite; the tower has not survived. According to legend, the structure was built upon the site where an early Khmer king, acting to protect the kingdom, had nightly congress with a dragon goddess (in some versions, a giant serpent) in the form of a beautiful woman.

The Khmers believed that the goddess could not be destroyed except by her own dragonfire, the only weapon that could harm her.

PROLOGUE

T HEY were friends once. The kind of special friends the
men of the hill tribes call "death friends" to distinguish
them from those with whom one merely shares rice and
talk. Nearly two decades later, the fact that they had
known each other at all became a critical element of the Dragonfire
operation, as the affair came to be called within the National Security Council.

Locked inside the "Black Vault," the innermost sanctum within
the CIA complex in Langley, there actually exists a photograph
of all of them together. All except Pranh, who snapped the shot.
Of course, no photograph of Pranh himself was ever needed,
because there was a time when, under the name Son Lot, you
could find his face on posters plastered all over Cambodia.

Still attached to the photo is a yellowing label typed by some
long-forgotten Army S-2 intelligence analyst. It reads: "U.S. Special Forces advisers attached to the 11th ARVN Ranger Battalion.
Parrot's Beak sector, Cambodia. 5 June 1970."

The photo itself is black and white. It shows four young men
sitting in relaxed poses atop an armored personnel carrier. They
are wearing camouflage fatigues dappled by the sunlight and are

cradling their weapons with the casual ease that comes with long familiarity. One of them, Parker, is caught in the act of flipping his cigarette in the direction of the camera.

He seems tanned, even cocky, wearing the kind of cynical sneer that only the truly innocent are capable of. In the middle is the agent later known only as Sawyer. The photo is the only physical evidence he ever existed, because after Dragonfire, his personnel file and all cross-references to his real identity were purged from the data banks of the CIA's Cray supercomputer.

In the picture, he is shirtless and so lean you can almost count the ribs. His green beret is draped over the muzzle of a captured AK-47, and he is squinting in the strong sunlight. He still had two good eyes then and, without the eye-patch that was to become his trademark, looks like a young Jack Kennedy. Next to him is Harold Johnson, nicknamed "Brother Rap," fist clenched in the Black Power salute. He sports a sparse, nineteen-year-old's mustache, a Black Power shoelace bracelet, love beads, and "Born to Kill" painted in white letters on his helmet liner. And squatting near the machine gun mount is Major Lu, wearing green fatigues and oversized aviator sunglasses that make him look like how the Buddha might look if he had been turned into a frog.

It was an ordinary photo. It captured only their faces, not their souls.

On the day after it was taken, their friendship was torn apart forever.

PART ONE

The dragon lies hidden
in the deep.

1

The deep yawns above the thunder.
Whoever hunts deer without a guide
Will lose his way in the depths of
the forest.
The superior man is aware of the
hidden dangers.

SHE was dressed in silk, red and gold, and atop her head was a gold crown spiraling to a point like a temple chedi. She stood alone in the spotlight, one foot gracefully raised in the classic lakhon dancer's pose. Her left hand gestured downward in a rejection of passion as it will be in the final dance on the last night of the world, when the stars fall from the sky and the mountains are engulfed in flame. Her right hand was upturned, signaling the acceptance of her lover and the primordial thrust of his desire. Her face was exquisite, her dark eyes impassive.

Now the rhythm of the pi-nai and the drum grew more insistent. She began to move her hips, swaying to and fro as though summoning an invisible lover. Two slave girls rushed from the wings and began to unwind her sarong. She wriggled out of her clothes in waves, like a snake molting its outer skin, until she stood completely naked. She bowed in a gesture of submission, her slender body glistening with sweat, her budlike breasts heaving, her buttocks moving in an enticing motion old as time.

The stage was wreathed in smoke from the joss sticks, mingled with opium and tobacco smoke. The smoke twisted and swirled in shafts of light like a living thing.

The drumbeat quickened as the slave girls threw off their robes and stood naked, but for big leather phalluses strapped to their loins. A collective male sigh escaped the audience. The drumming mounted to a crescendo as the two slave girls took turns playing the male. Their bodies tangled together, passion rippling through them. The drums went wild as they climaxed with savage cries, their black hair flying as they whipped their heads back and forth, then sank gracefully to the floor, limp and spent.

The crowd of Asian businessmen sprinkled with the occasional serviceman roared its approval. Green twenty-baht notes were tossed onto the stage. Smiling, the dancers came to the edge of the stage to pluck notes from upstretched hands using only the muscles between their legs.

In a dark corner booth, two men who had been engrossed in their conversation glanced over toward the stage. One was a portly graying Asian in a blue silk suit obviously made by a Hong Kong tailor who knew what he was doing. The other was a tall Occidental wearing the safari-style khakis inevitably affected by American officials and journalists in Indochina.

"There's the true seduction of Asia," Vasnasong said, gesturing at the naked dancers. "The promise that you can do anything . . . absolutely anything."

Parker raised his eyebrows.

"Are you talking about sex or power?"

"They are intertwined, like Yin and Yang. True power is ability to indulge every desire, every whim, no matter how bizarre. Is that not the ultimate aphrodisiac?" Vasnasong smiled.

"I thought you Buddhists frowned on sex."

"Although like most male Thais I spent time as naga, I am far from being bhikku monk. Besides, Lord Buddha did not teach physical passion bad. Only that to pass beyond suffering, you must also go beyond pleasure. Only then comes profit," Vasnasong replied, his eyes twinkling.

Parker jumped at the conversational opening. Otherwise, they'd be here trading Chinese fortune-cookie talk all night.

"Speaking of profit, of this thing with Bhun Sa, can it be arranged?" he asked.

Vasnasong sighed inwardly. Such rudeness was typical of a farang. Americans were the worst. Always in such a hurry that they heard only the words, never the nuances between the words where conversation really takes place. So be it, he thought. With such a one subtlety is meaningless anyway. But first he would exact a tiny revenge.

"Do you desire? It is house specialty," Vasnasong said, indicating the spicy water beetle paste with his chopsticks. He had seen that the farang was disgusted by it from the expression on his face when it was served.

Parker shook his head. Smiling, Vasnasong shoved it insistently toward him and was secretly delighted by Parker's obvious discomfort as he attempted a small polite nibble.

"Delicious," Parker said insincerely.

"Ah yes." Vasnasong smiled.

"Does that mean it can be arranged?" Parker said, looking around anxiously as though he was afraid of being overheard.

"Mai-pen-rai," Vasnasong shrugged. "In Bangkok, Hawkins-khrap, anything can be arranged—for a price."

Hawkins was Parker's cover name.

There was a burst of applause and Parker glanced toward the stage. In the spotlight a voluptuous woman was seated in a hanging bamboo basket, her naked bottom protruding from a hole in the basket. To the accompaniment of raucous cheers from the audience, she was slowly lowered onto a sailor from the audience who had volunteered.

Parker nodded and leaned forward across the table.

"How soon can I get upcountry to see Bhun Sa?" he whispered. No one but Vasnasong could hear him in all the audience noise. On stage, the sailor slowly twirled the basket. The woman revolved on his erection like a top.

Vasnasong looked curiously at the farang.

"Have you ever been in hill country of Golden Triangle, Hawkins-khrap?"

"No. Why?"

Vasnasong laid his finger alongside his nose in a gesture of warning.

"Hill country is most dangerous place, Hawkins-khrap. Most dangerous. And of all the hill people, Bhun Sa may be most dangerous of all," Vasnasong said uneasily.

"Yeah, well the world is full of tough guys," Parker shrugged. Did the prick think he was dealing with a Boy Scout? he wondered.

Vasnasong smiled politely. What was it his honored father used to say: "To reason with a fool is as to belch into the breath of a typhoon." He plucked delicately at a morsel of lemon chicken with his chopsticks, then genially raised his glass of Mae Khong whiskey.

"Then may you meet only good and overcome all your enemies, Hawkins-khrap," Vasnasong toasted, and they both drank.

"When can I make contact?" Parker said hoarsely, choking back the whiskey. Mae Khong was guaranteed by the manufacturer to never be more than two weeks old.

"Tonight. Very soon," Vasnasong said, consulting his gold Rolex. "And now, a thousand pardons, but I am old man and my bed calls," he added, delicately faking a yawn.

"Wait a minute," Parker began angrily. He started to grab at Vasnasong's sleeve, but instead found the torn half of a red hundred-baht note being pressed into his hand as part of a handshake.

"A beautiful girl will have matching half. Follow her and you will find what you seek," Vasnasong whispered, and stood.

Vasnasong glanced around, as if nervous for the first time, but all eyes were on the stage and the squealing basket girl. Parker surreptitiously touched the .45 automatic in the holster nestled in the small of his back.

"See you soon." Parker grinned, his fingers touching the gun grip.

"Sawat dee khrap," Vasnasong said, pressing his palms together in the wai sign.

A burst of applause came from the front, distracting Parker. The basket girl and the sailor were gone, replaced by a pretty girl who looked like she had barely reached her teens. She was trying to do something obscene with a snake.

When he turned back, Parker found himself staring at the most beautiful woman he had ever seen, standing where Vasnasong had stood just a few seconds before. It was like a conjurer's trick, and for a moment Parker couldn't believe his eyes. He was spellbound. He couldn't take his eyes off her.

She was tall for an Asian, with straight black hair that fell below her shoulders and dark almond eyes luminous with mystery and passion. They reminded him of the eyes of an ancient queen painted on the wall of a four-thousand-year-old tomb he had visited once in Egypt. She wore just a touch of lipstick and eye shadow on that exquisite face and smelled of jasmine. Her sarong was white silk, embroidered with gold and somehow tightly molded to her body in an effect that was at once modest and dazzlingly sensual.

She smiled, revealing captivating dimples and perfect white teeth, and like any bargirl, asked him if he wanted a good time, number-one time. But she was no bargirl. He was sure of that. His throat had gone dry and he had to swallow before he could ask her how much.

"Tao rye?"

"Nung roi kha," she replied, asking for the hundred.

As if in a trance, Parker handed her the torn half of the hundred-baht note. She unfolded another half and matched the two pieces. She looked around once to make sure no one was paying too much attention to what was, after all, an everyday transaction. All eyes were on the snake dancer.

"You follow," she whispered in English, and ducked through a bamboo curtain that led to a side exit. Parker tossed a bill on the table to cover the drinks, and by the time he reached the alley outside, she had already disappeared.

The alley was dark and strewn with garbage. But just a few feet away, Patpong Road was bright as day from all the neon lights. Parker hesitated. She had vanished as if she were a dream, or maybe one of those spirits the Thais built those little dollhouses for in the corner of every dwelling. Then he thought he caught a faint whiff of jasmine lingering on the hot sticky air characteristic of the nights before the southwest monsoon.

It's no dream, he told himself. She's your only link to Bhun Sa, so don't let her get away.

He ran out into the street. Traffic was heavy all along Patpong Road. Three-wheeled samlors, cyclos, and motorbikes narrowly weaved between the honking cars, barely scraping through by inches. Asian and European men, civilians and servicemen from half a dozen countries prowled the sidewalks, while girls in tight slacks and Western jeans called their siren song from brightly lit entrances to the bars and massage parlors. Rock music in a dozen languages blared from open doorways. Street vendors sold cigarettes and picture postcards from the top tray, pornographic photos, Thai sticks, and black balls of opium and hashish from the bottom tray.

At first Parker thought he had lost her in the crowd. Then he saw men staring after someone near the Silom Road intersection and just caught a glimpse of her white sarong rounding the corner. Ignoring Langley rules about never calling attention to yourself while on a tail, he ran after her. Rounding the corner, he was in time to see her duck into a side street near the corner of the Bangkok Christian Hospital.

She was very quick and very good, he thought, settling into a normal walking pattern about a hundred yards behind her. Even just walking, she moved with an animal-like grace that was incredibly sensual, and despite all his training, he found he couldn't take his eyes from the teasing sway of her skintight sarong.

She moved nimbly down side streets and darkened alleys, slipping between noodle stalls lit by kerosene lamps, a white figure flitting ahead of him in the darkness like a ghost. He knew he should contact his case officer to let him know he was entering the red zone. They had drilled that into him a hundred times. Always keep control posted. Better to miss an opportunity than to lose communication. But how, without losing her? She has to stop sometime, he thought, reassuring himself. When she did, he would find a phone before he made contact.

At the next corner, she paused to study the posters outside a movie house showing the latest karate epic from Hong Kong, glancing out of the corner of her eye to see if he was still with her. He made no effort to close the distance. He was grateful for this time to catch his breath. And he had to make sure they weren't being followed.

He studied the reflection of the street behind him in the darkened window of a closed goldsmith's shop. Traffic was bumper to bumper even at this late hour. Shoppers were filling wicker baskets in the fluorescent glare of a nearby market. At a sidewalk restaurant a prospective diner was sniffing at a cauldron as the owner held up a live crab for his inspection. Everything seemed normal enough except . . . Parker suddenly felt a terrible urge to urinate. His mouth had gone dry. *He was being watched.*

A big-muscled Thai in a suit that looked like it had been made for a much smaller man stood patiently waiting at the Number

71 bus stop. He wasn't looking at either Parker or the girl. But the buses in Bangkok didn't run after midnight.

There was another possible bulldog leaning against the noodle stall ahead. Also Thai. It looked like a front and back tail. He and the girl were boxed in.

And was it his nerves or did the passenger in a passing dark blue Nissan sedan take an excessive interest in him? The look had been held just a fraction too long, he decided. That meant they were mobile, as well.

Parker thought about aborting. There was sure to be a public phone back at the hospital on Silom Road. And what about the girl? Had she spotted the tails? He tried to think of a way to signal her, but it was too late.

She had started moving again.

He had no choice. He decided he would have to follow.

If only he knew where she was headed, he could try and flush the tails, he thought. She was heading south toward the Sathan Nua klong. Which way would she go when she reached the canal, left or right?

Then it hit him what she was up to. There was a water-bus dock near the Convent Road intersection. She had seen the tails! She was going to make a run for it on the water.

If he could eliminate at least one of the tails, they could still make the rendezvous. Assuming he was right, that is. If he was, the lead tail would stay with the girl, the second would peel off with him.

There was only one way to find out, he thought as he came abreast of the movie house ticket booth. He acted as if he were going to continue after the girl, then turned, bought a ticket from a sleepy-eyed young clerk and hurried into the darkened theater.

The tail would expect him to go out another exit according to standard flushing procedure. Instead, he took a seat in the last row near the aisle. When his eyes adjusted to the dark, he could see that only a few seats were occupied. Being able to see better than the tail, whose eyes would have less time to adjust, should give him an extra edge, he thought. He slipped the .45 automatic from its holster and clicked off the safety. He watched the curtained entrance while glancing at the movie out of the corner of his eye.

On the screen, the Chinese hero, clad in a black karate outfit, was spinning in the air, kicking out with devastating effect against at least a hundred white-suited adversaries from the karate school of a mad scientist. The sound effects man must have gone crazy because every blow sounded like a car crash. The kicks sent the hero's opponents flying like tenpins, despite missing them by at least a foot. All in all, one against a hundred seemed like a pretty fair fight, and Parker was wondering what the hero would do if he were in Parker's spot, when the curtain parted and the second tail burst in.

As he headed down the aisle, glancing left and right, Parker slipped behind him and, grabbing the back of his jacket, jammed the muzzle of the .45 into the Thai's broad back.

"Hold it, buster. Yoot!" Parker hissed.

The big Thai hesitated. Parker felt the Thai's muscles tense in preparation for a move and viciously jabbed the gun into the Thai's kidneys.

"Don't try it," Parker whispered.

The Thai barely flinched. But at least he stopped moving.

Parker prodded the Thai ahead of him back up the aisle and then to the small toilet cubicle off the threadbare lobby. The toilet itself was a foul-smelling hole in the ground where flies buzzed noisily. A single naked yellow bulb barely lit the darkness.

"Take off your belt," Parker demanded. When the Thai's pants were around his ankles, Parker used the leather belt to tie his hands behind him.

"You no understand," the Thai began.

Parker never let him finish the sentence. He coldcocked the Thai with the butt of the Colt, hitting him behind the right ear with all his might. The Thai sank to his knees, and Parker hit him twice more in the head. The big man sprawled unconscious over the filthy hole, his face in the muck. Parker didn't wait to see if he was still breathing. He had more important things to do.

Parker raced out of the movie house and down the street toward the klong, ignoring the astonished glances of passersby. He had to catch her.

There was still a crowd on the Sathan Nua landing, and at first he thought he might still be in time. But it was too late. The sleek white water bus, jammed as tightly as a rush-hour subway car, was already pulling away from the landing. Even if he could get through the crowd, it was too far to jump, and the gap of water was widening every second.

He stood there panting, watching the water bus pull away. He searched for her face in the crowd. He caught a glimpse of her looking back at him from the railing. It was a strange look. He tried to read her expression, but it was too dark, too fleeting to really see anything. But it was her all right. There was no mistaking the white sarong or that exquisite face. Further on down the railing, he thought he saw the lead tail.

Parker tried to decide what to do. Then he noticed a cluster of hang-yao, long-tailed water taxis, moored to the bank near the landing. Parker motioned to the first driver. He showed him a purple five-hundred-baht note and a minute later they were on the klong, bouncing in the wake of the water bus.

As they sped along the klong, getting wet from the spray thrown up by the water bus, Parker tried to figure it out. They had to try to reach the next landing at New Road before the water bus got there. But it was all happening too fast. The girl. The tails. Who sent them? Vasnasong? Bhun Sa? Or someone else? It made no sense. The mission had barely started and already it was coming apart. None of it ever made any sense, and he remembered something Jack had told him long ago, back in Da Nang.

They were having rum and cokes on the veranda of the Grand Hotel, looking out at the lights on the fishing junks bobbing on the oily slick that was the Tourane River. Around them grunts from the Americal Division sat at the tables drinking and openly shooting up skag bought for two bucks a vial just outside the base gate. The street boys and whores swarmed around the grunts like moths around a lamp, filling the air with cries of "Cheap Charlie" and "Fi' dollar" and "You Numbah-Ten Charlie." He had been complaining, Parker remembered. Nothing was working. Not their rules, their strategies, their technology. Nothing.

"You have to remember, this is Asia. Things are different here," Jack had said.

Parker felt a sudden longing for the green Virginia countryside outside Langley. The rolling hills, the white picket fences, the *cleanness* of it. How sane it was, especially compared to the squalor, the unending noise and intrigue, the sheer misery of Asia. He'd been out here too long, Parker thought. This, he decided, would be his last mission.

A change in the growl of the hang-yao's engine brought him out of his thoughts. They were coming into the New Road landing. The water bus had just tied up and begun to unload as the hang-yao bumped against the bank. Parker was already on his feet even before the driver could tie up. There was no time to waste. He had to catch her before she got off the boat.

Teetering like a man on a tightrope, he leaped from the prow onto the wet bank. His foot slipped and he had to scramble up the bank on all fours. By the time he was able to turn around, passengers were already streaming off the water bus, mingling with the crowd on the landing trying to board.

He couldn't find her in the crowd. He stood there searching until his training suddenly brought him up short. He couldn't be so damned obvious. Get cover and scan, he told himself.

He stepped over to a noodle stand on the quay and ordered a bowl of kow pat. Leaning against the stand, he casually turned and began a methodical scan of the landing, quartering the crowd in the market area, those heading for New Road, then the landing area and those still on the water bus. She wasn't in the crowd heading toward the bright lights of the New Road or in the market. He began to panic. He couldn't find her. But it was impossible. He couldn't have missed her. She had to be there.

Think, dammit, he told himself. What do you know about her, beyond the fact that she's beautiful? His mind raced. Her connection to Vasnasong. Bhun Sa, maybe. She's fast. A pro, spotting the tails like that and making for the water. A pro, under surveillance. What would she do?

She must have changed the image, he thought. Unconsciously, he hadn't been looking for her, but for the white sarong. He repeated the scan of the landing area, and this time he spotted her quickly. She had thrown a red silk shawl over her shoulders to cover some of the white. She was a pro, all right, he thought.

Parker nibbled idly at the kow pat as he watched her head away from the New Road and toward the market stalls and sampans along the banks of the Chao Phraya River. He got ready to follow her, but something in the back of his mind was sending him a warning signal. There was something wrong. There was . . .

She was no longer under surveillance. The lead tail had disappeared.

There were only two possibilities. One: her change of image

had worked and she had lost the tail. Or two: the tail had been switched and someone new was now tailing her.

He had to choose one. He decided she had lost the tail for two reasons: because he couldn't spot any sign of the Opposition now and because he wanted to stay with her. He wanted it!

He followed her as she weaved among the market stalls, moving purposefully as though she were nearing her destination. She paused by a fish stand for a final check. Half hidden under racks of dried squid, hanging like sheets of red parchment, she glanced back to make sure she hadn't lost him.

Parker took the opportunity for a final check of his own. He could see the lights along the Thonburi side of the river winking like fireflies as the boat lanterns bobbed in the wakes of the river traffic. The silhouettes of tall palms and temple spires could be dimly seen against the electric haze of the city lights. The steamy night smelled of mud and fish piled up on the river quay. There was no sign of the Opposition.

Why not?

There was no time to come up with an answer. She was moving again.

She made her way along the embankment, where the rice barges and the sampans were tethered. They had left the market area and it was darker here. The only light came from the kerosene boat lanterns. Then she stopped.

Parker waited. It was quiet but for the gentle lapping of the water. The occasional creak of a boat. A distant sound of a radio. And from somewhere nearby, the scent of a burning joss stick.

She had come to two sampans lashed together, tethered by a short rope to a stake on the muddy embankment. They were set apart, away from the other boats closer toward the market area. There was no one on the decks. They floated a few feet offshore, with enough water on all sides so that no one could enter or leave without being seen or heard. From a security aspect, whoever had set this up had chosen well, Parker thought.

She glanced for the briefest second back toward Parker, then with a slight tug on the rope, lightly leaped over the few feet of water onto the deck of one of the sampans. She hopped over the gunnel onto the other sampan and disappeared under the thatched arch that served as a roof.

The sampans floated on the water. They looked deserted and

oddly menacing. Nothing ventured, nothing gained, Parker told himself as he pulled the .45 automatic from his holster and cocked it. He took one deep breath, then moved.

In seconds he covered the dozen or so strides to the bank and leaped onto the deck of the sampan where the girl was. The deck bobbed under him as he ducked under the thatched roof, the .45 in the two-hand firing position.

Parker stared at the interior of the sampan, unable to believe his eyes. His gun hand dropped uselessly to his side. Thunderstruck, he looked around in a daze. It wasn't possible, he told himself. But impossible or not, it had happened.

The cabin was empty. The girl had vanished.

But there was no place to hide, he thought as he began to poke around. There were no signs of a struggle. The interior was lit by a Coleman lamp, and he found an American filter-tip cigarette with lipstick on it still burning in an ashtray on a low wicker table.

Parker felt as much as heard someone behind him. He whirled around, his gun ready, but there was no point to it. There were two of them. They carried Chinese-made SKS carbines and had him neatly bracketed between them. Even if he got one, the other would surely get him. They were young and they had that mindless wild-eyed look of trigger-itchy adolescents that in Asia means they might kill you even if ordered not to.

One of them shouted something, and although Parker didn't understand the language he was using, there was no mistaking the meaning.

Parker dropped his gun.

One of them sneered, then kicked him in the stomach. As he doubled over, gasping, they knocked him down with the butts of their rifles. Parker curled into a fetal position as they began a merciless beating, but at a barked command, they stopped as suddenly as they had started.

From his position on the deck, Parker could just make out a figure in the doorway, the face hidden in shadow. Parker struggled painfully to a sitting position. There was a sharp pain when he moved, and he wondered if they'd broken a rib. He started to wince, then stopped himself. Never show weakness to an Asian, ran the Langley credo. Bad face. Instead, always take the initiative.

"What's the meaning of this outrage? I'm an American official and I demand—" Parker began.

With a flick of his finger, the shadowy figure brushed aside his tirade as if it were a fly. The two guards grinned at him like gargoyles.

"Few things are more ridiculous than someone in your position making demands," the figure said in excellent, though accented, English.

"Where's the girl?"

"She served her purpose. Now you will serve yours," the figure said.

The voice was oddly familiar. Where had he heard it before? What the hell was going on? Parker wondered. Still, he had to try to establish some kind of control over the situation before it was too late. He licked his lips. They felt like sandpaper. He was suddenly very thirsty.

"Both the American government and General Bhamornprayoon are fully aware—" Parker began again.

"Ah, a general," the voice mocked. "I too am a general. There is no shortage of generals in Southeast Asia," the figure said as he stepped into the light.

When Parker saw the general's face he knew at once, with an overwhelming sense of sadness and certainty, that this truly was his last mission. He would never see the green hills of Virginia again. Because even after all these years, he immediately recognized the man in front of him.

"Hello, Pranh," Parker said.

2

*Water tends to move earthward
away from heaven above.
In a situation where there is
    strife
the man knows how important first
    steps are.*

SOMETIMES an entire era can be evoked by the name of
a local watering hole. The Deux Magots in Paris. Harry's
Bar in Venice. The Caravelle in Saigon. And Houlihan's in
Bangkok, Sawyer thought.

From the outside, it hadn't changed much since the rowdy
days when B-52 crews from bases with names like Udorn, Ta
Khli, and U-Tapao had nightly mingled with wild-eyed Marines
on R 'n' R, light-fingered bargirls, and Chinese black marketeers
who could sell you anything, including the contents of the over-
night bag you had left back at your hotel. In those days Houlihan's
had been a kind of discount store for used intelligence. Low-grade
stuff like the locations of military units and MACV leaks to journalists. Sawyer remembered how Barnes used to say that information was Houlihan's third most popular commodity after sex
and dope, in that order.

"What about booze?" Parker had demanded. He was falling-
down drunk at the time and pronounced it "boosh." A marine
sergeant at the next table, thinking Parker had said, "Buddhists,"
had yelled out "Fuck the Buddhists!" at which point the girl in

his lap with the see-through blouse tried to scratch his eyes out, starting a riot that almost closed the place down.

"Ah, booze, the stuff that takes the suffering away. Whiskey is the Catholic version of Buddhism, you might say. Not even a distant fourth," Barnes had replied, ignoring the mayhem around them and talking in a deep County Cork brogue that lacked nothing despite the fact that he wasn't Irish and had never spoken that way before.

Houlihan's.

Although the *H* in the neon sign was out, which meant that it was safe to approach, Sawyer lingered near the noodle stall on the corner.

He watched the three-wheeled samlors and motor scooters put-putting through the traffic, looking for anyone who spent more time looking at Houlihan's than at the mayhem of traffic around him. There were always a few low-level agents on scooters patrolling the red-light district, the grunts of the intelligence business. He took his time to check the windows and roofs of every building with a view of Houlihan's entrance. Safe was always better than sorry, he thought, remembering with a little inward grin Koenig's famous dictum about how paranoids would make good agents if they weren't so trusting.

The afternoon sun sent ripples of heat through the gasoline haze. The air felt thick and greasy. It lay over the city like a pool of stagnant water, smelling of Prek-kk-noo pepper and burning joss and diesel fumes, the scents that, even if you were blindfolded, would tell you you're in Asia. The neon lights from the bars and go-go joints, the cars moving in bumper-to-bumper convoys like schools of fish, the goggle-eyed tourists glancing left and right as they moved slowly through the oppressive heat, made Sawyer think of an aquarium. Soi Cowboy as a living exhibit of man's underside, Sawyer thought, and he wondered why he had been stupid enough to come back to Asia.

What was it the Japanese said? "Every man must climb Mount Fuji at least once; but only a fool has to climb it twice." What does that make me? he asked himself as he crossed the street to Houlihan's, having verified that there was no outside surveillance.

Inside the bar it was dark and cool as a cave. The meeting had been timed for the late afternoon lull, and the place was almost empty, except for a couple of bored bargirls plying drinks to a bleary-eyed British sailor, and Barnes himself at his old stand behind the bar, polishing a glass and listening to the kick-boxing returns on the radio.

One of the bargirls got up from the table and started to come toward him, and the Vietnamese words to beat it, "di di mau," almost popped out of his mouth. The feeling of déjà vu was very powerful, and he had to remind himself that the war had ended a long time ago. He hadn't thought the memories would be so strong. Sweat began to prickle along his entire body. But he should have expected it, he reminded himself. Memory is stimulated by environment. If you want to remember long-forgotten scenes from your childhood, go back to the old neighborhood. He shook her off and headed for the bar.

Barnes looked up as Sawyer approached, but his face showed no sign of surprise or even recognition. He was still a pro, Sawyer thought as he ordered a beer. He wondered if Barnes had recognized him right away, or had he changed so much? Sawyer stared at his own reflection in the peeling mirror behind the bar. He was wearing civvies now: a short-sleeved shirt and light-colored tropical slacks. That was different. And the black eye-patch of course, which made him look like a cross between a pirate and a shirt ad. But the dark hair and the aquiline looks hadn't changed. Or the odd green color of his good eye. Perhaps the lines around the mouth, he thought. Older, more cynical. He wondered if the idealistic young soldier he had been would like how he had turned out. Somehow he didn't think so.

Well, they all had changed.

He watched Barnes draw the beer with those big beefy hands that, according to legend, could squeeze coins into lumps of metal. He noticed that Barnes still wore the same hai-huang amulet on a CIA gold chain around his neck, breakable into separate links for instant currency. But Barnes had aged, he thought. His close-cropped hair had gone completely gray. His skin had also gone elephant gray. His eyes had a disconcerting glaze; the pupils were pin points, and Sawyer wondered what Barnes was smoking these days. Looking at him, it was hard to believe that in his time Barnes had been one of the greats. They'd called him "Mad Max" in those days because he had once charged his jeep into an NLF village—

armed only with GVN propaganda leaflets and, as he put it, "a .45 in my jockstrap."

In those days everyone in Nam with a "Get Out of Jail Free" card knew Barnes, Sawyer remembered. An ex-marine sergeant, Barnes was one of the CIA's early counterinsurgency agents. He had earned his spurs in the Philippines doing what the Company used to call "agitprop," which was a euphemism for a campaign of sabotage launched against the Hukbalahaps. That was back in the early fifties when Barnes, working for the already legendary Colonel Ted Lanigan, helped engineer Magsaysay's election. When Lanigan became CIA station chief in Saigon in '55, Barnes came with him.

Some of Barnes' feats in those days became CIA myths, like the time Barnes managed to contaminate the oil supply depot in Hanoi and ruin the engines of almost every truck and bus in North Vietnam. Later, after using massive bribes to subvert the Hoa Hao and Cao Dai sects, Barnes ran a double agent who led the Binh Xuyen, Bay Vien's bandit army, into an ambush, thereby bringing Ngo Dinh Diem to power in Saigon. "After Dien Bien Phu and the Emperor Bao Dai abdicated, Saigon was like a whorehouse without a madam. The Colonel and me, we *invented* South Vietnam, for Chrissakes," Barnes used to proclaim to skeptical newcomers sucking down gin and tonics at the Caravelle. Whether it was true or not, Sawyer knew for a fact that Barnes was the point man who seven years later launched the CIA-sponsored coup, led by Generals Don and Minh, that finally toppled that same Diem and the rest of the notorious Ngo family.

By then Lanigan was long gone, replaced by Donaldson and Secretary of Defense McNamara's new-style paramilitary CIA teams, whom Barnes used to privately call "McNamara's Ragtime Band," and even Barnes began to lose the faith.

There was a tinny growl from the radio as the crowd cheered. They must be broadcasting live from Lumpini stadium, Sawyer thought.

"May one purchase an Elephant lottery ticket here?" Sawyer asked Barnes, beginning the series.

According to Langley, the sequence was required even between agents who already know each other in order to verify that both are legitimately involved in the operation.

"You get better odds on the sporting wagers," Barnes replied.

"Who is favored in the main event?"

"Samsook, the Tiger of Raiburi, is unbeatable at four to one." Barnes shrugged.

"Yet even the unbeatable can be beaten."

"The will of heaven is inscrutable." Barnes grinned, letting Sawyer know that he recognized him by the twinkle in his eye.

He leaned confidentially across the bar.

"Watch your ass on this one, Brother Jack," he whispered.

"Jai yen yen," Sawyer agreed. Literally translated, the Thai saying meant "heart cool cool." To master one's emotions was more than a virtue in Asia. It was the only way to survive.

But Barnes still looked troubled.

"I mean it, amigo. Asia's not what it was."

"What is?"

Barnes nodded. He looked as if he wanted to say something more, then his face brightened artificially.

"Shit. Here comes the fucking Nippo leather set," he whispered sotto voce, a big shit-eating grin on his face.

"What'll it be, gents?" he called out loudly, moving to serve a pair of Japanese businessmen sporting the ever-present cameras dangling around their necks like a tribal folk emblem.

Sawyer hesitated to make sure no one was paying any attention to him, then went through the beaded curtain and up the stairs to Room 5 as indicated by Barnes (four plus one). Most of the girls hadn't shown up for work yet, and the corridor was empty. The unmistakable scent of opium seemed to permeate the walls, and the sound of a pi-nai came from behind the door. Sawyer knocked four times, then once, and went in.

The room smelled of stale perfume and sex and bamboo, from the matting on the wall, and over the empty bed in the corner was the inevitable calendar picture of the Swiss Alps that for some reason every bargirl in Asia seemed to cherish.

Harris was already waiting.

He glanced ostentatiously at his watch to remind Sawyer that he was late, then seemed to think better of it and gestured for him to sit down. As Sawyer sat at the rattan table, Harris poured them both cold glasses of Singha beer from sweating bottles. As a professional courtesy, Harris let Sawyer sit where he could watch the door. But he played it by the book, turning up the pi-nai music on the radio and running the tap in the sink. The plumbing chug-chugged like a boat engine that wouldn't start, then settled down to a slow gush of tobacco-colored water.

Harris mopped his forehead with a soggy handkerchief. There were big sweatstains under his arms, and Sawyer felt a secret delight at his discomfort. They couldn't stand each other, but being American males, they disguised their mutual dislike with elaborate attempts at sincerity.

"How's Rio? They still have those sexy cariocas in those teeny string bikinis?" Harris asked, putting the kind of leer into his voice men use when they want to prove they're one of the boys.

It was a lie, of course. Rio was for the record. In fact, Harris had yanked Sawyer from the Managua operation. Brazil was the official cover because of congressional resistance to anti-Sandinista operations in Nicaragua.

"Either the girls are getting bigger or the bikinis are getting smaller," Sawyer replied, grinning back at Harris. It was a game anyone could play.

Of any of them, Harris had changed the least, Sawyer thought. He still had the fair hair, tennis-court tan, and the kind of clean-cut features that ad directors identify with a "young American executive" look. A little sleeker, maybe. In his designer-label trop-ical suit, Harris could have been taken for a diplomat or a successful businessman. In fact, he was the CIA's Deputy Director for Covert Operations, and it was said that he never asked a question to which he didn't already know the answer.

It was also said that he never told the truth unless he thought no one would believe him.

"Do you like 'Sawyer'?" Harris asked.

He was really asking if the cover story was acceptable. It was light cover basically designed for initial entry, not deep penetra-tion. He was supposed to be an American Red Cross representative here to coordinate support for the refugee camps near the Cam-bodian border. They had supplied him with the usual documents, marked up and smudged work papers and so on. More than ad-equate for an initial scrutiny or airport check. All genuine; the Company was always good that way. The cover name "Sawyer" had been supplied by the computer back at Langley, and Sawyer suspected that the program was running through a children's literature data base, because his name came from Mark Twain and Harris' code name for this op was "Tin Man."

Sawyer shrugged.

"If it's not okay, give me a day and I can change it," Harris offered.

"It's okay."

"How was the flight?"

This kind of solicitousness was way out of character for Harris, and it irritated Sawyer more than Harris' usual know-it-all smirk. Sawyer suddenly felt like a mischievous kid about to kick over the milk pail. Anything to get Harris out of his "Pass Lady Bracknell the cucumber sandwiches" mode.

"I hope you didn't drag me all the way to Bangkok with a Cherokee just to make small talk," Sawyer snapped.

A Cherokee code in a cable was the highest urgency level for open communications, and because of it, Sawyer had left an operation in pieces and Ricardo would have to scramble on his own. Langley rules and nobody likes it, and during the long flight hours he had entertained himself by thinking up a dozen different ways to nail Harris' balls to the wall unless Harris had a damn good reason for all this.

Harris flushed, although Sawyer couldn't tell whether it was from anger or embarrassment.

"We have a little problem here," Harris admitted.

"First the Cherokee. Now this." Sawyer gestured vaguely at the room, because the fact that they'd had to use such a known location for the rdv meant they'd had to set things up in a hurry. "You're beginning to worry me, Bob. What happened? Somebody get it caught in the zipper?"

Harris winced. He obviously disapproved of Sawyer's lack of Company style. But he didn't object. That worried Sawyer even more.

He studied Harris carefully. Harris was an actor, he reminded himself. He didn't feel emotion. He used it.

If he was acting now, it was because something had gone wrong.

Even Barnes had warned him on this one. And Harris had flown out from Washington to brief him himself. That meant they were blown.

Basically, there were three kinds of mission failure. Counter-penetration. Public exposure. And the blow-up, which was the worst, not only because you also get the first two and more, but because the whole thing has fallen apart and the Opposition will be waiting to pick off anyone coming over the wall.

Salvage operations, as they were called, had almost a 100 percent mortality rate, and the Langley wisdom was that the only surer way to get rid of an agent than a Mafia hit squad was to send him out on a salvage mission.

"It's salvage, isn't it, Bob?" Sawyer asked quietly.

Harris was good, Sawyer thought. Instead of looking at Sawyer, he lifted his glass and studied it with the calculated intensity of a college Hamlet contemplating Yorick's skull. When he put it down, Harris was careful to keep both hands in sight. He must've gotten that from my file, Sawyer thought with a little inward smile. "Never make any move that might represent a threat to the subject. This agent is dangerous at all times, with or without a weapon."

"Like I said, Jack. We have a little problem here," Harris admitted at last.

Understatement was Harris' style—like the British habit of calling World War II the "late unpleasantness"—and hearing Harris admit to a little problem was the worst sign yet. Sawyer felt an icy shiver slide down his spine. When he was a child, they used to say that when you got that feeling someone had just stepped on your grave.

"I'm listening," he said.

Harris took his time, as if telling Sawyer wasn't a foregone conclusion. It was a little like watching a woman who's already invited you into her bedroom and changed into a sexy negligee debate with herself as to whether she was going to do it or not.

"One of our agents is missing," Harris said.

Salvage.

"You want me to find him?" Sawyer asked finally.

Harris looked directly into Sawyer's good eye for the first time. He was keeping it under control, but Sawyer could sense the desperation underneath. Harris hated his guts. He hadn't called Sawyer in because he liked him, but because his career was on the line.

"I want you to replace him," Harris said.

"Who was it?"

Harris shook his head.

"Need to know," he remarked primly.

In a way, Harris was within his rights, Sawyer reflected. A case officer was only supposed to give an agent enough data to do his job and not encumber him with information that might distract him or, worse, fall into enemy hands.

Except that Sawyer wasn't having any of it. It was bad enough to walk into a minefield, but he was damned if he was going to do it with his eye closed. He finished his beer and stood up. Over his head, the ceiling fan revolved slowly as the world, barely stirring the air.

"This isn't a briefing for CTP trainees, Bob. You don't want to tell me who it is, replace him yourself," Sawyer said.

Harris reddened. Sawyer wondered if he hadn't gone too far. Then he told himself that with someone like Harris, there was no such thing as too far.

Whatever Harris' real reaction, he obviously thought better of it. Harris' smile reminded Sawyer of the kind of smile an attorney whose client has been caught cold on tape might use when he tells the jury it was police entrapment.

"It was Parker. Mike Parker. Running under the cover name 'Hawkins.' He seems to have vanished into thin air," Harris said carefully. He concentrated on pouring the rest of the beer into his glass.

Sawyer felt the sudden urge for a cigarette. He hadn't touched one in ten years, and all at once the craving had returned.

"I believe you knew him, didn't you?" Harris asked a shade too casually, as if he hadn't gone over Sawyer's file with a fine-tooth comb before setting this up. As if Cambodia had never happened.

The sounds of the pi-nai on the radio faded like dying hopes in the hot still air.

"In the Parrot's Beak. I remember that real well," Sawyer said.

"Things are different now," Harris said, disapproval in his tone, as if memories, like warranties, were supposed to expire after a certain length of time.

Neither of them said anything. Outside, they could hear a furious street argument in singsong Thai. A woman cried out, and then the arguing was drowned out by the sound of a samlor with a bad muffler roaring by.

Harris waited, like a good salesman who knows that once he's made his pitch he has to let the customer argue himself into the deal. From somewhere came the tinny wail of a Chinese love song, and for no reason it reminded Sawyer of a line from Kipling. Something about "a fool who tried to hustle the East," and he knew he was hooked and that that son of a bitch Harris had known it all along. Because it was Asia. Because he had left a part of himself here. Maybe the best part. Asia. Like a schoolboy picking at a scab, we just can't leave it alone, he thought.

"What's the mission?" Sawyer asked at last.

Harris leaned forward, his forearms on the table. His eyes were very blue and very cold.

"We want you to start a war," Harris said.

3

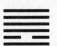

A fire beneath the open sky.
The superior man distinguishes
things according to their kinds
and classes.

THE dragon sailed slowly across the sky, its long red tail unfurled like a banner. It was a big male, a Chula, although so high up it was hard to tell how big. When it turned back toward them, they could see a smaller female Pakpao caught in its bamboo talons. Far below it, a second female kite, a petite Pakpao with a silvery tail, darted through the air currents like a fish desperately fleeing the inevitable. She flew into and then broadside to the wind, flaring to throw him off, but the Chula was not to be denied. He came around in ever tightening circles until the Pakpao had nowhere to go but up or down, riding the thermals like an elevator. Even then he waited, hovering high above her, unmoving, his paper wings and tail fully outstretched, as she began her last pathetic ascent.

The swoop, when it came, was hard and fast. The Chula dropped nearly a hundred feet in a few seconds, and just when it seemed he might miss the Pakpao altogether, his handlers brought his nose up sharply, snaring her with the bamboo hook. But the Pakpao suddenly somersaulted in the same direction. The tail, its embedded razors glittering in the hot sun, whipped across the

Chula's main control string. All at once she was free, soaring high in triumph as the big Chula tumbled out of the sky like a broken thing. It fell for what seemed like a long time before finally smashing itself on the muddy surface of the river.

The elegantly dressed guests assembled on the terrace broke into loud applause, and as the triumphant Pakpao team bowed and scrambled for coins thrown down to the quay, everyone began to move back under the gold-colored awning. Above the murmur of voices and the tinkle of cocktails, Sawyer could hear the god-awful voice of the Swiss chargé d'affaires' wife—the one in yards of rose tulle that made her look like a pink chicken—wondering if it was over and who won.

"Wonderful performance. Wonderful," the American press attaché gushed. He was a moon-faced little man named Schwartz, with the small feet and odd dancer's grace fat men sometimes have. "It's the Thai national sport. They take their kite fighting very seriously here," they overheard him explain to the local stringer for an international news magazine, a man whose only previous interest in sports was watching naked women wrestle in mud. Schwartz's round sweating face was beaming as he passed by, oblivious to the look thrown at him by Sir Geoffrey Hemmings, the British consul. They all watched Schwartz two-step over to the press table to make sure their glasses were filled and that they got their handouts.

"Extraordinary kite fight, that. In the end the female does a flip-flop and destroys the male. Almost a metaphor for the battle between the sexes, mightn't one say?" Sir Geoffrey asked, a polite smile failing to mask the wicked gleam in his eye.

"Don't be boring, Geoffrey. You think you're being provocative, but it isn't. It's just boring," Lady Caroline said, touching her tongue to her lip to check her lipstick.

"It's not boring, dearest. It's small talk. That's my job," he said wearily, and Sawyer caught in his voice the dead echo of a theme replayed over and over again in a marriage.

"Small men make small talk," Lady Caroline retorted, turning back toward Sawyer. "I take it you're a British subject too?" she asked, brushing close enough for her breasts to graze his arm. It was deliberate and she meant for her husband to see it. Not that anyone could have missed it. She was wearing a white silk number cut so low it would have been considered obscene if it hadn't carried the label of an Italian designer the cost of whose creations could pay off the national debt of a small Third World country.

"No, American actually," Sawyer replied. He hadn't meant to say "actually" and just threw it in at the last second to be consistent with the British character she had just bestowed upon him.

"American. Ah, that's so much cleverer to be these days," she said.

"For God's sake, Caroline," Sir Geoffrey sputtered, and for a moment they were all embarrassed for him.

"Don't swear, Geoffrey dear. You might be overheard and the Thais take offense so easily," she said, reddening. It made her look younger, and Sawyer could see how pretty she must have been once. She was still attractive, with the kind of well-used yet sleek blond lines that immediately suggested images of thoroughbred horses and fast white yachts and shuttered afternoons with a tennis instructor. She reminded Sawyer of the few women in his past whom he had known from the first were out of his league. And because he had known it—and maybe they did too—and because he was younger, he had treated them badly, worse than he had ever intended to, and oddly enough, that only made them want him even more. As he watched Lady Caroline bring her admittedly superb breasts to bear on him, he wondered with a touch of sadness if those women in his past had also finally gone sour, like wine kept in a bottle too long.

"You're looking at one of the great triumphs of modern technology," Barnes had said, pointing her out when they first arrived. "Lady Caroline Hemmings. Age fifty and not a wrinkle or a stretch mark anywhere. You name it. Eyes, chin, hair, tits, thighs, ass. There isn't a part of her that hasn't been redone at least once. There are whole Swiss plastic surgery clinics named after her."

At the moment, Barnes was leering expectantly at her like a man about to hear the punch line of a dirty joke, but she ignored him entirely to concentrate on Sawyer.

Sir Geoffrey coughed politely as though about to say something, and Sawyer decided that he was the diffident sort who would always do that. Except that his shyness might have been what the Company tacticians called "misdirection," because Sir

Geoffrey was also the local head of MI6 and was rumored to have once worked with Sir Robert Thompson's tough counterinsurgents in Malaya.

"You, uh, mustn't mind Caroline," Sir Geoffrey explained. "And please don't flatter yourself into thinking she's flirting with you personally. The only requirement she's ever had for anyone is that he wear a pair of trousers."

There was a burst of laughter from a nearby group, and the small Thai orchestra in native silks started up an excruciating rendition of an old Beatles song. For an instant the jangled rhythms and Asian quarter tones took Sawyer back in time to that French cabaret on Tu Do Street in Saigon and he almost missed the look that passed between Lady Caroline and her husband.

"Don't apologize for me, Geoffrey. Besides, it's all bloody nonsense. There isn't a farang man worth having in this whole bloody town."

"What about slant-eyed men?" Barnes put in crudely.

Lady Caroline smiled the kind of smile the English upper class reserves for members of the lower class who don't know their place.

"Don't be silly, darling. Asian men all have such tiny cocks," she said, nimbly plucking a glass of champagne from a tray carried by a white-coated waiter as she waltzed over to another circle of guests.

The three men were left standing there, each with his own thoughts, or maybe they all shared the same uncomfortable male thought. They sipped their gin and lime drinks, avoiding each other's eyes.

Sawyer watched Lady Caroline work the room. She was good, he thought, noting the way she deftly flirted with what passed for the cream of Bangkok society: diplomats, Western businessmen, wealthy Thais with political connections, and the occasional Chinaman who was just too rich to ignore. She was talking to one of them now, a pudgy old owl in gold-rimmed glasses, sweating in a gray silk suit. He was beaming at Lady Caroline like a Chinese Santa Claus, and next to him the inevitable dough-faced wife, a relic perhaps of the Chinaman's earlier, poorer days. He looked ordinary enough, but there was something about the Chinaman. An air—generals have it—of being able to order a competitor ruined, or a village destroyed and not lose a minute's sleep over it. He would hate to ever owe the Chinaman money, Sawyer thought, nudging Barnes.

"Who's the slope with Lady C?"

"Vasnasong. Muchee squeeze. Import-export. God, I hope that old bag doesn't come over," Barnes muttered under his breath, while grinning like a banshee across the room at the Swiss chargé d'affaires' wife, who was headed their way but who fortunately veered off toward a locally prominent silk merchant distantly related to the Thai royal family.

Sawyer nodded. Import-export was the classic cover for smuggling in every river port in the world. In Bangkok that meant jewels, rice, and opium. And even more profitable cargoes, like arms and people. He glanced at Vasnasong with heightened interest, and for a moment their eyes met across the room, neither of them showing anything more than polite curiosity, and they both turned away. But something bothered Sawyer. Something about the name. Then he had it.

"What is he, Max? Teochiu?" he asked Barnes.

Barnes winked.

"Head of the class, amigo. He's a Chink, all right. Got to be to do import-export in this part of the world."

"Then why the Thai name?"

"Daddy was a Thai. Momma-san was Chiu Chow. They say he started as a coolie."

"How does a coolie get so rich, Max?"

"How does anybody become rich?" Barnes shrugged, as if the making of wealth was a mystery he wished he could solve.

Sawyer was about to reply, then thought better of it. Instead, he nodded and went over to the bar to get his drink freshened, telling the bartender not to put in the ice cubes. It was best to get his stomach acclimatized gradually to the bacteria here, although if the bugs in Central America hadn't finished him off, nothing would. Leaning back against the bar, he casually checked the room one last time. The diversion would come anytime now.

When Sawyer returned from the bar, Sir Geoffrey was still watching his wife with an opaque expression that couldn't be read, the kind of bland look honed at a thousand committee meetings. Sawyer wondered what the bitch had on the old boy. Was it a little slant-eyed moose in a Silom Road walk-up with pink-flowered wallpaper peeling from the places where the roaches have eaten away the paste? Or maybe he liked young cowboys and a touch of leather. Whiff of the old public school, maybe. Whatever it was, watching the two of them was a little like catching a glimpse of something in an apartment window across the way that you wished you hadn't seen.

"One shouldn't, uh, take Caroline the wrong way. She's . . . um, well, there's more to her, you know. You know she, um, set up this whole benefit thing for the, uh, Cambodian refugees. She cares a great deal for the, um, refugees," Sir Geoffrey sputtered.

There were dark circles under his eyes. They gave him a kind of sad dignity. Sawyer almost felt sorry for him until he remembered who Sir Geoffrey was and wondered how much of it was real.

"She's obviously a woman of, uh, deep passions," Sawyer said carefully, as Barnes snorted into his gin and lime, trying to stifle his laughter. But the look Sir Geoffrey gave them was no laughing matter, and Sawyer wondered, not for the first time, what the hell he was doing there.

It wasn't his line of country at all. Too public. Harris might as well have taken out a full-page ad in the *Bangkok Post*, he thought irritably, feeling very exposed. As if to underscore the feeling, he spotted Schwartz hovering like an anxious hostess over a well-known American network television anchor passing through on his way back to New York from Beijing. The anchorman wore an Abercrombie and Fitch safari suit—the one with the big bullet loops over the pocket in case you ran across a charging elephant —de rigueur for American journalists in the tropics. Sawyer knew he had only stopped off in Thailand for a quickie "starving babies in refugee camps" on-the-scene exclusive, but still it made him antsy.

Mind you, the charity thing went with his cover as a Red Cross representative, Sawyer told himself, remembering the Farm doctrine that cover wasn't a story. Cover was who you are. He remembered how Koenig used to say it was the Eastern Europeans, clinging to dog-eared identity cards, who understood cover best, because in the Soviet bloc you literally are your papers; without them you don't exist. He saw Schwartz glance surreptitiously at his watch to make sure that he got the anchorman to the massage parlor on time, and felt marginally better. That meant the diversion would come at any moment now and they could get down to it. But Harris had been right about one thing. They were on very thin ice.

"You have to go carefully," Harris had stressed in that steaming whore's room over Houlihan's. "Very carefully. There are a lot of sensibilities here. Especially with the Thais."

At that moment Harris was lounging back in the wicker chair like an undergraduate; his feet, crossed at the ankles, were pointed toward Sawyer.

"You know you really shouldn't point your feet at anyone, Bob. The Thais consider it a mortal insult," Sawyer observed.

"I'm not interested in native superstitions!" Harris snapped, unaware of any irony. But then, after an uncomfortable moment, he uncrossed his legs and leaned forward. The sweatstains under his arms had grown almost to the hem of his jacket. A bead of sweat dangled from his chin like a wart and Sawyer watched it idly, wondering when it might fall.

"Christ, doesn't it ever cool off in this fucking place?" Harris wondered.

"This is the cool season," Sawyer lied, enjoying Harris' discomfort.

Harris nodded as if filing the information as an item for his expense report. He motioned Sawyer closer. It was an old-fashioned precaution, meaningless if the room had been bugged, Sawyer thought. As Koenig used to say, "There's no such thing as safe communication anymore. They've got bugs today that can pick up a cockroach's fart from a mile away." But then, Harris was a headquarters type. The kind whose idea of danger was a cutting remark at an embassy cocktail party, and the very fact that he was out here was more important than anything he had to say. It meant, as Harris himself put it, that it was "a political matter."

Harris tapped his finger on a local guidebook resting on the table. On the back cover was a crude map, and his finger touched the area near the Thai–Cambodian border.

"Three weeks ago a report surfaced at the NSC," Harris began, shaking his head to indicate that he wasn't about to reveal the source of the report. But Sawyer knew that as a matter of policy, the fact that the National Security Council had met and acted upon it meant that the data had to have been independently confirmed, usually by a second source.

Harris looked around uneasily at the dingy room as if half expecting to see enemy agents leaping out of the cracks in the wallpaper.

"God help us if this place has been bugged," he muttered. Sawyer understood his uneasiness. Harris was, in the jargon of the trade, about "to drop his pants." But this was more than standard paranoia. If Harris was worried about a safe house rdv being bugged, then he was as good as saying that it was a kamikaze mission, the kind where they show you your body bag even before you go out. And the very fact that Harris was lifting the edge of the curtain this way meant they were desperate.

"Maybe you'd better tell me what's hit the fan before I read about it in the papers," Sawyer said.

Although he had spoken softly, Harris stiffened. Harris gulped down his drink as though it contained something stronger than Singha beer.

"Okay," Harris began. "As you probably know, the Vietnamese have a vital interest in Cambodia and Laos. On the one hand it's critical to their security, but with China in the north and a crumbling economy at home they can't afford to keep their army there forever. And they can't wipe out the various rebel factions because the Cambodian guerrillas operate from sanctuaries on the Thai side of the border. That leaves Hanoi caught between a rock and a hard place, just like we were in Nam, which is perfectly okay with us."

Sawyer shifted irritably in his chair, the wicker creaking as he moved.

"You know, Bob, I'm sure this stuff impresses the hell out of the Georgetown crowd, but I could have read this kind of crap in *Time* magazine."

Harris flushed. When he looked back at Sawyer this time, it was easy to read the malice in his eyes. Sawyer liked it better that way. Like keeping the money on the table in a card game.

"All right, Sawyer. Let's get it out in the open," Harris said, his hands jammed into his pockets. "Let's not pretend we're old buddy-roo's, because we aren't. You probably think I'm a headquarters bureaucrat who's ass-kissed his way to the top and who doesn't know shit about what it's really like on the front lines. What were they called in Nam?"

"REMFs. Rear Echelon Mother Fuckers," Sawyer said. Once, he remembered, it had been Brother Rap's favorite word.

"Yeah. REMFs. Fair enough. And I know what I think of you. You're good, Sawyer. You're almost as good as you think you are. You're also a field agent who has maybe been out in the cold too long. You're undisciplined and a loner in a business that requires the utmost in teamwork. You also happen to have certain unique qualifications that your country desperately needs right now. So let's just get on with it, okay, because I really don't give a shit what you think of me."

Touché, Sawyer thought, raising his beer in a vague kind of toast. Harris took his hands out of his pockets and tapped the guidebook map again.

"Okay," Harris said. "Here's the part I hope to God you never get to read in *Time* magazine. We believe that the Vietnamese army is about to launch a full-scale invasion across the Thai border to root out all Cambodian resistance. That means war with Thailand. Now you might remember that the United States never signed the '54 Geneva accord on Indochina, nor did we ever have a single written or verbal obligation, yet we felt it was imperative to send troops to try to save South Vietnam, Laos, and Cambodia.

"Well, you know what happened. Everybody knows what happened. There's a black wall in Washington, D.C., with a lot of names on it in case maybe somebody's forgotten what happened," Harris said bitterly.

"Nobody's forgotten," Sawyer said.

Harris nodded.

"Okay, remember this: unlike South Vietnam, Thailand was, and is, a full-fledged member of SEATO and has a mutual defense treaty with the U.S. Diplomatically, politically, any way you slice it, we would have no choice. No choice at all."

"A second Vietnam war," Sawyer murmured, almost to himself.

"Worse," Harris snapped. "In those days we were fighting peasants in black pajamas carrying AK-47s, and the ground fighting was mostly confined to key areas south of the DMZ. This time the Vietnamese have the fourth-largest army in the world, fully equipped by the Russkies, and we can expect the theater of war to encompass almost all of Southeast Asia. A Rand report commissioned by the Joint Chiefs projects at least ten times as many American casualties as the first Vietnam war. The Company did its own independent study, of course. It found the Rand estimates too low," Harris concluded.

"What about nukes?"

Harris shook his head.

"Apart from all the other negatives, political damage to NATO, nuclear genie out of the bottle, and all that crap, there's something else. We have very firm information," Harris said, rolling his eyes heavenward to indicate the absolute impeccability of the source, "that if we used nukes in Asia, the Russians would use them against American installations in Europe. It seems the Politburo figures that without Vietnam threatening China's back door, the Chinese and Americans could close the noose around Mother Russia."

"Land war in Asia or World War III. I take it Washington didn't like either of those options," Sawyer ventured.

Harris leaned forward. Sweat dripped from his face down onto the table. The sound of the pi-nai on the radio grew stronger.

"There's a third option. A mission. One last chance before the balloon goes up."

"When are the Vietnamese supposed to move? Any idea?"

"The best time for them would be under cover of the monsoon season. We figured we didn't have much time left. There's even less now," Harris finished glumly.

"So the DCI authorized Parker's op?"

Harris shook his head and allowed himself a small smile as he showed his trump.

"Uh-uh. This one's straight from the Oval Office. You don't get to vote on this one, Sawyer," Harris said with a cold gleam in his eye that told Sawyer if he refused the mission, he'd never make it to Don Muang airport.

Sawyer's mouth went dry. They had to be desperate to lay it out that crudely.

"Which do you want? Me to find Parker or take his place?"

"Both. Parker obviously found a way in. We need you to find the same rabbit hole, go down it, and come out the other side."

"And if I have to choose—Parker or the mission. Which is it?"

"What do you think?"

Sawyer massaged the skin near the corner of his bad eye, a habit when he was thinking. Harris had a genius for stating the obvious, but this time he couldn't fault him. The whole thing was a little like a lottery, Sawyer thought. The odds were lousy but the stakes were too high not to play. For some reason he found it hard to breathe, and it took him a few seconds before he realized what it was.

He was afraid.

"What's it called, this little op of yours?" Sawyer asked finally.

"The operation has been code-named 'Dragonfire,' " Harris said.

Prince Ramindhorn's entrance was preceded by the banging of gongs to frighten away evil phi bop spirits and by the band's enthusiastic, if noisy, rendition of the Thai national anthem. Everyone bowed deeply as the Thai prince, preceded by two royal guards wearing the traditional white jackets, baggy black breeches, and gold caps, but carrying very untraditional loaded M-16s, came out onto the terrace. The prince, a handsome man in his thirties, tall for a Thai, wore sunglasses and the white, gold-braided uniform of a commander in the Royal Thai Air Force. He made the wai sign and beckoned them all to rise, as Lady Caroline came rushing over, smiling broadly at her social coup, for the promise of the prince's presence had been the main draw for the charity benefit.

In all the commotion no one noticed Sawyer slip behind an embroidered black silk screen and past busy waiters to a side door that led to the main corridor. He saw no one as he went down a flight of stairs and along another corridor to the last room on the side of the hotel facing the river. He knocked twice, then once, and pushed the door open. He had expected plainclothes guards, but the only person in the room was a small elderly Thai sitting in a chair that looked too big for him. The drapes had been drawn, and at first the room was too dim for Sawyer to make out the old man's features. Then Sawyer went closer, and as the old man made the wai sign, his fingertips coming up to his chin, the sign made to those of indeterminately inferior status, Sawyer saw that the old man was indeed Field Marshal Bhamornprayoon.

Sawyer made the wai sign in return, his fingertips reaching his nose, the sign made to superiors, and the old man smiled warmly. Face had been preserved and it would go well, which was a good thing, Sawyer thought, since the whole damn party upstairs, including the arrival of the prince, had been arranged solely to get the two of them together.

Sir Geoffrey had set it up to avoid the appearance of American involvement. "What else are the British good for?" Harris, who fancied himself a wit, had said, reflecting the persistent Langley prejudice that MI6 was largely populated by Old Boys who were either KGB moles or pansies or both, even though Harris really knew better. What Harris might have given Sir Geoffrey in return—probably the keys to the executive bathroom, Barnes had conjectured—was of less interest than the fact that Harris had even involved another service in what was, for the CIA, a salvage operation. That was curious, Sawyer thought. In fact, he was beginning to think that there were a lot of curious things going on in Bangkok.

The old man gestured for Sawyer to sit facing him. His face was the color of teak and hardly wrinkled, the eyes tranquil as a monk's, but his hands were old and gnarled.

"Sawat dee khrap. Sabai dee rue-ah, Your Excellency," Sawyer began.

The old man shook his head, a faint smile dancing in his eyes.

"Please, young sir. I am not here. This conversation is never happen."

"Dai prod. It is understood, Your Excellency."

"Your Thai is most good for a farang," Bhamornprayoon said approvingly.

Sawyer shook his head.

"The tones are weak. And I have difficulty with the honorifics."

"The tones of you are much similar to the Thai Yuan, which is spoken by the people of the north. That is of no matter. But you must practice. Much depends on it."

"Of a certainty, Excellency," Sawyer said, glancing around the hotel room. The old man caught his drift at once, a smile cracking his face.

"Let not the khwan of you to be disturbed. My men have, how you say, 'exterminated the insects from the house.' And they have left a device that none may hear us," Bhamornprayoon said, pointing toward a small sonic interferometer on a table near the door. Developed by the American DIA, it scrambled sound waves outside a given perimeter area for up to twenty meters, sufficient to disrupt most electronic eavesdropping.

"Khob khun krap. These are wise precautions in such times as these, Excellency," Sawyer said.

"Precautions are of importance. In my country we say, 'Dig the well before you are thirsty,' " the old man agreed. "But you will take some cha. It is jasmine tea, and the sahim are good." He gestured at a coffee table set for tea, with a plate of sticky Thai sweets covered with coconut milk syrup. Although tea was the last thing on Sawyer's mind, to refuse it would have shown poor kreng chai and both men would have lost face.

"Narm cha lorn," Sawyer said, munching a sweet.

"No milk?" the old man inquired politely. "Odd. The British always would to take their tea with milk and sugar."

"They also lost the Empire," Sawyer replied.

"That is so," the old man cackled. "Most good, Sawyer-khrap," he wheezed, raising his teacup with a hand that faintly trembled with age. As he drank, he surveyed Sawyer over the rim of his cup with the careful objectivity of a doctor evaluating a patient's potential for surviving surgery. Although he held no formal post in the Thai government, it was said that in Bangkok even the swallows could not light on the telephone lines along Yawaraj Road without Bhamornprayoon's approval.

"This thing you do is most dangerous," Bhamornprayoon said, carefully setting down his cup.

"It is of equal danger to wait and do nothing," Sawyer said.

"That is why we agreed. You are to establish a most unofficial communication with the Cambodian rebels. Of this, we of the Thai government know nothing."

"That is so," Sawyer nodded. "We will trade American arms and gold for opium. The arms will give the rebels the means to launch a preemptive attack against the Vietnamese in Cambodia, thus forestalling the Vietnamese invasion into Thailand. Essentially it is the principle we call a 'backfire': one sets a fire to stop a fire."

"Still, there is much danger. Sometimes the fire one sets can engulf one."

"Yes, Excellency. Fire is always most dangerous."

"I am most curious concerning the opium. Why does not rich America just to give the guns to the Cambodians?"

"Would you trust a farang who wished to give you something for nothing, Excellency? Also it will help the rebels gain favor with the local tribes by buying up their crops. And we may be able to enlist some of the local tribes against the Vietnamese. And we also gain. By buying up much of the Golden Triangle opium harvest, we can reduce the supply of heroin to the U.S. by one-half. There are many good reasons for such a transaction."

Bhamornprayoon raised his hands as if in admiration at the deviousness of the Western mind. From downstairs they could hear the faint sounds of khon music and applause. Lady Caroline had arranged for a traditional dance troupe to entertain the prince and her guests. They listened for a moment and sipped the sweet tea, the old man with eyes closed. With his eyelids down, he looked quite dead. When he opened his eyes there was a sadness in them.

"Tum mai, young peu-un? I say peu-un, which means 'friend,' but is truth? I have much fear America wish only to fight Communists to the last Asian. Now you say, is truth?"

Sawyer shrugged.

"I cannot say, Excellency. These are political matters. But surely it is better for Viets and Kampucheans to die than Thais."

"Thus spoke the first one, whom you call Hawken-khrap, though his true name Pakah. A brave man and of much confidence. Yet he is no more."

Bhamornprayoon held his palm up in a Thai Buddhist gesture that suggested the evaporation of dew in the hot tropic sun.

"It is to speak of Parker that I requested this meeting, Excellency."

The old man's face tightened. He gestured for Sawyer to proceed.

"My mission, Excellency, is the same as Parker's. To somehow reach the Cambodian leaders, not through any official channels, make the guns-for-opium deal, and get them to launch an offensive inside Cambodia that will prevent the Vietnamese invasion of your country. So much you know.

"We also know that Parker had found a way in. He had signaled his control that he'd made a contact and would be meeting with someone—we don't know who or where—that night. The fact that he disappeared only confirms that he was on to something. That's all we know."

"Nor do I know more, young peu-un," Bhamornprayoon objected and stood up. He looked around at the dim hotel room. "And now we must to say 'Lah gorn la krup' for we two have much to do, do we not?"

Sawyer remained seated, a faint glimmer of amusement in his good eye.

"Alas, Excellency. I fear you have not spoken all the truth to me."

Bhamornprayoon sat stiffly down. In his bearing was a lifetime of military parade grounds. His eyes were utterly opaque as they stared at Sawyer, who found himself wondering how many men this devout old Buddhist had ordered executed. Bhamornprayoon had initiated and survived at least a dozen coups and despite the Buddhist precepts against killing, his enemies had a nasty habit of being found floating facedown on the Chao Phraya.

"What you mean?" Bhamornprayoon demanded.

"Something's been bothering me all along about Parker's disappearance, Excellency. On a mission of this seriousness my people have given me the 'white tablet.' You understand? I can call up an air strike or an entire division of U.S. Marines if so needed. This much has been authorized by the president himself. So, with so much at stake, I ask myself why wasn't Parker shielded?

"Then too, why didn't my case officer on this mission offer me any such protection? True, he knows I would have refused, for I prefer to work alone, but standard procedure requires that he make the offer. But he didn't. Is that not most curious, Excellency?"

Bhamornprayoon shrugged with an eloquent gesture that somehow had all of Asia in it.

"Mai pen rai. For Asian peoples, peu-un, much of what the white man do is curious. Truly, how can I to know why American do anything?"

"Unless," Sawyer continued, "unless Parker *was* shielded,

whether he knew it or not. Just as I have been dirty since I returned to my hotel last night, Excellency."

"Dirty? Chun mai kao chai. What is this 'dirty' please?"

"Dirty is two tails, 'watchers' they are called in the trade. One in front, one behind. Both Thais and, unless I miss my guess, both from the Thai Central Security Police. If Parker had been covered, Excellency, it would have been with Thais. A farang stands out on an Asian street like a black man at a Mormon convention. It would also explain why Washington is going crazy over this. Because an agent disappearing is serious, but a shielded agent disappearing is a total disaster."

Bhamornprayoon poured himself another cup of tea and sipped it thoughtfully, the faint scent of jasmine tickling Sawyer's nostrils.

"This is most interesting, peu-un. But alas, even if truth, what all such things to do with your humble servant?"

"Because, Excellency," Sawyer said intently, "if Thais were used, you had to know about it. So now you tell me, Excellency. What happened to Parker?"

The old man sipped his tea calmly, giving nothing away. When he finished, he touched a napkin to his lips and looked up at Sawyer. It was a curious look and Sawyer wondered if he hadn't pushed the bounds of kreng chai too far. Then the old man smiled a strange half-smile, the kind emulated on a million statues of the Buddha.

"Among our people it is said, 'The father basks in the warmth of the good son.' Do you understand, peu-un? You are wise beyond the years of you. That is most good. More better than the confidence of such as this Nai Pakah-khrap you seek. So I will speak truth, khwan to khwan. We watch to Pakah-khrap, yes, but no to tell him. Song. Two watchers, as you say. This much, yes. But so sad, peu-un. Of what happen to Pakah-khrap, I know no thing," Bhamornprayoon said, touching his head, which is the seat of the khwan soul and may not be touched except when speaking the truth.

Sawyer's mouth went dry. He'd counted on getting a lead from the Thais. It also meant that things were worse than even Harris had led him to believe. He licked his lips.

"Chun mai kao chai. I don't understand, Excellency. How can your watchers not have reported what happened to Parker?"

"Because there is no report, peu-un. We find body of one 'watcher' in WC of cinema in Silom Road. His head clobbered, but that not kill him. Coroner find tiny poison flechette in leg. Most bad poison."

"What of the other watcher, Excellency?"

The old man shrugged again.

"Alas, he too has disappeared."

4

 Wind blows across the marsh.
The moon is nearly full.
One horse breaks his traces;
only one horse remains.

FOR a price the boat people of Bangkok will smile for the tourists and their cameras. But in the klongs off the Chao Phraya, questions go unanswered and the river keeps its secrets. So Sawyer, dressed like a tourist in a gaudy yellow shirt crisscrossed by a camera strap, munched a kow larm from a nearby street stall and asked no questions. Now and again he snapped a picture of a mama-san in blue pajamas and straw hat rowing a sampan against the backwash of a water taxi, or a monk in a curry-colored robe sitting cross-legged at a curb, oblivious to the traffic around him, but there was no film in the camera and his thoughts were elsewhere.

"Why we come here?" Sublieutenant Somsukiri had demanded just before Sawyer had left him sweltering behind the wheel of the car. Although the Thai's boyish face had been calm, his fingers were tapping nervously on the burning-hot steering wheel. He was clearly ill at ease out of uniform, Sawyer had noted, and probably more than a little pissed at being yanked away from his regular duty to nursemaid a farang who seemed to have nothing better to do than play tourist.

"Because missing farang come here, maybe," Sawyer had replied.

"How you know this?" Somsukiri demanded, the disbelief plain on his face.

"In order to hunt the tiger, you must know what a tiger is. One reason I was chosen for this is that I knew the missing farang and this may help in tracking him," Sawyer said, wondering if he sounded as fatuous as he felt. What he carefully had not mentioned was that by the same reasoning, it was because Somsukiri had been the best friend of Sergeant Tarasang, the missing second tail, that Sawyer had requested him. Of course, all Somsukiri had been told was that a farang official investigating the case had requested an undercover officer as a driver, no doubt because the farang did not know his way about the city and, as an American, was strangely unaccustomed to traffic on the left.

Glancing out of the corner of his eye from behind his big plastic sunglasses, Sawyer could see Somsukiri sitting rigidly in the parked car, sweat pouring down his face in the fiery morning heat. Let him simmer for a while longer, Sawyer thought with a little inward grin, turning his mind back to the question that had been gnawing at him since the mission began.

What happened to Parker?

"Dead reckoning" it was called in "the trade," itself an egocentric euphemism for the spy business, just as people in Beverly Hills call the movie business "the industry," as though there were no other. Dead reckoning—known as "Inductive Surveillance Analysis" in official CIA doublespeak, although some Company wags persisted in calling it "going up the yellow brick road"— was based on the same principle as old-fashioned navigation in the days before satellites. You took readings and then combined the data with the information in the charts and some basic mathematics to determine your location. For Sawyer that meant that by combining the few facts he had with his knowledge of Company field procedure and of Parker's "signature"—another trade term, meaning Parker's general modus operandi—he could somehow pick up Parker's trail. The technique was pooh-poohed by establishment types like Harris, who maintained that it was no more scientific than trying to find water with a divining rod. Sawyer himself conceded as much—and yet, those who were good at it were said to strike gushers regularly.

The problem was compounded by the fact that there was little point in questioning any of the locals who might have seen something. Nor would the Thai authorities fare much better. Either there would be no reply, in which case you came away with the notion that Bangkok was a vast city inhabited only by the blind, deaf, and dumb. Or else, if you pressed them, you would be told whatever they assumed you wanted to hear—this the invariable reaction of Asians dealing with outsiders or those in authority. It used to infuriate the Americans in Vietnam, but in a way you couldn't blame the natives. Barnes had taught him that, Sawyer remembered. It was at that Chinese restaurant in the Cholon section of Saigon, all of them long since pissed on 33 beer and plum wine, the curfew past, and nothing to do but drink and wait for the dawn.

"Confucius say: 'When the wind blows, the fucking grass gotta bend.' The auth-aaaarh-ities," Barnes belched loudly, extending it fortissimo as though playing an instrument, "are the wind. The peasants are the grass. And the grass don't get no choices. No choices at all. These here new MACV hotshots think the reason the peasants just tell 'em what they want to hear is 'cause they're dumb. That's bullshit, man. That ain't dumb; it's smart. Just remember," Barnes had said, playfully wagging an admonishing finger as he delivered one of those lines of his that embedded itself in the memory like a splinter, "there ain't no such thing as a dumb gook."

So that left Sawyer staring blankly at the river, trying to figure out which way Parker had gone from here, assuming he had even been here.

It had been Bhamornprayoon's remark about how and where the first tail had died that gave Sawyer the idea that dead reckoning might work in this case. Because there was a grain of truth in what he had told Sublieutenant Somsukiri. Although it had been a long time, Sawyer remembered Parker. Except for a dangerous tendency to shoot the works when he thought he had a shot at a coup, Parker's signature could have come right out of the Farm ops manual.

Dead reckoning.

A movie house was right out of the manual's section on how to flush a tail. It had been a front-and-back tail—Bhamornprayoon had confirmed that—and while Parker wouldn't have spotted something sophisticated like an "8-box"—for that matter an ex-perienced round-eye could spend a year on any street in Asia and still miss most of what was happening right in front of his nose —still Parker was certainly good enough to spot a simple front-and-back. And he hadn't been told they would be there; Harris hadn't known about it. That meant Parker hadn't known whether they were Friendlies or Opposition—and when in doubt, the book says, assume Opposition.

So Parker took the first tail out in the john. Again SOP. Except he wouldn't have killed him unless he was sure the tail was Opposition, or was under great pressure. That also went along with the coroner's report that the tail had been coldcocked from behind before he had been killed.

Sawyer was pretty sure Parker hadn't killed the tail. First, because the poison flechette wasn't standard issue. In fact, the only thing the Company had like it was something that came out of a ballpoint pen. All very James Bond, and the kind of thing that impressed the hell out of young CTP trainees, but to Sawyer's knowledge the thing had never actually been used in a real mission. Besides which, that wasn't Parker's job. Then too, why kill some-one if you've already taken him out of action? Especially if you're not sure who he is?

Another thing. Why didn't Parker flush the tail and then—again out of the manual—do a reverse to track the tail back to his base? That went along with the question of the missing second tail. Another mystery. For if there were two tails, what would Parker have gained by taking out only one of them? And while he was taking out the first, where was the second?

The second tail wasn't calling his control because Bhamorn-prayoon had told him there had been no report. That meant the second tail was someplace else. The only circumstance that Sawyer could think of to explain the missing second tail was—another trade term—a "split." In other words, there was someone else. Either Parker had met the "contact" he had called in about earlier that day, or Parker was himself tailing someone.

Standard police procedure everywhere is that when the target "splits," the watchers also split. So the second tail followed the "contact." The first stayed with Parker, who, still wanting to stay with the contact—that was his signature all right, to go for it, Sawyer mused—would have had to take his own tail out first.

Parker pulled it off, Sawyer decided. Otherwise there would have been no disappearances and no body in the movie house. Then, having eliminated the first tail, Parker either went after his contact again or to some predesignated rdv. Somebody else then came along later and finished the unconscious tail off with the flechette.

That left the three of them, Parker, the second tail, now known to be the missing Sergeant Tarasang, and the contact, maybe, all going somewhere. That was what had brought Sawyer to the New Road water-bus landing.

Where are you, you bastard? Sawyer asked himself, seeing Parker in his mind as he had been that night so many years ago, his handsome face twisted with fear in the dim light from the corridor. "It's the regs!" Parker had whispered, and Sawyer remembered grabbing him by his shirtfront and hissing something. Something.

Parker had called in a lead, a way in, earlier that day. But at the time he hadn't alerted them to an rdv, presumably because it hadn't been set yet. The contact would have let him know at the last minute, maybe playing telephone tag, leading him from one location to another. But neither Parker nor the presumed contact would have ever agreed to any kind of an rdv except in a public place. The same Parker who had said "It's the regs!" would have played it by the book. At that hour of the night, the most likely place was any one of the hundreds of joints in the Patpong or Soi Cowboy or Phet Buri districts. Loud, noisy, the neon turning the night to reddish day, and no one noticing or caring about a couple of men talking a little business over drinks.

Now if you drew a line between Patpong One Street and the movie house where the dead tail was found—Patpong One Street was closer to the theater than either Soi Cowboy or Phet Buri—then Parker could have gone either up toward Rama Four Road or down toward the klong. Sawyer figured the klong as more likely, because Parker knew he was under surveillance and that direction gave him more dark corners and byways to slip or flush the second tail. Also, if Sawyer was right about the sequence, then Parker came to the movie house after the Patpong rdv and would then have most likely continued in the same direction the extra few blocks to the water.

There was another reason for assuming he had come this way. Parker had most likely been snatched. It's much easier to pull a gun on someone when he comes on board a boat than to hustle him into a car with plenty of rubberneckers looking on. It's also easier to get rid of someone on the water, Sawyer noted. A muffled shot or maybe another flechette. Weight the body with stones and dump it overboard in the middle of the night. Very private and —in Bangkok, where a dozen bodies are fished out of the Chao Phraya every day—almost foolproof.

Whoever had snatched Parker had done it right under the noses of the Thai security police who were tailing Parker. That meant they knew what they were doing. They might have lured him or trapped him, but whatever happened, it wasn't a Chicago-style street-corner snatch, Sawyer's gut told him. So Parker was on the water that night. Probably a water bus or water taxi. And at that late hour, assuming he had boarded on the Sathan Nua klong, the water buses and taxis ran only to the New Road landing, which was where Sawyer stood at that instant, trying to figure out where to go next.

Sawyer leaned back against the kow larm stall, ripe with the scent of roast coconut, and watched the landing. A barge loaded high with sacks of rice moved slowly downstream, its wash almost tipping a sampan where a small boy balanced nimbly as a monkey as he squatted by the stern, brushing his teeth with river water. A young Thai woman in European clothes carrying a green and yellow umbrella to shade her from the sun dropped something into a monk's begging bowl as he sat meditating near the water's edge, his close-cropped hair and eyebrows making him look both sinister and innocent all at once, like a young trainee at a military academy. A Chinese businessman in a white shirt and flaming red tie stood stiffly, staring blankly at the brown river. He was probably waiting for the water bus to take him upriver to the Chinatown landing, Sawyer thought. Under a sagging palm tree blighted by automobile exhaust, a young street-boy of about eight-going-on-thirty in an oversized UCLA T-shirt, a cigarette dangling from his lips, hawked joss sticks that filled the air with incense.

What is it about Asia, this filthy, noisy, god-awful place, that tugs at us in the odd moments of the night like the memory of an old lover? Sawyer wondered.

And where in all this did you get to, you dumb son of a bitch? he thought, angrily addressing Parker in his head as though Parker had deliberately left no tracks for no other reason than to frustrate him. Because here dead reckoning failed him. There were just too many ways to go from here.

Parker could have headed up New Road, so-called despite the fact that it was one of the oldest streets in the city. There were plenty of offices, shops, restaurants up that way where he could have made contact. He could have stayed on the water, boarding another water bus, or water taxi, or maybe the ferry across to the Thonburi side of the river. He could have gone on foot, upriver toward the Oriental Hotel, legendary since the days of Somerset Maugham, or down toward the Krung Thep Bridge. He could have gone anywhere!

Sawyer was about to give it up. He had even started to head back to the car when a thought struck him. He had been looking through the telescope from the wrong end! Parker had been either hit or snatched. No, snatched, he decided. They would have wanted to sweat him for information before they terminated him. To figure out where the snatch had been done, he had to look at it from the snatcher's point of view.

If Sawyer wanted to set a snatch up from here, he wouldn't want to do it under the bright lights of New Road or the posher quarters near the Oriental. It would be better over on the Thonburi side, where the real slums are, or down toward the bridge, where the sampans cluster along the riverfront and the streetlights are few and far between.

If it was on the Thonburi side or if Parker had gone back on the river in either direction, forget it. The area was just too vast to cover and there were no tracks. No body. It would be like trying to find an invisible needle in a haystack the size of Mount Everest. Also if they had lured or forced Parker onto another boat, the timing would have been very tricky. Too many things that might go wrong while waiting for a water bus or ferry. That only left one option: Parker heading toward the Krung Thep Bridge on foot along the riverfront.

Sawyer turned and beckoned Sublieutenant Somsukiri, admitting to himself as he did so that the only real reason he had chosen this direction to investigate was because it was the only one he could investigate.

Sublieutenant Somsukiri was seething. Keep one's heart cool cool, he told himself again and again, for to show his anger would be a most terrible kreng chai. That the American farang was most inconsiderate, leaving him to swelter in the parked car, was unfortunately only to be expected. The Americans were like elephants crashing through the world and trampling little peoples without even noticing.

And though his superiors had told him that this assignment was of much importance, Somsukiri secretly suspected that he was being passed over for his heart's desire, an appointment to the Lumpini district, and that First Lieutenant Chaiyamajith had thrown him to the farang as one throws a gnawed and useless bone to a dog.

All this coming just at this time was most unfortunate karma, and alas, Somsukiri had to acknowledge his own fault in this. For he had been late this morning and had forgotten to show proper respect to the spirit house on the east corner of the apartment balcony. His mother had warned him against such foolishness, and he had no doubt offended the protective phi poota, although his karma had been so wonderful good of late. First, the beautiful Sumalee, who danced for the pig-faced Japanese in a club on Silom Road, had confided that her "agent" had demanded four thousand baht to let her out of her contract. A serious, but not impossible sum.

He tried to think of whom among his regulars he could squeeze, but then his dearest peu-un, Sergeant Tarasang, had come through. Tarasang—whom he had thought was a snake for not repaying him the eight, no, nine hundred baht he, Somsukiri, had invested upon Tarasang's advice in "Fists of Iron" Meang of Songkhla, whose iron fists, alas, were no proof against a cross-kick to the midsection in the fourth round at Ratchadamnoen—had not only appeared with newfound riches to repay the loss, but had given him another eight thousand besides. And then, most convenient, like the spirit in a hang shadow play, disappeared.

The eight thousand, Tarasang had confided, was to be bet on a black and red cock named Baby See Dum Daang, who had been bred and trained in great secrecy by his best "squeeze" to challenge the great champion, Prince Nung Pan Victory. At first skeptical, for odds of eight-and-more to one were being quoted for any challengers to the great champion cock, Somsukiri had himself seen the "Baby"—deliberately misnamed to lengthen the odds. He was a most large cock of incomparable speed and viciousness, and watching him peck the eyes out of a training bird made Somsukiri's heart to soar. The beautiful Sumalee and many baht besides were almost his.

And now this! Playing amah to a farang who seemed to have nothing better to do than to wander aimlessly around the city like a pai thiaw. Today of all days! For the cockfight was to be this very afternoon. Somsukiri squirmed on the hot car seat like a child that has to go to the bathroom, and vowed to burn a joss stick to the Lord Buddha at the Temple of the Dawn if only he could make the fight.

But the farang just stood at the water-bus landing snapping pictures like any tourist. No, not even a proper tourist, despite his dressing stupidly as the other farang tourists. They were a common sight on the tour boats from the big hotels, mostly fat and aged and the women with hair of a curious bluish color. They would enthusiastically snap pictures at the floating market at Thonburi as though it were a real market, instead of one that existed solely for the farang tourists, after which they would be led in platoons to whichever shop had bribed their guide the most, where they would squeal in excitement over bargain "authentic" antique carvings mass-produced in sweatshops all over the city and marked up twenty times their cost.

It was infuriating. He, Somsukiri, an important officer of the Security Police, and one of integrity, for he took far less squeeze than was his due, playing guide to a farang who, if he wanted to be a tourist, didn't even have enough sense to go to the important sights like the Royal Palace, or the Temple of the Golden Buddha. And in the evening, no doubt, he would want to be taken to a massage parlor. By rights, instead of a massage girl he should find the farang a kra toe, one of those provocatively dressed male transvestites—some of whom were beautiful enough to attract any man—who paraded nightly along Silom Road, and for a few moments Somsukiri amused himself by picturing the farang in various obscene postures with a kra toe. Alas, his reverie was suddenly ended by a signal from the farang to come down to the landing.

★ ★ ★

As Somsukiri hurried over, Sawyer could see he was upset. That was okay, Sawyer thought. Keep him emotional, not thinking.

"Most bad leave car. Bad peoples come. Steal car. Steal everything," Somsukiri declared unhappily.

"Mai pen rai. It is of no matter. I will tell them it was the fault of this farang and no fault of yours," Sawyer said, touching his own chest.

"Plenty bad peoples in Bangkok," Somsukiri insisted, pushing out his lower lip like a sulky child.

"Plenty bad peoples everywhere. Please to show me this way," Sawyer said, indicating the street along the embankment.

"What for you go this way? Go other way. See Grand Palace. Many wats most beautiful. Take many pictures," Somsukiri said, still hanging back.

Now, Sawyer thought. Now it was time to enlist him. In the jargon, "to turn him." It was for this moment that he had spent half of yesterday secretly closeted with First Lieutenant Chaiyamajith, learning everything he could about the missing Sergeant Tarasang and his best friend, Somsukiri. It was a spook's most delicate yet essential task, to use someone by making him think he's using you. First he had to shock Somsukiri, then seduce him. When Sawyer replied, the harshness in his voice was like a jolt of electricity.

"There's no damn film in the camera and I am not here for sightseeing and a little fuckee-fuckee on Patpong, Sublieutenant." Now the bribe, Sawyer thought. "You have been selected for a most important assignment. One of great opportunity. A man of lesser character than yourself could 'touch the dragon' with such an opportunity. This requires a man of metta and of most excellent kreng chai such as you are said to be."

Somsukiri almost visibly swelled. He had not offended the phi poota! Though, to be safe, he would still light a joss stick to Lord Buddha as he had promised. His karma was most good. The farang was not a fool tourist, but a man of power and significance. He, Somsukiri, had seen that at once. Everyone knew the Americans had money to burn, he thought, and when he smiled at the farang this time, there was a genuine desire to please in his eyes.

"Where we go now?" he asked enthusiastically.

"Water taxi," Sawyer said, hailing a hang-yao and telling the driver to head toward the Krung Thep Bridge, but slowly, so he could take pictures of the colorful Bangkok waterfront.

"What we do?" Somsukiri whispered over the asthmatic hammering of the ancient outboard engine.

"We watch," Sawyer replied enigmatically, gesturing at the shoreline.

Somsukiri smiled and gazed intently at the riverbank, although he hadn't the foggiest idea what he was supposed to be looking for.

No one spoke. The burning sun glittered on the muddy gray surface, and across the water came the faint whine of one of those endless Chinese love songs. The driver, a wizened old man, his lips and gums stained a permanent reddish-black from betel juice, hummed mindlessly along as they moved slowly downriver.

Sawyer reached into his pocket and handed Somsukiri a piece of paper. It fluttered slightly in the breeze of their passage like a living thing. When he saw it, Somsukiri's heart plummeted like a stone, and he mentally cursed himself for having once again underestimated this demon farang with his one devil's eye.

Because the paper was his beloved Sumalee's contract with her agent. He recognized her childlike scribble of a signature in the margin at once, and only a lifetime of jai yen yen kept the fear from showing in his face. Too late Somsukiri understood the strange look in First Lieutenant Chaiyamajith's eyes when he told him to go with the farang. He was under suspicion! Now, as the saying went, he held his khwan in his hands like a palmful of water. He touched the Buddha amulet that hung around his neck and stiffened himself to face the devil farang who sat in judgment in the prow of the boat like the Lord of Death himself.

"What should such as I do with this thing I purchased?" Sawyer said quietly, letting the contract flutter in the breeze like a flag. "Shall I," he went on, "use her as it pleases me, then throw her into the streets like a useless thing when I am done? Or perhaps sell this paper to another? And he to yet another? Or shall I," he said intently, "make you a gift of this thing as a gesture of my appreciation for your help in this investigation?"

Dry-mouthed, Somsukiri nodded, scarcely daring to believe his karma, yet still fearful what price the farang demon, for so he named him in his mind, might yet exact.

"Dee mark," Sawyer murmured, not permitting himself a

smile yet. Now came the tricky part. Convincing the young Thai that he knew more than he really did. "We need only to confirm some information," he said, tapping a folded piece of paper sticking out of his shirt pocket that was in fact only his laundry receipt. "Tell me, dai prod, where has Sergeant Tarasang gone, yes?"

The blood hammered in Somsukiri's temples. Sumalee was lost!

"I not to know," he blurted out.

Sawyer's heart sank. The Thai seemed to be telling the truth. But he smiled as if he had gotten the answer he had expected.

"We know this, Sublieutenant. We know you know your duty. This is not a question," Sawyer said, tapping an admonishing finger on the contract. "But perhaps there is some little thing, some change in Sergeant Tarasang just before he disappeared."

Somsukiri shook his head no. But there was a slight hesitation before he did, and Sawyer looked down to conceal his interest. The Thai was holding something back!

"No word? No thing of this assignment to his most best peu-un? No see good-time girl? Chase dragon, maybe? Or money maybe? Plenty baht?" Sawyer demanded.

Again the faintest hesitation before Somsukiri shook his head again. Money, Sawyer thought. Maybe somebody had Tarasang in his pocket. Bought and paid for. Because Tarasang was most likely alive. Otherwise they'd have already found him floating face-down in one of the klongs. Somsukiri was protecting Tarasang. Was that friendship or something else? Sawyer wondered. He might be hiding nothing more than a lousy hundred-baht squeeze, and Sawyer had to let the Thai know that he wasn't going to be taken to the woodshed for copping a mango from the corner pushcart.

"It is said that when the prince hunts the tiger, the deer may safely pass the bowmen," Sawyer said carefully. "All men have a thing to hide. A squeeze. A female companion the wife does not to know. Mai pen rai. Among men of metta, such things are of no consequence and need not to reach the ears of those on high," Sawyer smiled, one man of the world to another.

Somsukiri watched him as one watches a cobra. He wondered if the demon farang was setting a trap for him.

"Life in the streets is most difficult," Sawyer said wistfully. He started to stick the contract back into his pocket with an indifferent shrug, but his thoughts were seething. Come on, he thought. Shit or get off the pot!

Suddenly, Somsukiri stretched out his hand for the contract. His eyes were dark and determined.

"Before he go that night, Tarasang pay me money he owe me. Some four thousand baht," Somsukiri said, lowering the amount to keep as much of it as possible, though the demon farang would surely demand the tiger's portion. "He have plenty baht that night. Most excited. But he not to say of where money come or where he go."

"Squeeze maybe?"

"Plenty squeeze, maybe," Somsukiri agreed.

"But he not to say of where he go?" Sawyer asked, tapping the contract against his knee, just out of Somsukiri's reach.

No, Somsukiri shook his head firmly.

They were nearing the Krung Thep Bridge. Sawyer told the driver to turn around and head back. The old man took them in a wide circle around a big bridge piling, where the greasy water lapped like surf from the wake of a water bus. Land's end; dead end, Sawyer thought.

"Was maybe someplace of most importance to your peu-un Sergeant Tarasang? Family maybe? No. No family. If you have plenty money, maybe win big Elephant lottery, where you go, Sublieutenant?"

Somsukiri shrugged.

"Ban Phattaya, maybe," he offered, naming the big seaside resort on the Gulf of Thailand.

"And Sergeant Tarasang. Where he go if he have plenty baht?"

"Ban Phattaya. He say many funs there. All time talk Ban Phattaya." Somsukiri nodded enthusiastically as Sawyer handed him the contract.

"Khob khun khrap, peu-un," Sawyer smiled.

"Dai prod. What we do now?" Somsukiri said, smiling happily back. His karma had been most wonderful good, and he would light nung roi, yes, one hundred joss sticks to the Lord Buddha.

"We watch," Sawyer replied, gesturing at the riverbank slowly sliding by.

"Yes, Nai So-yah-khrap, but what we to look for?"

Sawyer made a face.

"I not to know, but I will to know when I to see it," he said, leaving Somsukiri staring blankly at the shore and telling himself that he would never understand the white man. Their thoughts were utterly incomprehensible.

As for Sawyer, if there was a clue to Parker's whereabouts along the riverfront, he couldn't see it. There were small stores, their most common advertisement a Pepsi sign; concrete landings for boats and rice barges, crowded with food stalls, flies buzzing among the big open metal pots; a wharf for a big white and blue tour boat with a sign in English that read: CRUISING TO THE SIAMESE GULF. KO SI-CHANG. KO LAN-PATTAYA. THE BIGGEST BRONZE BUDDHA IN THE WORLD AT SUPANBURI AND THOUSAND OF BIRDS; dilapidated white apartment buildings; naked children playing on the balconies; long warehouses with corroded metal shutters; and farther on, squatters' shacks perched on teakwood pilings just inches above the surface of the river. It was a pointless exercise really, Sawyer admitted to himself. He could be staring right at where they were keeping Parker—in the unlikely event he was still alive—and not know it. For instance, if you wanted to snatch someone, where they were passing at this very moment was as good a place as any.

It was a long concrete wharf for a huge two-story warehouse that belonged, according to a faded white sign over an open loading gate, to the Southeast Asia Rice and Trading Company. Big hundred-kilo sacks of rice were stacked all over the wharf, and through the open gate Sawyer could see a deep canyon between two rectangular mountains made of sacks of rice piled up to the ceiling.

It would have been dark here at night. A perfect place to take someone, or maybe lure him onto one of the sampans tethered near the far end of the wharf.

Sawyer shrugged. There were a million perfect places. This was Bangkok. A city where you could walk into any waterfront bar and hire a hit man for five hundred dollars U.S. He was wasting his time, he told himself, and had just started to signal the driver to head back to the New Road landing when he caught something out of the corner of his eye.

Dammit, that was the trouble with having only one eye, he cursed mechanically. After a while, you learned to compensate for the depth perception, but there was no way to make up for the fractional loss of peripheral vision or the partial blinder that your nose becomes on the bad side.

What he had seen was a hand-lettered sign on a small door in a metal shutter that closed off part of the warehouse, no doubt leading to an office. It had caught his attention because it looked like it was in French.

Turning casually as if to take a snapshot, he angled himself to get a better view, pointing the camera full into the sun like an idiot as he clicked. He turned away and told the driver to take them back to the landing. As they headed back, Sawyer hoped Somsukiri couldn't spot his excitement. Because the sign had read: COMITÉ NATIONAL POUR L'AIDE AUX RÉFUGIÉS KAMPUCHEANS.

And although he couldn't pin it down, the name rang a bell. Sawyer was sure he had heard it before somewhere. More to the point, Kampuchea—*Cambodia*—was what this thing was all about.

Of course, it might have meant nothing at all, he thought, trying to play devil's advocate, the position he was sure Harris, who hated hunch plays, would take. So somebody rented a little extra office space to a Cambodian refugee outfit. Bangkok was full of them. So what?

So nothing. Maybe it was just a coincidence, Sawyer thought, remembering how Koenig used to lecture them in that Quonset hut on the Farm. "There are no coincidences in this business. None," he used to say, slapping his ruler against the side of his leg as though it were a riding crop. "The minute you spot something that even smells like a coincidence, you've either struck pay dirt, or it's about to strike you. Either way, you'd better haul ass."

The hang-yao came into the landing with a faint bump. Sawyer paid the driver and followed Somsukiri up onto the landing. As they hurried back toward the car, Sawyer thought that it might be very interesting to find out who owned the Southeast Asia Rice and Trading Company.

The contact was set for a souvenir stall in the courtyard of Wat Po, the huge Temple of the Reclining Buddha. The stall sold good-luck amulets, joss sticks, carved elephants, and other such trinkets and was indistinguishable from the dozens of similar stalls clustered near the gate to the inner temple. The gate was made of stone and defended for eternity by intricately carved gilded Yaks, the fearsome spirit guards of the Other World. A teak elephant encrusted with bits of glass and tin hung from the left side of the woven awning over the stall, indicating that it was safe to approach, but still Sawyer hung back. There was something wrong, but he couldn't quite pin it down.

He had felt it before, this sense that somewhere just ahead was a booby trap with his name on it. Some called it "mission feel," but it had nothing to do with tradecraft. It's the thing that makes you jump when you're alone in the house at night and you hear a noise, and no one has to learn it. His instinct had picked up a danger signal too well hidden for his conscious mind to catch, and he didn't need Harris' warnings to keep clear of all established rdv's and safe houses to let him know he was in the red zone on this one. Which was why, when he had called the Snake Farm from a public phone in the Oriental Hotel lobby to get them working on the Southeast Asia Rice and Trading Company and the Kampuchean Committee, they had set up the rdv at the temple. Standard procedure, and as a big public attraction, it went with the tourist cover he had adopted for today. He should have been able to just walk in, exchange countersigns with the stall keeper and get the data. Everyday stuff. Except that the stall signaled that the approach was clear, but Sawyer's instinct told him it was hot.

It can't be hot, he reasoned with himself. He hadn't knocked on any doors yet. Except for Harris and Friends, no one even knew he was in Bangkok, and just to be on the safe side he had changed the image, swapping his eye-patch for sunglasses and tourist garb. And although the call to the Snake Farm had been an open call, it had been routed from there on a secure scrambled line to wherever the hell Barnes was. Max had handled it himself, because Sawyer had recognized his voice even through the faint distortion of the scrambler. So it was safe. All he was feeling was "buck fever." Sooner or later it happened to everyone, even old-timers on their hundredth mission into Indian Country, he told himself.

Except it was all horseshit, because his instinct—Sawyer always called it "the Reptile" because he had a pet theory that it was a part of the brain that had developed long before man was man, or even before we were mammals—was sounding the alarm for all it was worth.

So he did what they had learned to do in Nam. Stop. Look. Listen. Find the invisible trip-wire in the foliage, glistening with dew like a spider thread; because if you missed it, half your body could say good-bye to the other half, and if you were lucky, you wouldn't survive to see the letter your mother got from the president of the United States.

Although the Reptile was telling him to get out now, Sawyer methodically divided the courtyard into sectors and began to quarter each sector, first at ground level, then up. Back toward Jetupon Road the halls and huge towers, called prangs, swarmed like hives with monk trainees, vendors, and sightseers. From here he could see the great bell-shaped chedis that housed the ashes of the Chakri Royal House, encrusted with green and blue and white mosaic glistening in the afternoon sun. Near the paved walkway a monk and several Thais from the city in their white shirts and slacks meditated in the shade of a holy Bodhi tree, said to be descended from a seed of the original tree in whose shade Buddha attained enlightenment. Vendors along the walls and galleries sheltering hundreds of sitting Buddhas were selling joss sticks and amulets said to be especially efficacious for gamblers—Somsukiri had bought a handful of joss sticks there and was on his way over—and frustrated lovers.

In the center of the courtyard stood a large black lingam, its phallic shape symbolizing the Hindu god Shiva and the Yang force that is far more ancient than Buddhism. It was said to inspire fertility and was covered with orchids and paper prayer flags placed by childless women, one of whom knelt before it even now. Beyond the lingam, a guide was ushering a Japanese tour group, with their plastic badges and cameras, their drip-dry suits wilting in the heat, past the bronze lions guarding the gold-roofed bot, from which the sound of monks' chanting could be heard.

Everything was as it should be, Sawyer thought. There was no one more interested in him than in saving a few satang on the price of a plastic Buddha, nor was any local at a noodle stall more interested in his copy of *Siam Rath* than he should be. It was clean, dammit, and yet, if anything, the Reptile's signal was getting stronger. He had to do something. Not even mad dogs and Englishmen would just stand there in the blazing afternoon sun taking snapshots of the pigeons clustering on the carved eaves of the gateposts near the rice stalls. As was the custom, Sawyer had purchased a handful of rice and dropped it in the begging bowl of a young apprentice monk sitting in the lotus position near the contact stall. As he dropped it in, the monk had murmured "Khob khun khrap" and—

Sawyer's blood froze.

A Buddhist monk never thanks anyone! By accepting alms he allows the giver to acquire merit.

Sawyer started to turn back toward the monk, but it was too late. The monk was already pulling an air pistol out of the folds in his robe. Sawyer cried a warning as he dived sideways, but it was like watching an accident happen—everything seeming in slow motion, yet no way to stop it—as Somsukiri came up to him, smiling and holding his lucky joss sticks. Somsukiri suddenly straightened at the sting of the dart in his back. He whirled and started to slap at it, as at a mosquito. Then they were both running toward the monk, who raising the skirt of his robe, scampered on bare legs toward the inner temple gate.

Somsukiri started to head him off, still trying to clutch at his back and then Sawyer saw him slow, still pumping hard, but the legs moving heavily as if he were wading. Almost at the gate, Sawyer watched him try to draw his gun, not realizing he hadn't worn it, the legs caving, and then he was down. As the monk leaped over him toward the gate, Somsukiri was still trying to crawl. Sawyer wondered what was keeping him going. Somsukiri started drifting sideways, his movements out of synch like a broken toy. And then he just stopped and lay down on his side.

Somsukiri's eyes were already glazing over in the second or two that it took Sawyer to reach him. They held the dark certainty that he was about to die, and Sawyer didn't try to sugarcoat it by telling him he'd be okay, which Somsukiri wouldn't have believed anyway. He owed the young Thai that much. Somsukiri's lips moved, but no sound came out. His eyes looked desperately down. He was going. Sawyer felt like an idiot for not knowing what he wanted. In desperation he tore at the Thai's shirt because that was where he had looked. And then he saw it. Hoping he had enough time, he grabbed the little hai-huang Buddha amulet that hung around Somsukiri's neck and put it into the Thai's mouth.

Somsukiri felt it and looked gratefully up at Sawyer. At least he would not go to the Lord of Death emptyhanded. And then he died. Before he had stopped breathing, Sawyer was already up and sprinting through the temple gate where the monk had disappeared.

Just before he entered the Hall of the Reclining Buddha, he remembered to kick off his shoes—he didn't need a Buddhist lynch mob after him for desecrating the shrine—and dropped down to a crawling position. Fortunately, because as he came through the door he heard the whispered snick of another flechette splitting the air where his chest would have otherwise been. Before the monk could reload, Sawyer scuttled sideways on all fours like a crab, then dived behind a massive stone pillar. Hidden in the shadow, he tried to catch his breath and figure something out.

That was pretty goddamn stupid, he cursed himself, trying to blink the sweat out of his eye. Just because he's a punk kid doesn't mean he can't take you out. That was the mistake some of the green American troops used to make in Nam. Because they were big and strong and had muscles like John Wayne, they couldn't believe that some runty teenaged gook in oversized black pajamas could blow them away before breakfast. He's already killed Somsukiri and probably the first tail too, so he's plenty good and you'd better watch your ass, Sawyer thought, starting to edge his way around the pillar.

Take him alive, Sawyer told himself. He's the way in if you can sweat him—and if he doesn't get you first. Moving carefully now, head low, trying to think only of tactics and not about the question starting to nag at him: What kind of Thai—no, he couldn't be Thai—of Southeast Asian wouldn't have known how a monk is supposed to behave?

Don't think about that now, Sawyer thought. He's had time to reload that thing. Peering around the pillar for a second, just long enough for his good eye to catch a glimpse of the vast half-lit hall shuttered against the afternoon heat. At the far end was one of the most awe-inspiring sights on earth, the great Reclining Buddha, half the length of a football field in size and covered in gold leaf, bathed in golden rays of light seeping through the lattices and filling the hall with its glow. Despite its massive size, the stupendous figure seemed almost to float above the ground. Although stylized, as all Buddhas were, it was strangely lifelike, every fold of its robe artfully designed to convey the reality of the exquisite moment when the Enlightened One glided into nirvana. But Sawyer's thoughts were far from enlightenment. He had picked out the monk's silhouette lurking in the shadows near the giant soles of the Buddha's sandals.

There were a few monks and other worshipers all around the hall in various postures of meditation, and along the walls, dim bas-reliefs from the *Ramakien*, the Thai version of the Hindu *Ramayana*. The rest was empty space. But getting close wasn't the problem, Sawyer figured. The effective range of the air gun couldn't be more than twenty feet or so. The kid—no, don't think of him that way; "We're in an inhuman business," Koenig used to say. "Humanize your enemy and he'll blow your brains out"—the phony monk would let him get close. He wouldn't have time to reload for a second shot, so he'd want to be sure.

Except it didn't matter, because the monk was good. He'd already proved that. He wouldn't miss the first shot. So the problem wasn't getting close. The problem was how to cross an open space and get so close he couldn't get a shot off before he realized what was happening. What made it even harder, of course, was that the monk was just waiting there like a spider for Sawyer to come within his killing range.

The only way was to come in contrary to the monk's expectations, Sawyer decided. The monk would probably fire low to be sure of a body shot, so he would come in high. He would anticipate him coming straight on, so he would have to come in around the corner. And he would have to change his image. If he could make the monk hesitate for even a fraction of a second over whether he was shooting the real target, it might make all the difference. And just to make life interesting, he added, he had to do it without attracting attention to himself. Both because the monk would zero in on him otherwise and because he was on holy ground in a kingdom that took religion more seriously than American football coaches take winning.

Sawyer briefly debated going back outside and buying a change of shirt from a vendor, but rejected the idea. Right now he had the monk spotted. Once he left, the bastard might go anywhere. So that was out. But he had to change the image somehow.

He looked around the hall, but no one was paying attention to him. The Thais were meditating in the tranquil dimness, the golden light suggesting an eternal twilight. Nearby, an old man in ragged clothes sat on his haunches facing the Eternal. His eyes were downcast. His hands made the wai sign to his forehead. He was motionless as a statue. Behind him he had placed a weather-beaten straw hat. Sawyer took the hat, leaving a five-hundred-baht note in its place. Perhaps the old man would take it as a sign that his prayers had been heard, Sawyer thought.

He took off his sunglasses and left the eye-patch off. Then he took off his gaudy yellow shirt that he had worn loose, turned it inside out and put it back on, tucking it in this time, and put on the hat. When he was ready, he took a deep breath and moved from behind the pillar toward the distant head of the Buddha in an obeisant crouch, his head bowed and his hands in the wai sign over his face.

He padded forward, glancing left and right, but no one paid him any attention. In his stocking feet he hardly made a sound. As he approached, the staggering size of the Buddha began to fill his range of vision. He was the only thing moving. He felt very exposed.

Just then he caught a movement in the dim recesses near the Buddha's feet. He'd been spotted. The Reptile was telling him to dive for cover, but he ignored it and kept going. A crouched-over figure in a straw hat was all the monk could have seen, Sawyer told himself. The monk was just popping out to check. He couldn't be sure yet.

Now he was at the great golden head, craning his neck to stare up at the caste mark on the Buddha's forehead in the place where the third eye is said to be. An iron spike-topped fence ran around the statue, preventing anyone from getting close enough to defile the great Buddha by touching it. It ran back to the rear wall of the bot, so he couldn't try to come around behind the statue. He would have to come all the way across the front of the statue from left to right. But how could he cover the open distance down the entire length without the monk seeing him?

Then he remembered something. The monk wasn't a true Buddhist. It was impossible that he not see Sawyer, but he might not know what he was seeing. It wasn't great, but he couldn't think of anything better. And he had to do something fast. Som-sukiri's body was no doubt attracting attention out there the way garbage attracts flies, and before too long he'd have to spend a week playing tic-tac-toe with the Bangkok police and never get a shot at a Company-style interrogation of the monk.

Sawyer took a deep kokyu no henko breath to calm his emotions, because it was like jumping from an airplane. Once you took that first step, there was no going back.

Sawyer shuffled in an obeisant crouch toward the Buddha's feet for a few meters, then sank down in a head-to-earth bow. He waited for a minute, then got up and repeated the process, working his way down the Buddha's length as if in fulfillment of some private vow. It wasn't normal Buddhist practice, but the phony monk might not know that. He'd already made one mistake about that. Sawyer fervently hoped so, because he was already at a fold in the Buddha's robe somewhere around the midsection.

Head bowed in meditation, he glanced out of the corner of his eye, but could see nothing near the feet. There was no way of knowing if the monk had changed position or had begun to notice him. Others had, though. He caught a glimpse of a monk staring wide-eyed at him, and others were beginning to watch. But no one made a move to interfere. Perhaps because of kreng chai, or because the essence of Theraveda Buddhism is that each man must find his own enlightenment and perhaps this was one individual's way along the Eightfold Path. But they watched as he got up and went on.

There was still no sign of movement from the monk. By now, Sawyer was near the folds draped over the Buddha's knees and there was no way he hadn't been seen. Something's wrong, he thought, getting up and moving a few meters closer to the giant soles of the Buddha's feet, each of them a good five meters long. Why hasn't he made a move? Sawyer wondered, his face beaded with sweat as though he had broken out in some horrible skin disease. Come on, you motherfucker. Where are you?

Don't kneel, charge, the Reptile was hissing in his ear as he sank down near the Buddha's ankles. He was within the air gun's range now, a sitting duck if the monk made his move. He bowed his head again, unable to keep his right side from twitching as it anticipated the prick of the poison dart. He waited, unmoving, counting each breath.

Still nothing. A sudden excitement began to stir in Sawyer. He's buying it, he thought, getting up and moving almost to the

Buddha's toes. The next move would take him around the corner and he'd know for sure, one way or the other.

Head bowed for the last time, he rehearsed the sequence in his head: how he would use the fence and a diversion, because ready or not, it would be a matter of hundredths of a second either way. He heard a quiet sigh that might have come from anywhere in the vast hall or from the great Buddha himself. He felt a prickling at the back of his neck. The tiny hairs were standing on end.

And then it didn't matter because he was moving at a flat run around the Buddha's toes, and in a single instant he saw it all, the lone ray of light from a crack in the ceiling lattice embedded in the floor at the monk's feet like a spear, the 108 symbols inlaid on the Buddha's giant soles in mother-of-pearl, and the monk's death's-head grin as he stood ready, a good ten feet away, not fooled for a second by the stupid farang, his gun aimed right at Sawyer's belly.

Sawyer didn't have even an instant for despair—there was no time for it or for anything except the sequence. He feinted to the right with a slight lurch, sailing the straw hat at the monk like a frisbee, anything to distract his aim, even as he leaped up to the left, using the fence spike to lever himself up and kicking out with his right foot in a flying tiuchaki. The blood was roaring in his ears and he never heard the pop of the air gun, only the slight tug at his pant leg as the flechette hit the fabric.

He wasn't sure whether he'd been hit or not. All he could do was finish the kick and—

He saw the flechette. It hadn't hit his leg. The bastard had anticipated him going down, not up, and had aimed low, Sawyer thought exultantly.

But he missed the kick and stumbled as he fell forward, the monk dancing out of the way. For a moment Sawyer teetered on one foot, almost losing it and always conscious of the flechette embedded in the fabric, twisted sideways and plucked it out and away as he fell over and rolled toward the monk. Then they were both up, the monk backed against the iron fence, his black eyes darting back and forth like a cornered animal. He pointed the gun at Sawyer's chest. Sawyer held his hands up as if believing the threat and starting to back away, left foot behind his right and into the feint that Koichi always used to say was Sawyer's best, pivoting on the right foot and whirling into a spinning back kick to the monk's knee.

The monk went down. Sawyer scrambled on top of him. The monk tried to club Sawyer with the gun butt, and Sawyer just brushed it away with a forearm block. No clever tae kwan doe moves now. He simply jammed his thumbs into the monk's throat and pounded his head against the stone floor, the killing rage on him and only somewhere a faint voice reminding him not to waste the little bastard.

The monk's face had swollen tomato red, and Sawyer was just about to haul the son of a bitch to his feet when he was hit with a savage blow to the side of the head. The great Buddha started to topple over. An octopus wrenched him off the monk. Sawyer held up his arms to shield himself and clear his head. Then all at once the world righted itself for a second, and he realized that a crowd of Thais were beating him for attacking a holy monk.

Others helped the monk to his feet. He stood shakily for a moment, gathering his robe around him. His eyes were slits. His face was an impassive mask; a mottled red necklace showed where Sawyer's fingers had been. Some in the crowd were calling for the police, and there were dark mutters against the farang who had desecrated the shrine.

Sawyer tasted blood in his mouth as two husky Thais hauled him roughly to his feet. For an instant, through the crowd his eyes met those of the monk's, gleaming with triumph, and Sawyer, feeling sick to his stomach, knew the little bastard was right. He had blown the mission even before it had begun.

A Bangkok policeman came over and, puffing his chest out like a pigeon to assert his authority, began to jabber something to the monk, both of them looking suspiciously over at Sawyer and then at a teenaged boy who had picked up the air gun and was examining it with great curiosity. The policeman held out his hand for the gun, but before the boy could hand it over, the monk darted away and grabbed it out of the boy's hand. The monk ran straight for the temple gate, shoving bystanders out of the way, the gun clutched to his chest.

The crowd buzzed, confused. They stared after the monk. For the moment no one was paying attention to Sawyer, who was still held by the two Thais. Someone said something. The policeman started to come over, and Sawyer knew it was the only chance he was going to get.

Sawyer sidekicked the knee of the man on his right, knocking him over like a bowling pin. His right hand freed, Sawyer hooked his fist into the midsection of the man on his left. The policeman tried to stop him, but Sawyer just barreled over him like a running back on fourth and goal to go, and then he was running like crazy through the crowd, too quickly for them to react.

He blinked blindly in the brilliant light outside, hesitating for a second over which way to go. Then he saw people looking over toward the great prangs and chedis as if watching after someone. As he pounded across the burning hot stone pavement in his stocking feet, Sawyer spotted a crowd clustered around the place where Somsukiri still lay.

The little bastard was fast, Sawyer thought, weaving across the courtyard toward the corner of the great golden bot. He was starting to get winded and hoped to God the monk would trip or something because otherwise . . . He rounded a corner fence post, intricately carved and leafed over with gold, and saw something that made him stop dead in his tracks.

A long line of young monks in identical curry-colored robes was filing into the massive golden chedi of King Rama the Third. It reminded Sawyer of Koenig's famous "purloined letter" lecture, the one that ended with the line about how the best place to hide a suitcase was in the luggage department. What better place for a monk to hide than a monastery? Sawyer thought. After all, he had seen the monk only twice, very briefly, and in those instants his attention had been focused on the gun. If the monk played it cool, Sawyer wasn't sure he'd be able to pick him out of all the other monks.

Except he won't play it cool, Sawyer thought. He's an impulse player; the business with the gun proved that. You don't have to identify him; he'll identify himself once he sees you. Just check near the end of the queue. Suppose he's had a chance to reload and you walk right up to him? What then? the Reptile whispered, and Sawyer didn't have any answer for that.

Nothing happened. Sawyer didn't spot the monk and the monk never broke ranks. But the crowd from the Hall of the Reclining Buddha was heading this way, and he had to do something fast. Sawyer, trying to look as inconspicuous as a five-foot-ten-inch farang can look at the end of a line of Buddhist monks all under five foot five, filed past carved teak doors inlaid with pearls and into the chedi.

Hundreds of chanting monks were seated in the huge circular hall like a field of talking yellow flowers. Along the curving walls, frescoes showed scenes from Buddha's life. A golden Buddha sat enthroned on an altar rising like a miniature mountain peak from the clouds of smoke from hundreds of burning joss sticks. Sawyer sensed a stirring as, one by one, the monks began to look his way. He began to back away and look for a side exit, because not only was he an intruder, but not even Sherlock Holmes could have found one monk among so many.

But if he couldn't spot the monk, he was himself spotted. There was a slight commotion near the side door that led to the towering white stone prang adjoining the chedi. And then Sawyer spotted the monk, still clutching the gun, barging through the doorway.

You couldn't hold your water, could you, you green son of a bitch? Sawyer thought, leaping over a seated monk lost in meditation. He ran around the circumference of the hall. Behind him the chedi began to buzz, but Sawyer by then was through the doorway. He charged up the circular stone staircase that wound around a giant central pillar that must have been at least fifty meters high.

His breath was getting shorter as he pounded up the stairs, round and round in the dizzying heat. Watch it! He's had a chance to reload, he told himself, stopping now and again to catch his breath and to listen for footsteps above. But either he was too far behind, or he couldn't hear over his own heavy breathing.

And then he heard something. A tapping sound. But coming downstairs instead of up, getting closer, as if something were rolling down the—

Sawyer began moving back down the stairs in great leaps. He bounced off the circular outside walls, pushing off with his hands, tripping and recovering, racing down, relentlessly pursued by that clicking just around the corner behind him and coming faster.

The explosion was almost deafening in the confined space

of the stairwell. Burning hot fragments of the grenade rattled against the stone stairs and walls like hail, one of them skipping off the step Sawyer was on. He waited only a second. His ears still ringing, Sawyer began the long climb back up. This time he did it slowly. When he started to think again, he had realized that once the monk got to the top of the tower, where could he run?

Now he paused more frequently, husbanding his strength and listening for a footfall on the stair around the corner. The one good thing was that in his stocking feet he made virtually no sound at all. Suddenly he stopped.

He sensed something just around the next turn. It wasn't a sound. He heard nothing, not even breathing. Only the distant buzz of voices somewhere far below. And then he realized what it was. A slight bump in the shadow of the pillar against the outer wall.

Sawyer's heart pounded against his chest as if it wanted to come out. The monk was waiting there with that thing cocked.

With a savage growl, Sawyer popped around the turn like a jack-in-the-box, catching a blurred glimpse of the waiting monk, the air gun, the motes of dust floating in the light slanting through the scrollwork on the outer wall, before he jumped back down. The dart clattered against the outer stonework, and Sawyer was already pounding back up the stairs, taking them two and three at a time, feeling it in his thighs and hoping they wouldn't give way. The monk's feet were just ahead of him. He grabbed for the ankles, missed, fell down and got back up again. Coming around the next turn, he found the monk, his chest heaving, trapped against the wall next to an arched opening to a narrow ledge outside. The ledge led nowhere. It was a good hundred feet high. Through the sunny opening Sawyer could see the spires and carved eaves of the entire temple complex and, far below, the toylike people and gray paving stones shimmering in the appalling heat. The two men looked at each other.

Sawyer moved into a fighting stance.

The monk's eyes were black with hate. They had the look of a snake when it's pinned by a forked stick. All at once, the monk's expression changed. His eyes acquired a strange shine, as if seeing something that had been hidden from them before.

Sawyer had seen that look before. He started to move forward. The word "Yoot" escaped his lips, but it was already too late.

The monk had dived straight through the opening. Sawyer got there just in time to see him rocket headfirst onto the paving stones below. The head disintegrated with a horrible *splat*, and even as it happened, Sawyer knew that he would be hearing that sound, like a sack of wet clothes hitting the ground, in the silences of the night for a long time to come.

5

*Thunder within the mountain
explodes from the volcano.
The superior man controls his
    mouth;
what comes out of it
and what he puts into it.*

B Y the time Eddie Macbeth missed the second rdv at Mother
Grace's, Sawyer knew he was in trouble. Langley rules
were that if a scheduled rdv is missed, you try again at
the same place exactly one hour and ten minutes later.
And if you don't connect then, you abort.

Except that Langley rules weren't made for someone like
Eddie, who had stringy hair that hadn't been washed for a year
down to his shoulders, one gold earring that he fancied made him
look like a pirate but actually made him look like a vaguely psy-
chotic homosexual, a thin nervous face that might have been handsome if you added twenty pounds and subtracted as many years,
and a brain three-quarters fried by some of the purest heroin known
to man.

Besides, Mother Grace's bar in the Village in Ban Phattaya
was the closest thing to an address Eddie had. So instead of aborting, Sawyer decided to stick around, figuring that if Eddie was
still functioning, sooner or later he would show.

Sawyer signaled the Chinese bartender for another Singha
beer and stared gloomily at his reflection in the mirror behind the
bar. In the red neon light the eye-patch made him look sinister,

which was almost normal here, he thought, using the mirror to check the room. One of the bargirls started to get up hopefully, but he shook his head and she went over to join her friends at the table of two young American sailors in civvies, their fresh red faces, peach fuzz haircuts, and service shoes making them dead giveaways. They were looking for a story to tell their shipmates, and Sawyer was sure they'd have one because it was five to one that, come morning, they'd never see their wallets again.

An American flag hung behind the bar, the neon light turning the red stripes purple. The uncanny tug of déjà vu made him very uneasy. It was like the Vietnam days when all the married guys on R 'n' R wanting beach went to Hawaii and all the single ones came to Ban Phattaya. Or maybe it was the young Thai with the tray of what looked like Christmas-colored candy, saying "Fi' dollah, you see dragon," that brought it all back. At the other end of the bar were a couple of American vets, deposited on the beach like wreckage after a naval battle, living off their VA checks and still arguing about whether General Westmoreland knew about the NLF build-up before Tet in 'sixty-eight.

Reruns, Sawyer thought. All they're showing are reruns, and if there was anyone interested in him except the girls who hadn't made their quota for the night, he couldn't spot it. But he had to assume they were looking for him, despite everything Harris and Bhamornprayoon had done to smooth over the incident at Wat Po.

All the damage had been blamed on the phony monk, and as for the mysterious farang desecrator, they had even found a fall guy in the person of a middle-aged American tourist sentenced to a year in a Bangkok jail for the inexcusably stupid act of tearing up a twenty-baht note in a fit of pique over an excessive taxi fare, thereby insulting the king of Thailand, whose sacred picture was printed on the money. In exchange for confessing to the crime at Wat Po temple—committed while he was in jail—the American tourist was sentenced to be deported to San Francisco, where presumably he would entertain his friends with the story of how it was possible to become a major criminal simply by getting into the wrong taxi.

But although Sawyer's part in the affair at Wat Po had been covered up, Harris had been furious. His hands clasped behind his back like Napoleon reviewing his troops, he stood rigidly at the window of the Pasteur Institute office at the Snake Farm, watching a quick-handed attendant milk a banded krait into a glass vial.

"Irresponsible. Absolutely irresponsible. Especially in light of the situation here," Harris said, not looking at Sawyer.

"The stall was flying the safe sign," Sawyer said.

That shut Harris up. It was Harris' screw-up at the temple and they both knew it. The safe sign is supposed to be sacrosanct. Making sure it was safe was how a senior case officer earned his salary. And it couldn't have happened unless communications were leaking like a sieve, also Harris' responsibility.

Sawyer got up and stood beside Harris. For a moment, the two of them stared through the glass at the cobras and kraits gliding lethargically over each other in the stifling temperature. When Harris turned to Sawyer, his sweating face was beet red, although Sawyer couldn't tell if it was embarrassment or just the heat.

"We're working on that," Harris admitted.

"Terrific. That's like the captain of the *Titanic* saying he's going to send out a party with bailing buckets."

Harris turned even redder. But he was smart enough not to say anything. He stared at the tangled snakes as though they formed a knot that could somehow be unraveled. His shoulders sagged, and when he looked back at Sawyer, his eyes were shiny with sincerity.

"We're stymied, Sawyer. Did you ever feel like you were in a chess game where your opponent says, 'You can't move that piece.' "

Sawyer massaged the skin at the side of his bad eye and tried to think. They were handing it to him, and he wasn't sure he wanted it. Be careful, he warned himself. With Harris, honesty is just another ploy. Finally, he just threw it out.

"The whole thing is cockeyed, Bob. We don't even know who the Opposition is, or what they want. Or what kind of an Asian is it who knows how to use poison flechettes, but not how a Buddhist monk behaves?" Sawyer said.

Harris sighed heavily, like a husband whose wife has her heart set on a dress he knows he can't afford and knows he's going to have to buy anyway.

"What do you want, Sawyer?"

"I'm on my own from here on out."

Harris looked at him curiously.

"It's what you wanted all along, isn't it? The file is right about you, Sawyer. You're just not a team player."

"It helps to know who's on my team," Sawyer said, and was gratified to see Harris redden at that.

"What else?"

"We've got a leak. So from now on, no standard communications drops or rdv's. No embassy, no Snake Farm, no more so-called intermediary lines. Just you and me. Private line."

Harris nodded again.

"Anything else?"

"Yeah. Who owns the Southeast Asia Rice and Trading Company?"

Harris' face expressed impatience.

"Look, why don't you just get on with the damn mission instead of going off on these wild-goose chases? We don't have time for this shit."

"You mean like Parker did, huh?"

Harris recoiled, as though he had been slapped. Then he looked away, obviously not convinced.

"And you still haven't answered my question," Sawyer added.

Harris exaggerated a sigh.

"We're working on it. It's a tangle. Holding companies owned by other holding companies. We've tracked it from Bangkok to Hong Kong to Macao back to Bangkok so far, and we have to be careful with our inquiries, you know."

This time it was Sawyer who sighed theatrically.

"Save the bedtime stories for the kiddies, Bob. Just tell me who owns the fucking company."

Harris smiled unwillingly, as though in spite of himself he had chosen the right bloodhound for the job.

"It looks like a wealthy businessman. Name of Vasnasong. As a matter of fact, I think you might've seen him at Lady Caroline's party. But I think you're barking up the wrong tree, Sawyer," Harris burst out.

"Oh?"

"Don't give me that crap, Sawyer. We checked out Vasnasong long ago. He's pro-Western, pro-Thai monarchy. Wealthy pro-

Capitalist. Very well connected. Done favors for MI6 and us, I might add. Besides, what's his motive? He has everything, and anything he doesn't have we'd be happy to give him."

"You know, Bob, some people in our business might call that 'deep cover,'" Sawyer said mildly.

Harris looked sharply at Sawyer. He tapped his forefinger thoughtfully against his lip. All at once, Sawyer could see in him the Ivy League wunderkind he was supposed to have been.

"It's possible. We'll have to look into that," Harris muttered, still tapping his lip.

"No, don't! We can't afford it," Sawyer said.

Harris looked straight into Sawyer's good eye and nodded once. The nod meant he not only understood what Sawyer was driving at but that he had reversed his position and agreed. The advantages were obvious. Because what Sawyer was implying—which was that the local CIA Bangkok station apparatus could no longer be considered reliable—not only explained everything that had happened, it also took Harris off the hook for the screw-up.

"What about that Cambodian refugee outfit?" Sawyer asked.

"This is the first we've heard about them," Harris admitted, looking troubled.

There was something wrong with that, Sawyer thought. He knew it was wrong the way you know something's changed when your lover kisses you and it's different, although you can't say what the difference is. Only he couldn't say it because he wasn't even sure at this point if Harris was a part of it or not. So he contented himself with an admission of his own.

"It's all bits and pieces. It's not a mission; it's like the wreckage of a mission. I feel like one of those paleontologists, trying to piece together a dinosaur from odds and ends. A tooth here, a bit of toe there. There's a missing piece somewhere and that's the way in," Sawyer said.

Harris nodded slowly.

"How will you know?"

"By finding out who got to the missing second tail, Sergeant Tarasang," Sawyer said.

The attendant suddenly slapped the snake he was milking and jerked his head back. There was something about the way he did it that made Harris smile.

"You'll need a local contact in Phattaya," Harris said, still watching the attendant and the snake.

"Max suggested Eddie Macbeth."

Harris' handsome face looked pained, as though he had just stepped in something left behind by a dog.

"You know him?"

"Just keep him on a tight leash. Don't let him do any thinking, if slime like that is capable of thought," Harris said.

"How'd he get the nickname 'Macbeth'?" Sawyer asked, wondering at Harris' reaction. Who the hell did Harris expect to find in a honky-tonk Asian beach town, Snow White?

Harris raised his eyebrows in surprise.

"I thought everyone in Nam had heard that one. It even made the papers briefly before the marine brass could squash it."

"Must've happened after I left," Sawyer shrugged.

Harris nodded.

"It was a Stars and Striper in Eye Corps who came up with the nickname. You know the type. English major. Copy sprinkled with literary allusions. Anyway, the story was that when Eddie was a second looie, he fragged his captain to take over command of the company. Just like in Shakespeare."

"How come he wasn't court-martialed?"

Harris shrugged again.

"The Corps was dying to nail him, but there wasn't a thing they could do. The whole company swore that at the time somebody dropped a grenade in the captain's hootch, Eddie was in the CP with nothing more lethal in his hand than a can of Coke."

"Maybe he didn't do it."

"Oh, he did it all right. Everybody knew he did it. But it was touchy. Very touchy. A lot of people felt the captain deserved it."

"What happened?"

"The company had just taken eighty-five percent casualties after three days of murderous fighting to take some hill near the Rockpile. The VC had honeycombed the place with caves and tunnels like an anthill. It was a mess and by the time the marines took it, Eddie was the only officer still walking. Then the choppers came and airlifted what was left of the company off the top of the hill. Two days later this captain ordered Eddie to take the survivors and some green replacements and retake the same fucking hill. It seems that after the marines had been evac'd out, the VC just infiltrated back. I guess Eddie just couldn't see the point," Harris said.

"After a while it got a little hard for anybody to see the point," Sawyer agreed, staring through the glass at a cobra twining around another rearing cobra as though creating a medical symbol.

"Anyhow, there wasn't another officer available, so they had to give the company to Eddie. That's when the Stars and Striper coined the nickname and it stuck. It was in all the papers."

"Are you saying not to use him?" Sawyer demanded.

"I'm saying if something happens to Macbeth, nobody's going to lose any sleep over it," Harris said in a tone that gave Sawyer the creeps.

They watched the snakes through the glass. Finished, the attendant cautiously backed away. As he passed, the snakes stirred softly upright, swaying in the heat like silent deadly flowers.

Sawyer wiped the beer froth from his mouth and tried to remember if there had been anything in his meeting with Macbeth at the cockfight earlier that evening, anything to justify Eddie not making the rdv at Mother Grace's. Christ knows he had made it clear from the start that he was keeping Eddie on a very short string.

"I'll be there, Sawyer. Don't be an old lady." Eddie had grinned, showing a gaping mouthful of discolored teeth, stained and tilted haphazardly like tombstones in an old cemetery.

"That's a comfort, Eddie," Sawyer replied, a roar from the crowd distracting him for a moment. In the pit the two cocks, one a pure black, the other a black speckled with green, flew at each other in a flurry of feathers. The black's spur got twisted as he landed, and he tried to hop out of striking distance. The crowd buzzed as the green leaped again, bloodying the black. It was only a matter of time.

Although the fight hadn't ended, the betting for the next match had already started. Sawyer glanced around the ring as if looking for a wager, then down at the neatly slicked hair on the back of Sergeant Tarasang's head, three rows below him. Tarasang got up and turned so Sawyer could see his face. Tarasang was smiling broadly and waving a thick wad of bahts at the Chinese bookie standing in the aisle. Tarasang seemed to have no idea they were interested in him.

All around, the stands were filled with Thais and Chinese shouting bets, kids peddling cigarettes and drinks, and women in warpaint peddling something else. The heat was intense enough to melt metal, and the air was thick with noise and smoke and cock crows, the endless tumult of Asia.

"I said I'll be there. I always come through, don't I?" Eddie said truculently. His pupils were needle points. A nerve along the side of his jaw began to twitch, and Sawyer wondered how soon it would be before Eddie would have to have his next fix.

"I found Tarasang, didn't I?" Eddie insisted. When Sawyer didn't reply, the nerve in Eddie's jaw began pulsing like a line on an oscilloscope.

"You've got a big mouth, Eddie. In our business, that's not an asset," Sawyer observed.

In the pit the green was pecking viciously at the black's eyes to finish him off. The crowd roared its encouragement. Eddie looked straight at Sawyer, but his mind was up a dark alley some-where else.

"Don't threaten me, Sawyer. Everybody knows you can't threaten Macbeth," Eddie replied, his hand going to his pocket where Sawyer knew he kept a switchblade.

Sawyer didn't even tense. In Eddie's vacant eyes he had al-ready seen that whatever had flamed inside the young marine lieu-tenant had long since burned out on Phattaya beach.

Time to jerk the string, Sawyer thought. He needed to know where Tarasang was getting his money. Who had bought him off? It wasn't complicated and it wasn't difficult. God knows, it had been easy enough to find Tarasang. Ban Phattaya was too small a town for a newcomer like Tarasang not to be noticed. And it was a town for noticing people. Even the fat Germans turning lobster red around the palm-lined pool at the Phattaya Palace and endlessly complaining about the verdammt slow service were noticed.

Eddie Macbeth's job was to find out what was the crooked cop's hot button. Dope, girls, money. Odds-on, money, Sawyer had coached Eddie. Tarasang would probably ask around and find out that Macbeth was what used to be called a "serviceable farang." Then all Eddie had to do was lead him like a Judas goat—"Tell him it's a quick couple of thousand American and have him meet you," Sawyer had told Eddie—to someplace where Sawyer could sweat him. And show up on time, Sawyer thought irritably.

Down around the pit, there were good-humored catcalls and frenetic wagering as the disgusted owner dragged out the dead black and handlers showed the next pair of cocks to each other to get their blood up.

"What're you gonna do, Eddie? Frag me?" Sawyer said, deliberately provoking a dangerous spark in Eddie's eyes. "Don't you get it, asshole? Somebody like you breaks the law a hundred different ways just by breathing in and out. The last time they cold-turkey'd a junkie in the farang section of the Bangkok prison, he thought he was being attacked by a million spiders and gouged his own eyes out with his bare thumbs."

A roar went up from the crowd as the handlers swung the cocks toward each other like trapeze artists, then let them fly at each other, clawing savagely as they fluttered to the ground.

"You don't have to be such a hard guy, Sawyer. I'll be there," Eddie Macbeth whined, pulling his head defensively down to his shoulders like a tortoise into his shell. It was hard not to feel sorry for him, Sawyer thought. He had been a good soldier once, and maybe he had even thought he was being a good soldier, saving what was left of his outfit from an asshole CO, the day he became Macbeth. And then going home a junkie and getting it from the other side from a wife he couldn't talk to and pretty girls with long hair who wanted to know how many babies he had napalmed. But feeling sorry for Eddie was like mourning the deaths at Pompeii, Sawyer reminded himself. He had burnt away a long time ago, and the only thing that mattered anymore was that he do what they were paying him to do.

Except that Eddie Macbeth hadn't shown up at Mother Grace's, and Sawyer was starting to get a very bad feeling, even as he sat there nursing a Singha beer and watching the girls work the navy.

He motioned the bartender over. He was a small Chinaman with a set of absurdly white false teeth that gave him a headwaiter's smile. Sawyer ordered another Singha and put two five-hundred-baht notes on the bar.

"Have you seen Eddie Macbeth tonight?" he asked in English, raising his voice over the din of hard rock music from the disco next door.

"Who 'dis Eddie?" the bartender shrugged.

"Eddie Macbeth," Sawyer repeated, suggestively tapping the money.

"Eddie—you flend?" the bartender squinted suspiciously at Sawyer.

"Eddie's everybody's friend." Sawyer grinned and the bartender giggled. As they were laughing, the bartender pocketed the money slick as a gypsy.

"He good flend evelybody 'cept self him maybe." The bartender giggled again at his own wit. His false teeth were exactly even all the way across. They gleamed in the neon light like pink piano keys.

"Have you seen him tonight?"

"Him no come tonight."

"Maybe later?"

"Him no come tonight," the bartender shook his head firmly. He started to move down the bar.

"If he comes, tell him Morrison was looking for him," Sawyer called after him. They had chosen the name Morrison because Eddie, whose brain was still lost in the sixties, had been a big fan of Jim Morrison and the Doors.

The bartender came back.

"You Mollison?" he muttered suspiciously.

Sawyer nodded.

"Eddie say tell Mollison meet him by beach."

An icy chill shivered through Sawyer. Eddie Macbeth was breaking every rule in the book by passing messages in the clear through a civilian. Either Macbeth had lost the few marbles he still had left, in which case Sawyer would have his balls for breakfast, or he had been desperate.

"Who brought the message?" Sawyer asked.

But at this the Chinaman's face shuttered closed and he walked on down to the other end of the bar. By the time he reached it, Sawyer was already out the door.

The buzzing of the flies should have warned him. He had heard them clearly as he crouched behind a palm tree near the thatched

beach hut where Eddie sometimes crashed and where he was supposed to lure Tarasang. And Sawyer had known going in that it
could be—almost had to be—a trap. Padding along the shore in
his bare feet, his shoes in one hand and a ridiculously inadequate
NATO-issue 7.62mm Beretta with a silencer in the other—he'd
have to talk to Harris about getting him the Ingram M-10—
Sawyer had tried to find some excuse not to go in. Except that
there was a slim chance that the message had been a bona fide
distress signal from Macbeth, leaving him no real choice.

The beach was deserted so late at night, and despite the feeling
that he was exposed, he knew he was virtually invisible in the
darkness. The sand was still warm under his feet, and any noise
he might have made was masked by the sound of the waves. If
the Opposition was there, he was counting on being able to hear
them before they could hear him.

The night hung heavy with the suffocating heat that comes
in the last days before the monsoon. A crescent moon was a sliver
that cast almost no reflection on the sea. Along the surf line, small
breakers were rolling in like logs. Just beyond the reach of the
water lay overturned sunfish and wind-surfing boards, beached
like giant shells from the Mesozoic era. Dense dark foliage and
palms shielded the beach from the traffic along the shore road. In
the distance, he could see the lights of the Merlin shimmering in
the heat, as though the world was a normal place where the worst
a farang had to fear in these parts was sunburn or a case of "Thai
tummy." But just to be on the safe side, he crept into the foliage
to approach the hut from the tree side.

That's when he heard the flies. Maybe he would have waited
and figured it all out if he hadn't heard the crashing sounds of the
hut being ransacked and known he had to move—because there
still might be a chance for Eddie.

Coming around the tree, Sawyer saw two dark figures, gro-
tesquely elongated shadows in the smoky light of an old kerosene
lantern. They were pulling things apart, obviously searching for
something, and then one of them hissed something and straightened up. Whatever it was, he had found it. Coming through the
foliage, Sawyer knew he was making too much noise. He was
still hoping to surprise them. But they heard him.

In the split second as he approached the opening to the hut,
he saw one of them already heading out into the darkness on the

beach side as the other, the one who had found what he was looking for, was swinging around toward Sawyer, a Mark VII machine pistol in his hand. There were two other shadowy figures that Sawyer hadn't seen till now, lounging across a table from each other like cardplayers. There was no time to dodge or retreat with the Mark VII coming up, and as the first shots were fired, Sawyer rolled on the sand under the eaves. The Mark VII's shots were loud enough to wake the dead. They shredded the thatching above Sawyer's head. He rolled into a prone position, close enough to see the briefest flicker of panic in the Asian's eyes, and fired twice.

The Asian's head jerked back. The bullet had hit him in the eye, blasting a glob of blood and matter out of the back of the skull. The Asian crumpled backward, twitched once, and was still. Once again, the only sound was Sawyer's breathing, loud in his ears, and the nearby rumble of the surf.

Sawyer got slowly to his feet, wiping the sweat and sand from his good eye against his sleeve. Then he was up and could see it all and wished he couldn't.

The two seated figures were Eddie Macbeth and the missing Sergeant Tarasang. At least that's who Sawyer thought they were from their clothes, general appearance, and hair. Because there was no way to tell from the bloody masks swarming with flies that they wore instead of faces. Even if they weren't both dead, they couldn't have talked, Sawyer thought bitterly, because their tongues were among the various pieces of flesh displayed on the brass-topped table from Calcutta that had once been Eddie's pride and joy.

Sawyer felt sweat prickling all over his body. Bile rose in his throat, and all he wanted to do was get out of there. Then he remembered that the dead Asian had found what he had been looking for. He knelt over the Asian and pulled a crumpled piece of paper from fingers still warm and sticky with Eddie's blood.

It was with a sense of anticlimax that he unfolded the paper and read it in the dim light, as though he had known all along what it would be. It was a sight draft for twenty-five thousand baht made out to Sergeant Tarasang. It was drawn on a Bangkok bank and the payer was the Southeast Asia Rice and Trading Company.

Perhaps if he hadn't been so engrossed in trying to spell out the spidery Thai letters, he would have heard them sooner. From the shore road came the sound of a police siren, and he could hear the sounds of muffled orders outside the hut. It had been a trap after all.

Through the gaps in the thatch he could see dancing beams from flashlights as the police moved into position around the hut.

6

The sky above, the marsh below.
He has one eye and thinks he can
*   see well;*
he is lame and thinks he can walk
*   well.*
He treads on the tail of the tiger.

THE sampan stirred in the current like a restless sleeper. In the distance a temple bell tinkled once and was still. Night hung over the river; the air thick with the heat. Sawyer checked his watch one more time. The dial gave a zodiac glow in the darkness. The temple bell tinkled again, giving the illusion of wind. But it was just hot air rising, Sawyer thought. There would be no more wind till the coming of the monsoon.

He scanned the shadows along the wharf for the guard he had spotted earlier, and wondered if he wasn't pushing his luck too far. It was only by the skin of his teeth that he had escaped from the burning hut and the police.

"So you managed to get away. That was very clever of you," Vasnasong had said. He was grinning hugely as though it were all a big joke on him.

For an instant the mental image of the police surrounding the hut leaped into Sawyer's mind. He saw himself smashing the kerosene lamp against the wicker chair, the leaping flames, confusion and shouting in the darkness, as he slithered through the dense foliage. It didn't seem all that clever to him. Not very clever at all, he thought.

"Most excellent clever," Vasnasong repeated, still working hard on his smile like a maître d' trying to entice an uncertain couple into an otherwise empty restaurant. "You are better, I think, than the first one, this so-called Hawken-khrap."

Vasnasong was far too clever to try to pretend he knew nothing of Parker. But then, Vasnasong hadn't become one of the wealthiest men in Asia by being stupid, Sawyer reminded himself. He glanced around the teak-paneled office, almost shivering in the exquisite coolness of the air conditioning. The paneling, Danish modern leather-topped desks, and brass lamps gave the office the feel of a successful East Coast lawyer's office. But few law offices could have afforded the collection of Ming vases displayed on a teak credenza from one of Vasnasong's furniture factories. A pair of planters in the center of the room, a giant fern in the corner, and fresh-cut orchids in rare green Celadon ceramic vases helped soften the masculine austerity. Dominating the room was a stone bas-relief mounted on one wall. It was an apsara, a celestial dancer. The figure was nude from the waist up, except for an intricately carved necklace and crown, and possessed of that rare combination of willowy sensuality and otherworldliness characteristic of the best Khmer art. It was priceless, yet private. A voyeur's fantasy.

A number of framed photographs hung on the wall behind Vasnasong's desk. They were of Vasnasong and various heads of state, including one with de Gaulle, one with a former U.S. Secretary of State and one of Vasnasong being greeted by a smiling Chou En Lai and a troop of Chinese schoolgirls waving red flags of welcome. Apart, and in a place of honor, was a large picture of Vasnasong, head bowed in an impeccable posture of correctness, standing next to King Bhumibol. As Barnes had said, Vasnasong had "muchee squeeze."

One entire wall of the office was a single floor-to-ceiling plate glass window covered by a white gauzy curtain, with heavy gray silk curtains gathered at each end. Through the window, Sawyer could see the incredible vista of the teeming city stretching all the way to the horizon and, some twenty stories below, the river glittering like metal in the sun.

Sawyer looked down at the toylike figures of coolies loading a rice barge, as Vasnasong no doubt did from time to time, and thought of Vasnasong's painful inch-by-inch climb from the muck down there up to this office. "Started as a coolie," Barnes had remarked. It must have taken a relentless intelligence, none of which was remotely visible on the good-natured bespectacled face before him. Vasnasong seemed relaxed, his pudgy hands clasped comfortably on the mound of his belly. Sawyer was fascinated by his hands. When he talked, he would gesture with the grace of a temple dancer. His lips were fleshy and sensual. They wore an easy, almost self-satisfied smile that seemed to imply that it was a very fine thing to be a millionaire. Except that you couldn't let the modern skyscrapers fool you. This was Asia, Sawyer reminded himself. In the West we create our images in order to impress others; in Asia one creates one's image only to conceal.

Or was it only the expression around Vasnasong's eyes that were lined with good humor? The eyes themselves were unblinking as a carving, Sawyer noted, trying to put any sign of wariness out of his own eye. He thought about what they had done to Tarasang and Eddie Macbeth. Vasnasong would no more have a qualm about killing him than a tiger would feel a tinge of regret for his prey.

The two men faced each other with deadly attention completely masked by an air of lounging relaxation. They were both carnivores.

"So-called?" Sawyer asked, his eyebrows raised.

"His real name Pakah, yes?" Vasnasong smiled blandly, as though he was merely repeating what everyone in Bangkok already knew.

Sawyer kept the surprise out of his face. He'd used the technique of implying that he knew more than he really did too many times himself to give it away free to this son of a bitch.

"So you did see Parker that night," Sawyer said.

"Ah yes. We met at the Roxy Club. A very good fellow this Pakah-khrap, but also perhaps impetuous. I tried to warn him that the Golden Triangle was a most dangerous place, but he seemed not to mind. Mai pen rai, you understand?" Vasnasong said, tsk-tsking like a Chinese grandmother.

"Where is the superior man who lacks all faults?" Sawyer said carefully.

A hint of amusement flickered in Vasnasong's eyes.

"Let us be candid, Soyah-khrap. The man you seek was a fool," Vasnasong said, not bothering to complete the rest of the thought, which was the implied question, Are you going to be one as well?

"Unfortunately, Parker was engaged in matters of interest to our organization," Sawyer said, holding to the tattered shreds of his Red Cross cover.

"The Red Cross, of course." Vasnasong smiled.

"Of course." Sawyer smiled back. Vasnasong was good, he thought. So good he didn't bother to dispense with Sawyer's cover, though they both knew that nobody was fooling anybody.

"Tell me about Parker. What happened to him?"

Vasnasong leaned forward, sincerity shining in his eyes like faith in the eyes of a true believer.

"Of this I know nothing. Your Pakah-khrap is, as it is said when one knows nothing of another's fate, in the hands of the Lord Buddha."

"But you set up the contact."

"Excuse, dai prod?"

"Whom did you arrange for Parker to meet that night?"

"A most beautiful woman. One not to be forgotten easily, not even by old man like myself." Vasnasong smiled, his fleshy lips parting for a moment, then snapping shut like a trap.

It wasn't what he said, but the way he said it that jarred Sawyer. There was something obscene about it. For some reason it reminded Sawyer of that rdv in a Colombian brothel when he opened the wrong door and saw the pale faces of young children crouched in the darkness waiting to be summoned. Sawyer thought he had masked the thought, but Vasnasong picked up on it immediately.

"Ah, you disapprove, Soyah-khrap?"

Sawyer mentally cursed himself. You've got to do better, he thought, remembering Koenig's endless lectures: "Being a spook is like being an actor. Only if the critics don't like your performance, they'll kill you," he used to say.

"Mai pen rai. It is not for me to approve or disapprove anything. Besides, it is of no matter to me how any man takes his pleasure." Sawyer shrugged.

Vasnasong's eyes glittered.

"I fear you lie, Soyah-khrap. To you'self if not to myself. Ah yes," he continued, holding up an admonishing finger, "you see me and you think it is bad thing, this old man and beautiful young girl, like slug crawling on lotus flower. Such self-righteous! Such foolishness! How little you Europeans understand sex passion."

"Ah, the ancient wisdom of the mysterious Orient," Sawyer mocked, damned if he was going to let Vasnasong get to him.

"Not at all." Vasnasong smiled. "It is you Europeans who make mystery of man and woman. I remembered colored cards shaped like hearts I used to import for GI to send home to America. With little poems. I love you this. I love you that. What nonsense, Soyah-khrap. What is this to do with man and woman matters?"

"Come on, Vasnasong-khrap. Let's not make a religion out of something you can buy for a few hundred baht on any street in Bangkok," Sawyer said, grinning impudently.

Vasnasong sighed, patiently tapping the desk with his finger like a teacher with an obstinate pupil.

"You laugh, Soyah-khrap, but I see you heart. You are not of those who can rest content with half-truth, no matter how comfortable. You are of those who for truth would leave the world shattered behind you, gasping for breath like fish on the shore. Truly Soyah-khrap," Vasnasong said, looking sidelong at him, "you are dangerous man."

"And what is this great truth I feel sure you're about to impart?" Sawyer half-smiled. But Vasnasong was almost solemn.

"For herself, beautiful woman is one such as you or I. But for men, she is also image of all we desire, a living cinema; what our Lord Buddha calls 'tanha,' " Vasnasong paused. He looked sharply at Sawyer. "One thing you must to remember, Soyah-khrap. Sex is older than mankind."

"Chun mai kao chai."

"You understand most very good, Soyah-khrap. There is more truth in drake who pins duck by her neck to ground as he mounts her than in all the songs of love and colored heart-shape cards."

"Then if it's truth we're talking, tell me about the girl—and Parker," Sawyer said, an edge coming into his voice.

Vasnasong splayed his pudgy fingers in a helpless gesture.

"It was arranged she come to Roxy that night after I have gone. I myself left before she come. So you see, I am mystified as you, though why you not come to me from the first, this I do not understand." Vasnasong shrugged.

"We had no idea who Parker was meeting with that night," Sawyer admitted, hoping he sounded casual enough. Because the terrible implications of not knowing before about Vasnasong and Parker were beginning to harden his suspicions into a certainty. He opened another line of questioning to allay any suspicion Vasnasong might have that he was onto the scent.

"What about the girl? Who is she?"

"Ah, the girl." Vasnasong smiled. "That is some girl, believe me, Soyah-khrap. Her name—Suong. This means 'springtime.' Only this Springtime most special. She say she can put Pakah-khrap in touch with the warlord of the Shan, Bhun Sa, and also the Cambodian rebel leader, Mith Yon."

"Why Bhun Sa?"

"He has an army. Also much opium passes through he hands. Some say he have mountain of morphine base, all the opium of the third and best cutting, hidden across border. Maybe Burma-side. Maybe Lao-side. No one knows for certain. Most interesting, mm-hai?"

"Most interesting," Sawyer agreed. So Parker was going to work the deal through Bhun Sa, he thought. It made sense given the fact that Bhun Sa was rumored to control much of the opium trade in the Golden Triangle. He could cross borders at will, and a secret cache of morphine base of the size Vasnasong was talking about would be worth billions. It could finance the whole operation. And if he could add Bhun Sa's army to that of the Cambodian rebels, it would be a force that would keep the Vietnamese so tied up in Cambodia they wouldn't be able to even think of mounting an invasion against the Thais. No wonder Parker decided to go for broke, Sawyer thought excitedly.

"How did you find the girl?"

Vasnasong glanced at Sawyer with the kind of half-pitying, half-disgusted look corporate vice presidents use when a junior executive has just very publicly stuck his foot in his mouth.

"I don't find people, Soyah-khrap. They find me," Vasnasong said.

Sawyer lowered his head to make Vasnasong think he was acknowledging having lost face. The veil had dropped a fraction. He had caught a glimpse of the real Vasnasong.

"You mean a strange female calls you up, an important man like you, spins you some fairy tale about warlords in the

Golden Triangle, and you agree to face-to-face meetings just like that?"

"Ah yes, Soyah-khrap. I always listen," Vasnasong said, nodding agreeably.

"A female," Sawyer said, implying that it was most curious in patriarchal Asia for Vasnasong to do business with any female, especially one not of his own family.

"Ah yes," Vasnasong repeated, this time allowing condescension to show through his smile. "I will tell you story, Soyah-khrap, and perhaps you will understand.

"I began most poor, Soyah-khrap. Most poor. Europeans do not know of this kind of poor. But then the Lord Buddha smiled upon myself, and I began, with much difficulty, to acquire money.

"One day a female who is dear to me and is later to be wife to me tells me story. She has befriended farang acquaintance"— reading between the lines, Sawyer surmised that Vasnasong's wife had probably started as a Suriwongse-style hostess—"who is having most terrible difficulties with the Thai bureaucracy. This farang wishes to arrange for supply of Coca-Cola and other such things for United States soldiers when they come to Thailand for air bases and also for holiday time from war in Vietnam. Now it is well known, Soyah-khrap, that peoples in strange lands hunger for the food and drink of their native land. With help of this female, I persuade this farang for me to be agent, handle Thai bureaucrats who I know how to deal with," Vasnasong said, rubbing his thumb against his first two fingers in the universal sign for payoff money. "With result that soon I earn commission on every bottle of Coke, Pepsi, et cetera, sold in Thailand. Then we expand. Pretty soon we handle hamburgers, toothpaste, all manner of things for soldiers. Vietnam was very big war. Many soldiers, Soyah-khrap. Many Cokes and Pepsis.

"So you see, Soyah-khrap, I make many profits from listening to female who have story to tell," Vasnasong concluded solemnly.

"And I suppose you have no idea what happened to little Miss Springtime either?" Sawyer persisted.

Vasnasong shook his head, his eyes filled with an infinite sadness like those of Christ contemplating the sorry human spectacle.

"No, I don't, Soyah-khrap. But I fear you are not believe me."

Sawyer lounged insolently back in his chair.

"What about the late Sergeant Tarasang? Why was he on your payroll?"

A dangerous gleam appeared in Vasnasong's eyes, and Sawyer knew he had pushed it too far. Then Vasnasong smiled and the gleam disappeared as though it had merely been a trick of the light.

"I have many people I pay money to, Soyah-khrap. For information—and other things. But someone must have purchased this Sergeant Tarasang's loyalty before I. This Tarasang make no report for me. As for the draft from my company, it was, as you know, never cashed." Vasnasong shrugged.

He acted like none of it had anything to do with him, but this time Sawyer wasn't having any of it.

"Forgive my skepticism, Vasnasong-khrap, but that still doesn't explain Le Comité National Pour L'Aide Aux Réfugiés Kampucheans."

At this, Vasnasong looked confused and that really threw Sawyer off. He had said it just to rattle the tree and see what might fall out, but if he didn't know better, he could have sworn that he had finally shaken the old bastard, though he wasn't sure why. Whatever the reason, his question had acted like a slamming door on the conversation.

"Perhaps you should ask your own people such questions, Soyah-khrap," Vasnasong said, his face drawn tight as he stood and abruptly offered his hand Western-style. "A pity you must go now. I am so sad not to be of more help, Soyah-khrap."

"So am I, Vasnasong-khrap," Sawyer said, making the wai sign, his thoughts churning. "So am I."

Sawyer slowly pulled the sampan up to the wharf. Going in the front door had been of no help, maybe he could find out what was going on by the back door. Whatever it was, it had to be soon, because if what he suspected was true, he had very little time left. He wondered if he wasn't being used for bait. Because he *had* asked his own people about the Cambodian refugee outfit, dammit! You better not think about where that's leading, he told himself. You better get the goddamn facts first. Timing it carefully, he jumped up, landing catlike onto the concrete.

He crouched in the shadows waiting for the hidden guard to move and reveal his position. He hadn't seen a rifle, so the most the guard had would be a pistol, probably holstered, and in his black shirt and pants and rubber-soled shoes, Sawyer figured he could probably sit right next to the guard without being spotted.

A cigarette glowed about ten feet to the right of the stanchion where he crouched and he started to move.

He had the sequence rehearsed in his mind. The chokehold from behind. Forget the Hollywood movie bullshit where people get tapped on the head and go nicely to sleep. It was very difficult to hit someone with the precise degree of force needed to cause sufficient brain hemorrhaging to render him instantly unconscious without killing him or causing permanent brain damage. And although the rules changed—depending on who was DCI that year—in general, Company policy frowned on terminating civilians not clearly identified as Opposition. The chokehold was the best nondrug approach that would allow him to keep the guard alive.

Except he must have made some sound because at the last moment he saw the guard's eyes go wide, and instead of the head move first as he had planned, he spun into a sidekick to the midsection, knocking the wind out of him to prevent him from crying out, followed by a smash to the face to bring his head back up. The guard gasped and tried to reach the holster, but Sawyer was already behind him with the chokehold, pulling the guard backward to keep him off balance.

Sawyer pinned the holster with his leg, blocking the guard's hand from reaching it. They swayed in a desperate dance of kicking feet and clawing hands, the guard tearing at the rock-hard forearm Sawyer had jammed into his windpipe. Sawyer held on grimly as the fingernails dug deeply into his arm. The guard hit him with an elbow chop to the ribs that Sawyer knew he would feel later on, followed by three enormous jerks of the guard's entire body, almost wrenching him free. The guard's thrashing began to subside after what seemed much longer than the thirty to forty seconds it was supposed to take. All at once, the guard was dead weight, and Sawyer sagged to the ground with him, still holding his death's grip even tighter, at first in case it was a ruse, and then, as the seconds ticked away, because he had to bring the guard close to the edge of death to keep him out for more than a minute or so. And there was no real way to tell where the line between life and death was.

When he finally let go, Sawyer's hands were slick with sweat. It took him a minute to find the guard's pulse; fluttery, but it was there. Sawyer retrieved the guard's pistol from the holster and heaved it far out over the river. In the blackness, the distant splash might have been a fish breaking the surface.

The lock in the corroded metal door to the warehouse was one of those heavy iron tumbler devices of ancient design that would have taken the balding "flaps and seals" instructor in Langley less time than to tie his shoes. As it was, it took Sawyer an agonizing four or five minutes with the pick until it clicked open and he stepped inside.

It was a city of rice. Tall cubed buildings made of big sacks of rice stacked like bricks and between them ran rectilinear aisles like narrow streets. The warehouse was cavernous and gloomy, yellowish light from a few bug-spattered bulbs not penetrating down to the dark aisles. You could hide an army in here, Sawyer thought, holding his breath to listen. The silence was thick as the gloom, but all around there were faint, almost imperceptible scratching sounds. Rats, burrowing insects, Sawyer thought, turning a corner, the Beretta in his hand.

At the far end of a very long straight aisle was a mountain of unsacked rice. It towered over the stacked cubes like Vesuvius over Naples. Something about it beckoned Sawyer closer. A signal from his Reptile, perhaps, Sawyer thought as he tiptoed down the long corridor, pausing at each intersection to check for anything that might come at him out of the shadows. But there was nothing but the tiny chewing sounds of things that lived in the dark. And then Sawyer realized what had attracted his attention. Almost concealed by the mountain of rice was the partial outline of a ventilator panel.

Parker! The image of Parker bound and gagged in a little room crackled in his mind like electricity. It would be a perfect hideout. A few shovelfuls of rice was all it would take to completely seal the door from view behind the rice mountain, Sawyer thought.

He took off his shoes and socks. The rice was pale as snow in the gloomy light. It felt firm and granulated under his bare feet. Moving carefully, one step at a time to make as little sound as possible, he began to climb the rice mountain. At each step, a tiny avalanche of rice grains tumbled a short way down the slope. He made no more sound that a large rat as his head came up to the open ventilator panel.

Slowly, Sawyer raised himself up. He held his breath and peered over the top of the panel.

He could see nothing. It was pitch black down there. A sharp chemical smell filled his nostrils. He had smelled it before, but he couldn't remember where. Sweet Christ, what have they done to him? he thought. Then he realized that if Parker was down there, he would be unguarded. They wouldn't have left a guard without a light.

Sawyer reached into his back pocket and took out a small pencil flashlight. The narrow circle of light revealed a tiny room filled with small wooden boxes and a table on which were some iron pots, glass jars, and a couple of bricks made of something that looked like white chalk. No Parker, of course.

Sawyer felt like kicking himself. He recognized the chemical smell now all right. It was acetic anhydride. The white bricks were morphine base. They'd had something to hide, but it wasn't Parker. It was a small heroin factory.

He had just started to turn around when he was blinded by powerful floodlights. He blinked desperately to clear his eye, his gun already in position, but it was pointless. They had him covered on three sides with AK-47s. He tossed his gun down the rice slope and raised his hands over his head. As he stared down into their grim unblinking Asian eyes, he knew that it was over. He had tried it one time too many.

The one in the middle barked something Sawyer didn't understand in a language that might have been Cambodian. The one in the middle, whom Sawyer took for the leader, shouted again, this time in French, for him to descend with the hands on high. So they were Cambodians all right. His throat went dry as he came down. He remembered all the stories from the war, the ones that always sounded too Hollywood chain-saw massacre to be true. Then he thought about what they had done to Tarasang and Eddie Macbeth.

The leader kept his AK-47 trained on Sawyer's chest all the way down. When Sawyer got closer he could see the leader's face drawn tight, the eyes red-rimmed, and then everything looked red because the leader had smashed the muzzle of his rifle across

Sawyer's good eye. Sawyer staggered back, his hands coming up to protect his face, and the leader screamed at him in a high unnatural voice to make the hands come down, behind his back. His voice carried the strange, almost hysterical note of orders shouted during a bombardment, though the warehouse was dead quiet. As they roughly tied his hands behind him, Sawyer tried to blink the red film of blood from his eye. He could see, but everything stayed red: the stacks of rice, the long aisle, and the three Cambodians with the smoky-eyed look of guard dogs straining to slip the leash.

"Who are you?" demanded the leader, waving his rifle in Sawyer's face. He only had one chance, he knew. That they weren't acting under orders about him specifically. Otherwise they would just kill him now and dump him in the river. It was the perfect place for it, and the only question then was whether they would do it quickly or take their time. He tried to take a breath, but it wouldn't come. Keep authority in your voice, he told himself.

"These are affairs of interest only to myself and your commandant. Take me to him at once, or I assure you, he will make you regret it."

"Answer me at once, or it is you who will regret," the leader said, his voice thick with rage. One of the other two Cambodians picked up Sawyer's pistol, cocked it, and put the muzzle to Sawyer's temple.

Their eyes had the vacant stare of those to whom killing was nothing. He had only an instant.

"I am called Sawyer. International Red Cross representative," he managed to mutter.

The leader reached into Sawyer's back pocket and took out his diplomatic passport. He squinted at the lettering and held the photograph up to Sawyer's face. When he was satisfied, he put Sawyer's passport in his own pocket and grinned at Sawyer as though what he was about to say was going to give him great pleasure. His breath stank of fish. His teeth were bad, and in the reddish haze through which Sawyer saw everything, his smile was that of a demon.

"We know who you are, Monsieur Sauyair. You are not from the Red Cross International. You are an American spy and my orders are to kill you," said the grinning demon mask.

Sawyer looked into the leader's burning eyes and saw that he meant it. The only question left was fast or slow. If it was slow, he would try to make a break for it, hopefully forcing them to shoot him, he decided, already beginning to look around and calculate angles. But they were starting to back away from him and raise their AK-47s, so they weren't going to waste any more time and it didn't matter whether he ran for it or not.

"I must speak with your commandant. I have vital information for him."

"Please, monsieur. Let us not insult each other with these nonsenses. Only to stand there—comme ça!"

"Your commandant will punish you when he hears what—"

"No, monsieur, he will not. But in any case you will not be here to know." The Cambodian shrugged and nodded to his men to make ready.

So this is where it ends, Sawyer thought. He looked around the gloomy warehouse as if there was some meaning to be extracted from the last thing he would ever see, but there was nothing. They'd been expecting him. Vasnasong had outsmarted him, and he was paying the prescribed penalty for a mistake in this business. He had blundered into it like a fly into a spider's web, and the worst part was knowing that he deserved it for having been so stupid. All out of vanity. Because he was good at what he did and knew it. But not good enough, you prick, he cursed himself. Because it was all in front of him and he had missed it, like the way he had forgotten where he had heard of the Cambodian Refugee Committee before.

And just like that he remembered where he had heard it before. A desperate gift from his subconscious on the brink of death. And he saw them all clear as day, exactly as they had been at Lady Caroline's reception that day: Sir Geoffrey, Barnes, Lady Caroline, Bhamornprayoon, and Vasnasong, of course. Let's not forget Vasnasong, he thought bitterly, moving them around in his mind like chess figures—all the pieces finally falling into place now that it was too late. And all he needed was for Harris to make one call to London to confirm. Only now it would never be made.

The Cambodian shouted something and they raised their AK-47s like a firing squad. Too late, Sawyer thought. He had understood it all too late. Because he had been a child all along. Because deep in his soul he had still held on to that naive American notion that things would somehow turn out all right in the end. But now, in this last moment before dying, the leader counting "One . . . two . . . ," Sawyer knew it was all bullshit. He had lived believing in a fairy tale his whole life and never knew it until this instant. There would be another Vietnam war and thousands would die because he had been a goddamn fool.

He blinked his eye open to see the last thing he would ever see. The demon face of the Cambodian sighting his AK-47 at his head.

But there was something else. Floating dreamlike in the darkness, like the image of the moon on still water, was the face of the most beautiful woman he had ever seen.

He wondered if he was hallucinating, or was he already dying? His chest tightened. The sound of his own breathing was loud as a bellows. He saw the mouth of the Cambodian cry, "Three," but he couldn't hear it over the roaring in his ears.

The night exploded in bursts of automatic rifle fire.

7

 The sun shines above the earth.
The man advances horns first.
He uses them against rebels
within his own city.

FONG WU rolled the black ball in his palm, then held it up between his thumb and forefinger so the man could see its size. The man nodded and Fong Wu tamped the opium into the pipe bowl and lit it. He waited while the man's cheeks hollowed to make sure that the pipe was drawing well. When the man had sucked the smoke up the long stem for the first good puffs, Fong Wu turned to the woman.

Like the man, the woman was also European. She lay curled on her side facing the man's bunk. She wore heavy makeup, as though she were a common Suriwongse whore, and an expensive Western-style evening dress that almost completely exposed her sluttish bosom. As he knelt close to prepare the pipe for her, Fong Wu could smell the musky scent of recent fornication on her. It mingled with the thick perfume she had splashed on to mask the offensive body odor of the European. Fong Wu ogled her huge breasts, bigger than any Chinese girl, allowing himself a brief fantasy of coupling with her. But the woman, foolish as all her kind, noticed nothing. She merely murmured a polite "Khob khun kha" in a disgusting English accent. All this with a grateful little smile as she looked across at the man, her eyes warm and soft.

As always, these two had come here after coupling, and even now they reached out and held each other's hand in an unseemly display of affection.

Busying himself with final preparations before leaving them in their private teak-lined cubicle with the two cots, the tea on the low table, the lamp turned down just so to ensure an easy entry into dreams, Fong Wu still hadn't decided whether he should warn the man on the bunk or not.

The other European, the one-eyed man with the fierce expression of the hawk, had given him a five-hundred-baht note, which was most excellent good joss. In his mind Fong Wu could already see the expressions of the other players when he tossed the note on the table of the mah-jongg game of his mother's brother's son, Chin. They would covet it, but he would outbid them and win back some of his losings. Thus would he silence the endless grumblings of his foolish wife.

But if he should warn this European, perhaps he could get a second five hundred baht. And what if the one-eyed man meant to do evil to this European? These were farangs. Who could say what a farang might do?

Fong Wu prepared to leave. If he were to say something, now was the moment. But the man and woman ignored him as though he weren't there. The man said something in their barbarous tongue and the woman pursed her lips and made a kiss at him. The slut!

Fong Wu deliberately made a sound as he lifted the tray. The man frowned, then relaxed, his eyes already growing dreamy from the opium. The man dropped a ten safang coin in Fong Wu's hand.

So be it, Fong Wu decided. One who tips so miserly will never part with five hundred baht, he thought as he bowed and backed away through the beaded curtain. Let the farangs kill each other. What were the farangs to him?

As he passed the one-eyed man, lurking in the shadows of the big room where the smokers lay side by side, Fong Wu nodded.

After the Chinaman passed, Sawyer stood there in the darkness listening. He listened to the sounds of those who were sleeping and the sounds of those who were still awake. Occasionally there would be a flare in the darkness as someone relit his pipe, followed by deep sucking sounds. Then the darkness, composed of small restless turnings and sighs, would again settle over the room.

Time to go, Sawyer thought. He glanced over toward the side exit door that led to the alley in back, setting its location in his mind, just in case. He hefted the Beretta in his hand, checking to be sure the safety was off. He hoped to God he wouldn't have to use it this time. Not this time.

He moved silently down the dark corridor, stopping in front of the beaded curtain over the doorway. The beads parted with faint insect clicks, and before the two smokers could look up from their pipes, he had the muzzle pressed against the man's head.

"Hello, Max," Sawyer said.

Barnes blinked stupidly up at Sawyer. He looked confused, as though he couldn't remember where he had put something. Then his eyes narrowed as he felt the muzzle against his temple and realized what it was.

"I don't like people pointing guns at me, kiddo," Barnes said.

"That's too bad," Sawyer replied, running his free hand over Barnes. When he was sure Barnes was clean, he moved away. He sat near the foot of Lady Caroline's cot, but he kept the gun on Barnes.

"How'd you find us?" Barnes asked, eyeing the Beretta.

"It wasn't hard," Sawyer shrugged. "I knew you wouldn't take my fair lady here"—nodding at Lady Caroline—"to any old dive. Everybody knows that Fong Wu's is the best fumerie in Chinatown."

"Perhaps I should just leave you gentlemen to conduct your business," Lady Caroline said carefully. She started to get up.

Sawyer motioned her back with the gun.

"Oh," she said, and sat back against the wall, her knees drawn up, arms around them like a young girl in a window seat. "I'm afraid I don't understand," she said, not looking at Sawyer and not taking her eyes off the gun.

"Not bad." Sawyer grinned. "In fact, you're both pretty good."

"What's the beef, Jack? So we both like to kick the gong a little, the lady and me. So what? After all these years in the Orient, you wouldn't figure me for a candidate for a Baptist choir anyway, would you?" Barnes said, putting down the opium pipe and shaking his head to clear it as he sat up.

"Oh Christ, Max. Save the horseshit for the Washington crowd, will you?" Sawyer said.

"Well, this is ridiculous, Mister Whatever-Your-Name-Is. I never thought Geoffrey would stoop so low as to have us followed by some little man with a gun. Well, what do you want, little man? Money?" she snapped contemptuously, her eyes blazing. She looked older as she glared at him. Not so pretty, Sawyer thought.

"She's even better than you are," Sawyer said, grinning over at Barnes.

"Well, you can put up with this tuppenny-ha'penny extortion if you want to, Max, but I'm leaving—right now," she said, reaching for her handbag and tossing her hair like a young actress at a Beverly Hills bistro when a movie producer sits down at a nearby table.

Sawyer cocked the hammer and pointed the Beretta in her face.

"Make another move, lady, and I'll blow your fucking head off," Sawyer said quietly.

Lady Caroline slumped back. She stared up at him with a dark expression that could not be read.

"Come on, Jack. Take it easy, huh? I mean, okay, you got us. So Caroline and me are having an affair. So what? Is that supposed to shake the Anglo-American alliance, or what? I got to tell you, amigo," Barnes said, pursing his lips. "She wasn't exactly a virgin when I got her. Come to think of it, neither was I." He shrugged, screwing his face up in a slap-happy grin.

"Why'd you do it, Max?" Sawyer asked sadly.

Barnes pulled himself heavily to a sitting position at the edge of the bunk. He looked at Sawyer as if calculating something. Then he looked at the gun and obviously thought better of it. He folded his arms across his chest, his forearms with their Marine Corps tattoos bulging like a stevedore's, the massive knuckles white. His brow furrowed, bringing his eyebrows close together so they almost formed a ridge, giving him the appearance of an intelligent Neanderthal.

"Why'd I do what, Sawyer? Fall in love with the most fabulous beautiful woman I've ever known? A classy lady like her and a monkey like me—you've got to be kidding. Call it 'attraction of opposites.' Call it anything you like, but I'll tell you one damn thing, Jack old buddy. She's the best goddamn thing that ever happened to me," Barnes said, shaking his head. "Go ahead. Be a rat. Tell Sir Geoffrey." Barnes shrugged. "I don't give a shit. Maybe it's better this way, out in the open," he said, looking across at Lady Caroline, his eyes shining.

"Oh, Max," she said, biting her lip.

For a moment the three of them just sat there. From beyond the wall came a racking smoker's cough that started a round of coughing, followed by stillness and a faint echo of Chinese music on the radio.

An odd sound came from Sawyer. They both looked up and he shook his head, trying to stifle his laughter.

"Jesus, you two are really something."

"Watch it, Jack," Barnes warned.

"I don't mean this fucking joke of an affair, Max. Although I'm not sure whether you're lying to me, or to yourself, or both. I'm not sure anybody, not even Sir Geoffrey, really gives a damn who you or the lady smoke with, sleep with, or anything else with," Sawyer said.

He watched the hate kindle in Barnes' eyes. He saw the muscles bunch as for a rush and began the slow imperceptible pressure on the trigger. Barnes saw it and his muscles sagged. He looked up at Sawyer, shaking his head sadly from side to side.

"You don't understand, amigo. You just don't understand."

"No, I don't understand, Max. Explain it to me. Explain how you and Vasnasong cooked up this whole thing. Explain about Parker. What happened to him? And Sergeant Tarasang and Eddie Macbeth. Remember him? And how you tried to terminate me not once, but three fucking times, amigo. Tell me about it, old buddy-roo," Sawyer snapped.

Barnes looked confused.

"Jeez, Jack. What makes you think I had anything . . . I swear. . . ." Barnes said, looking at both of them.

Sawyer made a face.

"Come on, Max. You're better than that. Someone on the inside had to set Parker up for Vasnasong. Someone who knew the terrain and the op and Parker. Like you, Max. Then there was the mysterious Cambodian refugee committee that lady bountiful over here did her benefit for—that was my own dumb mistake," Sawyer said, turning to Lady Caroline for a moment. "The committee name was on the invitation in English and I should have remembered it, even when I saw it in French. The committee was tied both to Vasnasong—their office is at his warehouse, and he was at the reception too—and to your ladylove, Max. And you, right in the middle. So you knew about it, Max. Christ, everybody in Bangkok knew about the goddamn committee except Harris. And the only way that could've happened was because you didn't tell him. Not very nice, Max. Definitely not according to Hoyle.

"Then there was the attempted hit at the temple. The booth was flying the safe sign, and it was your voice I heard at the other end of the line, amigo. You set me up, Max. Only you ran into some tough luck, and Sublieutenant Somsukiri bought it instead of me.

"I should have suspected you then, Max. You were the logical candidate. But I didn't. You know why? Because I liked you, dammit. I didn't even want to think of you as a double. But it was you, all right.

"You knew about the rdv at the temple. You also tried to warn me off the op right from the beginning. And then the Good Housekeeping Seal of Approval for Vasnasong. Harris got that from you. Christ, you'd have thought Harris was going to nominate Vasnasong for man of the year. All to try and lead me off the scent. And then no data available on the Southeast Asia Rice and Trading Company, or anything about its connection with Vasnasong. The only way Harris could have got it so wrong was because of an inexcusable failure on the part of the local station watchdog. Or because maybe someone was deliberately trying to mislead him, eh, Max?"

"You've no proof. . . ." Barnes began.

Sawyer looked at him ironically.

"Don't you get it, Max? You're like the hound in Sherlock Holmes. The one that should have barked and didn't."

"Listen, Jack. . . ." Barnes tried again, running his tongue along his lips as though sealing an envelope.

Sawyer waved the interruption away with the gun.

"But now I was getting too close, wasn't I? So you tried again at the beach in Ban Phattaya. Vasnasong had bought off Sergeant Tarasang so they could set up Parker. The bank draft proved that. But I showed up, so Vasnasong had to get rid of Tarasang. Poor Eddie Macbeth got in the way. So you and Vasnasong set a trap

to frame me for what those goons left of Tarasang and Eddie.
Only I arrived a little too early, just before the police, alerted by
an anonymous phone call, just happened to show.

"Third time was the charm. You almost got me in the warehouse, Max." Sawyer winked.

"How'd you get away?" Barnes asked, looking strangely up
at Sawyer.

"Girl saved me. She came charging in like Annie Oakley with
a squad of Cambodians packing M-16s. Killed the guards. Bing.
Bing. Bing. Just like that. Like Vasnasong said, that's some girl."

"What do you want, Sawyer?" Barnes said in a strangled
voice. It didn't sound like Barnes' voice. A change had come over
his face too. His eyes were shadows in his skull.

He was watching Barnes die inside, Sawyer thought.

Lady Caroline watched them both with a kind of horrified
fascination, as though she were watching a very beautiful, very
deadly snake stalk a mouse.

"Where's Parker, Max?"

"They've got him. I don't know where," Max said, a deadness
in his voice.

"Who's got him?"

"The Khmer Rouge. Pranh. Pranh's got him."

Sawyer went very quiet. So quiet they thought he might have
gone away and left his body behind. So quiet Barnes thought
Sawyer was going to kill him then and there.

"What a shit you are, Max. They'll think he knows something. They're probably killing him by inches. Inches," Sawyer
said, his voice so soft Barnes had to strain to hear him.

"It wasn't me. It was Vasnasong," Barnes said.

"Sure it was Vasnasong. Him and his goddamn Cambodian
sculptures hanging on the wall right in front of my eyes. You
were just along for the ride, weren't you? Parker was bait. Vasnasong was using him to get to the Khmer Rouge. To let Pranh
know about the arms-for-opium trade. Vasnasong wanted to let
Pranh know that he had something to deal and that Pranh should
deal through him and not the Americans. Only how did the Khmer
Rouge come into the picture?"

"Grow up, Jack," Barnes said, a trace of the old annoyance
showing in his voice. "There's a rumor up in the hill country that
Bhun Sa and Pranh are working together. Between them they

control most of the opium in the Golden Triangle and together they're the only fighting force with a real chance of keeping the Vietnamese out of Thailand."

"Shake hands with the devil," Sawyer murmured, almost to himself.

"Grow up, kiddo," Barnes repeated. "This is business. We're talking three, maybe four metric tons of one-hundred-percent-pure heroin, worth over two billion dollars—*wholesale!*"

"Why'd you need the money, Max? Her?" Sawyer asked, looking at Lady Caroline.

Barnes' face worked.

"How can I make you understand, amigo? Her husband treats her like shit. He's . . . well, sexual abuse. All kinds of stuff I don't even want to get into. But what can a mug like me offer her? The few bucks I can get out of Houlihan's and a Marine Corps pension? Are you kidding? One of her goddamn Hermes handbags costs as much as I make in a couple of months. We're too old to start over with nothing, her and me. Sure, the money. You're goddamn right the money," Barnes said bitterly.

"Love. The holy grail. Is that it, Max?"

"A new start, kiddo. For her and me," Barnes said, his eyes shining in the lamplight.

"Maybe you should grow up, Max. Do you really think the local head of MI6 doesn't know where his wife spends her nights? Take a good look at her, you pathetic bastard. Do you really think she's going to wait around for the next twenty years till you get out of the federal penitentiary?"

"You don't understand. We love each other," Barnes insisted stubbornly.

"Look at her, Max! I can't believe you didn't see through that phony dog and pony show she and her husband put on at the reception. For the Cambodian committee, you jerk! Suong, the girl who saved me—she's with a splinter group of Mith Yon's KPNLF. They're trying to make the connection between the Americans and Bhun Sa. Don't you get it? Lady Caroline's the one who put the girl and Vasnasong together!" Sawyer said, shaking his head as if he couldn't believe Barnes didn't see it. "They led you up the garden trail, Max. Harris finally admitted that London was the source on the Vietnamese, for Chrissakes. It originally came from their Bangkok station. God save the Empire!

And what a coup for Sir Geoffrey! The cap on a brilliant career and home to England and the society where she belongs—where everyone has goddamn Hermes handbags, or whatever the hell it is Sloan Rangers are wearing these days."

"You're wrong," Barnes said, not looking up.

Sawyer stood up.

"I'm not going to shoot you, Max. Call it auld lang syne. You have a few minutes till I get to a phone to go to ground. It's either that or go back to Washington, where they still think treason is a dirty word."

Barnes just sat there as though he hadn't been listening. His face was gray and wasted.

"As for the lady, I think she's coming with me. It's her only way out," Sawyer said, offering her his arm.

"She won't go, Jack. She loves me," Barnes said, his voice so hollow it seemed to carry its own echo.

Lady Caroline got up with a silken swish of her dress and took Sawyer's arm. She wouldn't look at Barnes.

"Go away, Max. Hide. Don't let them find you," Sawyer said.

They walked out and down the dark corridor together. When they got outside, Sawyer detached himself from her. The street was deserted and silent in the night. He watched her face, looking for something, but he wasn't sure what. In the red glow from a neon sign her face looked enameled, like her nails.

"Where can I find the girl, Suong?" Sawyer asked.

She looked amused.

"Don't tell me you've misplaced her?"

"They had a hang-yao waiting. Left me standing on the wharf. She was afraid. Didn't know who to trust."

"Oh, that's bloody funny. The great American whose got us all figured out—outsmarted by a woman!" She gave a forced laugh. It pealed in the dark street like a cry for help.

Sawyer stuck his hands in his pockets. How do they get that way? he wondered. These brittle upper-class women who could be as tireless a predator on one man as the vulture that daily fed on Prometheus' liver. He felt grateful that it was Max and not him who subscribed to the fantasy of rich and beautiful. He waited for the mockery to fade from her expression before he spoke.

"An American agent is being tortured right this minute by

people who have so few qualms they put three million of their own countrymen to death, lady. And Max isn't here to cover for you anymore. So if you want to walk away from this in one piece, just answer the question."

She bit her lip. He could see the awareness of her position starting to dawn on her. In Whitehall they used to say that when Washington sneezes, London catches cold.

"Aranyaprathet. The refugee camp," she said in a low voice.

Sawyer nodded and started to walk away.

"Wait a minute," she said, grabbing his arm. She squeezed close, her breasts pressed against him. "Where are you going?"

Her eyes had a desperate bruised look, and it suddenly occurred to Sawyer that she was one of those women who know how to use men superbly, but not how to function without them.

"As far away from you as I can," he said, shaking her off. He began to walk down the street.

"Sawyer! Your turn will come, you bloody bastard!" she cried after him, her voice echoing in the night.

"Why not? Everyone else's has," he tossed back over his shoulder.

"Sawyer!" he could hear her shriek as he turned the corner into Yawaraj Road. Streamers of swallows were perched on sagging telephone lines. It should have told him something, but he wasn't paying attention. Up ahead he could see the lights of an all-night market. The proprietor would have a phone he could use, he thought.

Just then something hit his forehead. It felt warm and wet, and he had automatically started to brush it away like an insect before he realized what it was. He looked up. Bloated drops of rain were starting to fall through the light of a streetlamp.

A solid curtain of rain swept down the street as it does only in the tropics, instantly soaking him to the skin. He had left it too late.

The monsoon had begun.

PART TWO

*The dragon rises from
the deep.*

8

The earth covers the deep.
The superior man educates the
people
making soldiers of the multitude.
The soldiers set forth under
orders.

T HE village lay hidden in a fold in the hills. It was a Meo village by the look of it and a big one. Sawyer counted almost a hundred wooden huts on stilts, their roofs slanting steeply to turn the rain. It was well situated on an incline so the water would run down to a narrow gorge, at the bottom of which, hundreds of feet below, wound the river, muddy and swollen with rain. A snaking trail led down one side of the gorge to the only road, which ran alongside the river.

Sawyer studied the village with his binoculars through a gap in the pines. They had done it well, he thought. Leaving trees interspersed among the huts so the only way you could see it from the air was if you already knew it was there. Below the village enclosure were stepped fields cut into the slopes. The poppies were green and yellow; the time of the fourth cutting. The white petals that in the spring turned the fields into carpets of snow had long since fallen away. Now the hills were deep green and a heavy sky the color of pewter without the shine lay over the village like a roof.

A black-clad sentry, who had foolishly given away his

position by lighting a cheroot, sat behind a tree on a rise near the bamboo fence that enclosed the village.

"See, there," the girl said, pointing at the sentry. From up here they could smell the rising smoke of his cheroot. Among the hill tribes it was said that a man with a good nose could smell cheroot smoke from across the Salween and name the village where the tobacco was grown.

"Meo. Two of them," Sawyer whispered back, pointing his M-16 at a well-camouflaged tree platform up the slope from the first sentry.

The girl nodded.

"Always two," she agreed. "But do not call them 'Meo,' " she corrected him, her eyes serious. "This means 'barbarian' and is a name given to them by the Chinese long ago. Ce n'est pas gentil, tu comprends? They call themselves 'Hmong.' This means 'free men.' You must make attention. Since the Thai border patrol came last year and burned the poppy fields to stop the opium trade, they do not like strangers."

That was true enough, Sawyer thought. Even though the rains had already made the roads nearly impassable, the villagers had blocked the road with giant logs in half a dozen places. And they had rigged traps of sharpened pungi sticks and strung vines neck-high along the hill trail.

"Is that your opium trader?" Sawyer asked, indicating the bamboo corral, where perhaps twenty mules and half as many plump Karen ponies were grazing.

She reached for the binoculars and adjusted the focus.

"Yes. Those are Burma-side ponies. And see there—the smoke from the hut of the headman. That means they are finished bargaining and are ready for rice and cha."

She stood up and brushed the brown pine needles from the red and white checkered krama that she wore over her shoulders like a shawl.

"Wait here. I go ahead to tell them of your coming. A woman is less likely to be shot at than a farang with an M-16."

Sawyer nodded. And from here, with the telescopic sight, he could cover her if she got into trouble.

She had started toward the trail when he called softly after her. She looked back at him with those strange two-color eyes, deep blue at the center surrounded by black, and he tried to remember his excuse for calling. The real reason was to see her face again.

"This Thai opium smuggler. Can he be trusted?"

"Who can be trusted?" she replied softly and was gone.

He watched her climb gracefully down the steep slope, now and then raising the hem of her black phasin to step over a root or a pungi trap. She moved with confidence, finding her way as though she had been raised in this village, and Sawyer, watching her lithe figure through the binoculars, found it hard to believe that she was the same glamorous woman who'd sat across from him at dinner the night before last at the hotel in Chiang Mai.

"I knew you would find me," she had said, the reflection of the table candles in the restaurant window shining around her hair like stars against the misty lights of the city below. She wore blue silk that matched her eyes, and Sawyer felt that curious mixture of self-satisfaction and unease a man feels when he's with not merely the most beautiful woman in the room, but one who will not soon be forgotten by any man who saw her that night.

"How did you know?"

"I knew. Didn't you ever just know something without knowing how?"

"Yes," he admitted. "But it wasn't knowing. It was wanting."

"Do you have to hear the words? Is that it? That I wanted you? Ah, les hommes." She smiled, showing sharp, perfect little teeth.

And later that night in the dark hotel room, the sound of the rain against the window barely audible over the hum of the air conditioning, the whisper of silk as she came to him, putting her finger to his lips to keep him from speaking. She pressed her soft white breasts against his chest and stretched her legs against his. They swayed together, watching themselves and each other in the full-length mirror, enjoying the contrast of her ivory skin against his sun-darkened body. His lips glided over every part of her, and Sawyer thought he had never touched anything so silky in his life. And then she was over him, her sleek black hair enclosing them like a tent, moving and then moving faster, crying out "Vite, ah, vite," and later there were sounds and no words at all.

Afterward, her head on his shoulder, her throaty voice murmuring in his ear like a conscience, "C'est vrai, tu sais. When I saw you again at the camp, I knew."

"Why me?"

She looked amused.

"Do you not understand women, my So-yah? We are drawn to power like iron filings to the magnet. You should have seen yourself when you entered the hut in the camp, dripping with rain, black patch for one eye, the other eye like fire and gun ready for killing, like a hawk among squabs. What woman could resist?"

"Some have managed," he admitted.

"Pah! Scaredy women!" She snorted. "A woman in a fire wants safety of the nest. A woman safe in the nest wants to play with fire. True man, who can offer both nest and fire, can have any woman in the world."

"Is that what your look meant?" he asked, remembering how she had looked up at him when he had entered the hut, the light from the lamp shining like candles in her eyes. He had searched the muddy refugee camps till, in the Khao-I-Dang camp, a small boy who had lost a foot to a mine led him to the right hut for ten baht and a cigarette.

"My look mean I see you and I see my karma," she said.

Sawyer held her close, thinking how lucky it was that she had felt something, because when he entered the hut, there were about a dozen of them already putting down their rice bowls and reaching for their weapons. "No!" she said sharply in Khmer, all the while looking at him with that strange wild look of hers that was like no one else. And yet strangely familiar. An earlier life, the Buddhists would say.

A young man with hard eyes, whom Sawyer later learned was the rebel leader, Mith Yon, pointed an AKM straight at Sawyer's belly. He must have gotten the gun from a dead enemy, because it still had the symbol of the RPK painted on the stock. For a moment, no one moved. They listened to the rain clattering on the tin roof like pebbles.

"Vous vous êtes trompé—" the young man began, when the girl interrupted with a torrent of Khmer that Sawyer couldn't understand except for the odd phrase. Something about "the one" and "the warehouse" maybe.

Sawyer saw recognition come into the young man's eyes. But the rifle was still pointed at him.

"I owe you a life. If I owe you more than one, you will have to wait till the next life for repayment," Sawyer said, going from French to Thai.

"That is truth," someone said.

"With joss that is too long to wait," another cackled, and the others began to smile. The young man shook his head obstinately.

"If my brother wishes to become old, he will learn not to give trust so easily," the young man snapped over his shoulder.

But he wasn't going to shoot anymore. They could all feel it, and one of them even picked up his rice bowl again.

"Why did you run away at the warehouse?" Sawyer asked the girl.

"To be certain you were the one," she said, coming between the AKM and Sawyer. She touched the young man's arm and he lowered the weapon. There was something proprietary in the touch that made Sawyer wonder if they were sleeping together and if maybe part of what was happening was jealousy. Sawyer deliberately resisted looking at her so as not to provoke him. A jealous twenty-five-year-old with a gun was no joke. "How else could we know that you were the one we had been told to expect? That Vasnasong-kha had already lied about the first American farang. And look what happened to him! Il est tombé entre les mains des Khmers Rouges," she said, and despite the danger he couldn't help looking at her. "We knew only a true CIA man could find me," she added, as though it were not only a test to confirm his bona fides but an article of faith—like "Only the true prince can pull the sword from the stone"—and he knew then that they would be lovers. But he had to defuse the young man's jealousy, if that's what it was.

"We have a common enemy in the Vietnamese. That is a good basis for friendship," Sawyer said to Mith Yon.

"That is truth," the same voice from before called out.

Mith Yon lowered his rifle, all at once looking very young. But his eyes were still suspicious.

"You will to sii bay with us," gesturing for Sawyer to come and sit.

The girl scooped a bowl of rice from the pot and they made a place for him.

"I will take you to Bhun Sa," she said, her strange eyes unreadable as she handed him the rice.

That night Sawyer had a final rdv with Harris before going back to the camp in a rented Isuzu to pick up Suong. The meeting had to be hastily arranged, and the best they could do was the back room of a Honda motor scooter shop in Aranyaprathet whose Cambodian owner, a swarthy former army officer who had managed to get away before the debacle, accepted payment only in gold, rubies, opium, chickens, and sexual favors, the currencies of life here.

Harris gave Sawyer the pack and the equipment he had requested. As Sawyer went over it, the concealed transmitter, the gold links and dust, the stubby Ingram M-10—he had dumped the Beretta in the Chao Phraya River at the first chance—and sound suppressor, the M-16, Harris briefed him on the latest updates in the "Three C's": Communications, Codes, and Cut-outs. He told Harris about the girl. Harris told him about the SR-71 Blackbird they now had flying unseen, unheard, twenty miles straight up, almost directly overhead. The Blackbird's infrared cameras and sophisticated radio equipment had reported a sharp increase in Vietnamese military activity across the border.

The rain drummed against a small window they had covered with a black rag. Harris told him they would keep a Blackbird up on a round-the-clock basis to monitor the situation and to pick up any message Sawyer could get out in case of emergency. For backup, they had secretly moved the Delta Force to an out-of-bounds area of Clark Field in the Philippines. They were now on standby alert.

They're scared, Sawyer thought. They're really scared.

"What about the Limeys? Sir Whatsis and Countess Dracula?" Sawyer asked.

"Don't worry. They won't get near the 'coconuts,' " as Harris mulishly insisted on calling the heroin, as though that kind of crap would fool a CTP trainee.

"And Vasnasong?" looking curiously at Harris.

"We're leaving him in place for the time being. There are reasons. . . ." Harris said—a little too casually, Sawyer thought, and he started to get a bad feeling. But he pushed it away. Harris was within his rights as the senior case officer for the op. They never did tell you everything. Less baggage to carry.

"What about Barnes?"

Harris made a face.

"You think we're all a bunch of wimps back in Washington, don't you?" Harris said quietly. It sent chills down Sawyer's spine.

Sawyer didn't say anything.

"Houlihan's won't be the same without him," Harris sighed. "Everyone was shocked. But they gave him quite a send-off. Like the old days. Asian go-go girls! The works! Shame you had to miss it."

That was how he learned that Barnes was dead.

The next day after using every switch in the book through the murderous Bangkok traffic to flush any tails—just to be safe, though Sawyer knew that where they were going no tail could follow unnoticed—they sat by the window of the first-class couchettes express to Chiang Mai, watching the jade green hills and rice paddies racketing by. He waited until he had checked out their compartment and the rest of the car before he finally asked what he couldn't delay asking any longer.

"You led Parker to the sampan, didn't you?"

"To meet someone who would take him to Bhun Sa," she nodded. "But when I saw no one aboard I feared betrayal and hid myself."

"Where?"

"In a space behind un faux side of boat. It is common in sampan for smuggling."

"A false bulkhead?"

"Oui, c'est ça."

"How did you find it?"

A smile dimpled her cheeks.

"I was born on sampan, elder brother. My father was French rice merchant, my mother sampan girl, but so pretty, he keep her like wife in big apartment in Phnom Penh."

"And Parker?"

"I heard him come on sampan. Then others came and took him away. They were Khmer Rouge."

"How do you know they were KR?"

She turned toward the window. The train rattled past a village. Bamboo huts, rustic pagoda, a peasant boy riding a water buffalo flashed by the window and were gone. She didn't look at him when she finally spoke.

"Once you have heard the voice of angkar, elder brother, you do not forget."

That night, drowsy from the rhythm of the train, he fell asleep on his sleeper bunk beneath hers. Some sound, something woke him. Instantly the Ingram was in his hand. He found himself pointing it in her face.

"I am unarmed. See for yourself," she said, dropping her slip to the floor and standing naked before him, swaying to the movement of the train. She was tall for an Asian, perhaps five foot six, and perfectly made. Unbound, her hair was long and sleek and very black against the whiteness of her skin. White and black. Ivory and onyx, he thought as she came to him for the first time, and even then, he knew it was how he would always think of her, ivory and onyx. She stepped into the circle of his arms, soft, pliant, her eyes shining, and he knew he could do anything he wanted with her. Then telling himself he was a fool, but knowing he couldn't afford to make a mistake, he forced himself to push her away.

"What of Mith Yon?"

She raised her head and looked at him curiously.

"What is that to us?"

"He acted jealous. I thought you . . . and he . . ." he finished lamely.

She made a face.

"I love Mith Yon like elder brother. If he wanted me for pleasure, I would give him. Gladly. This he knows, but it makes nothing. Mith Yon is a man, but he cannot be a man with a woman. The angkar, they did things to him, tu comprends?"

"What things?"

"You do not want to know," she said, not looking at him.

She shivered. He held her tightly against him until the shivering subsided. They stood naked, moving with the motion of the train. Raindrops skidded slanting across the window. The train rocked them against each other, the touch of flesh making warmth, and then it began. The old tickle and she made an awkward move and then the exquisite sliding, locking them together. The rhythm of the train became their rhythm and both of them conscious of every sensation, the air moist and warm as a kiss, the sound of the rain and the wheels moving under them, the jasmine smell of her skin, and then the moving growing wilder, more intense, and they tumbled onto the bunk, hard now, pounding against her, no more tenderness, only the ache to be deeper and deeper inside her.

She pulled him to her, tearing at his skin with her nails, and he felt the scorching heat of her. The tempo rose rhythmic and harder, and she moved desperately against him as if she could never have enough of him, both of them moving faster, wilder, the tingle at the peak and she cried out as they slid down the far side, still grinding away at each other as if to drain the very last drop, until they were still at last.

"I have to know," he said later, and when she asked "Why?" he just shrugged. She smiled ruefully.

"Thoughts spoken are like wine corks, my So-yah. Once aired, they will no longer fit back in the bottle," she said, and finally told him of Mith Yon and Tuol Sleng prison. How they attached electrodes to that which made him a man but left his hand free to work a switch that controlled electric wires attached to his mother, stripped naked and spread-eagled like a whore. They forced him to stare at her sagging breasts and her face dark with shame. They told him the only way to avoid the pain was to give it to her. And why should he not? the cadre demanded. Familial ties have no place in the new Kampuchea.

To this, Mith Yon said nothing, but in his heart, he later told Suong, he could only stare at the cadre, a boy of eighteen perhaps, and wonder how the boy had so quickly managed to forget what it is to be human. "I am the imperialist agent. Not this old woman who knows nothing," Mith Yon told them with quiet dignity.

Suong frowned. This because Mith Yon's words, she said, had the ring not of words said, but of words he wished he had said. But no matter what he really said, the cadre merely smiled, as though at a child's meaningless babble. Mith Yon remembered the smile.

Everyone in Tuol Sleng knew of Mith Yon. How he withstood hours of it, till he was screaming if the cadre so much as smiled, until at last his twitching hand, almost by itself, gave her the first small shock, and how it ended by him electrocuting his own mother.

For a long time neither of them said anything. They listened to the wheels on the tracks, and when they kissed it was because they had to, like climbers on a ledge desperately clutching each other because there is nothing else to grab. They might have slept. Sawyer wasn't sure.

"Why have you come, my So-yah?" she asked finally, her head on his chest, listening to the strong beat of his heart.

"My job. To help freedom fighters."

"Ah, freedom fighters. What is that?" she teased.

"Anyone who kills Communists is a freedom fighter. Anyone who kills non-Communists is a terrorist," he teased back.

"Why not say the truth? Your job is to make one group of —how you say?—'gook' kill other 'gook' for benefit of American. No?"

"Yes, but it's never difficult to get people to kill each other. We just add technology to make it more efficient. For the benefit of America, as you say," he agreed, letting his fingers trace the outline of her breasts, feeling the nipples grow taut and erect.

"No wait," she said, stopping his hand for a moment. "You do not answer my question. I do not ask why America help us. I ask why you do this job."

Sawyer paused. He wasn't given to introspection and he didn't have an answer ready. Finally he began haltingly, as if groping his way in the dark.

"It sounds . . . I don't know . . . naive. But then, one person's politics always sound ridiculous to someone who doesn't share his point of view. America may be civilization's last hope . . . but like all democracies, America has a fatal flaw. We don't solve problems, we debate them. Like Hamlet, we never act until it's too late. Sometimes, someone just has to do something."

"You lie to yourself, if you think that," she said.

He reddened and was glad it was too dark for her to see it.

"Oh," she said, clapping her hand to her mouth. "That is most terrible kreng chai. Your little sister is silly fool and begs forgiveness," bowing her head.

He took her chin in his hand and raised her head.

"You can drop the little Asian girl crap, Suong. It isn't what you want of me. It isn't what I want of you. And besides, neither of us believes it, do we?"

She shook her head, not looking at him.

"Now, why don't you tell me what you really think?" he said, turning her chin to force her to look at him. A passing signal light lit her face like a flare.

"You are most vain, my So-yah. The world makes you sad.

So you seek to prove to God that you could make the world better than He. That is why you have come," she said, her words striking home with enough force for him to feel truth in them.

"A fool's errand, then?"

"No. Not a fool. You see most clearly, my one-eyed lord," she said fiercely, her mouth upon his.

Now, watching her as she scampered into the open and made the wai sign to the Hmong sentry with the cheroot, he could still taste her on his lips. She spoke to the sentry, and after a time, he stood up and elaborately scratched his crotch before gesturing for her to enter the village enclosure. He followed behind her, his eyes never straying from the sway of her hips till they disappeared into the headman's hut.

It began to drizzle. Sawyer made an instant lean-to out of two sticks covered by a giant alocassia leaf. He lay prone on the pine needles and zeroed in on the headman's hut with his sight. After a while, she came out again. With her was a man in black peasant's pants and a dark shirt over a white T-shirt, wearing a curious knitted cap with an upturned brim that reminded Sawyer of a porkpie hat. He wore an American-made M-79 grenade launcher slung across his back. Sawyer assumed he was the Thai smuggler.

He could see her clearly through the sight, not having to switch to the binoculars. The Thai was squat and bandy-legged. He had a round face with thick eyebrows that pointed out and up from the center like those of the devil. He had a round head set close on broad round shoulders, and his hands were black with dirt or opium paste and looked very strong. His eyes were protruding, and although his thick sensual lips were smiling broadly at the girl, the eyes were not smiling at all.

Then she turned and made a beckoning gesture to Sawyer. The man looked up in his direction, and Sawyer got reluctantly to his feet, wishing she hadn't done it and knowing that once she had, he could no longer stay where he was. He slung both their packs over one shoulder and carrying the M-16 with the safety off in his free hand, made his way down to the corral where they stood waiting.

"This is the trader we speak of. His name Toonsang. He is much known in these parts. Most good trader. He says he goes to trade with Bhun Sa now. He takes us with him for eight chi of gold plus four chi for use of ponies. Half now, half when we see Bhun Sa," she said.

Hearing this, the trader nodded his head in agreement, displaying his betel-stained teeth in a broad smile that made Sawyer want to check his pocket to see if his wallet was still there.

"Why you want go see Bhun Sa, hey?" Toonsang asked, still grinning. He spoke the Northern Thai, called Thai Isan.

"To trade, what else?" Sawyer grinned back.

Toonsang thought this a huge joke and slapped the corral rail in appreciation.

Well, this is a jolly one, Sawyer thought, his uneasiness growing. Toonsang's laugh subsided and his eyes narrowed.

"The price is agreed?" he demanded.

Sawyer calculated mentally. A chi was 3.75 grams of gold, so twelve chi was about five hundred dollars' worth, but if he didn't object, they would be suspicious.

"The price is outrageous and this one will not pay," Sawyer said, slapping his chest in mock outrage.

"Not pay! Not pay!" cried the aggrieved trader in a high-pitched tone, looking wildly around as if unable to believe his ears. "By the phi, you will pay what is agreed!"

"By the chao, I will not," Sawyer said, letting the M-16 hang loosely down, not to threaten, simply to remind Toonsang that it was there.

Toonsang's eyes blinked once like a camera shutter.

"Your woman agreed to the price," Toonsang muttered sullenly, not taking his eyes off the M-16.

"Did you?" Sawyer turned angrily on Suong.

She hung her head.

"Yes, my lord. Forgive this worthless one."

"Your word will make a pauper of me," Sawyer growled. Then to Toonsang: "I will honor this worthless female's word, though by the phi, it goes hard. But only half now, as was said. Have you scales?" pulling a small leather sack of gold links and dust from around his neck.

"Inside. All is inside, younger brother. Also kow and cha for guest," Toonsang said, grinning widely as before and bowing them ahead of him. Not "honored guest," Sawyer noted, which a Thai used even if he were just lighting a stranger's cigarette. "Younger brother," which was always used for an inferior.

"I am more elder than you," Sawyer said in a joking way, not to force the issue, but to let Toonsang know that he understood the insult.

"Nay, nay. Only a young stallion can service such a mare," Toonsang cackled, roguishly rolling his eyes at Suong as he urged them up the bamboo ladder to the headman's hut.

The headman's hut, which also doubled as a guesthouse and tavern, was a single long room, of bamboo and teak, with a high, steeply sloping thatched roof. The hut had one side open to a porch on the east side to permit light yet provide shade from the afternoon heat. A large iron pot containing the stick Lao-style rice of the northern hills sat on a hearth near the center, and around it, a half-dozen of Toonsang's ruffians were eating rice and washing it down with rice beer. These were of different races, Thai, Karen, Akha, one with a Kachin turban, a tattooed Shan, but of one type. They were all heavily armed with automatic weapons and bandoliers of ammunition crisscrossed on their chests.

The headman himself was seated at a low bamboo table near the west wall. The headman had an amiable face that, like many of the Hmong, could have been pure Chinese. He wore a black robe and skullcap and, around his waist, his "trading day" white sash. He was drinking cha served by a female dressed in the black turban and red sash of the Hmong women. Also on the table were an abacus and a balance scale for weighing gold.

Another female served rice beer to four young Hmong men in black squatting by the western wall, not seeming to be doing anything, but with their rifles close to hand, making Sawyer feel a touch less conspicuous with his M-16. He laid the packs on the ground near the table, slung the carbine across his shoulder, and made the wai sign to the headman.

"Sawat dee, khrap," Sawyer said.

"And to you, honored guest," the headman said, gesturing for Sawyer to sit and take cha.

Sawyer sat facing Toonsang's men, implicitly placing himself under the headman's protection. The Hmong would never attack while he was under their roof. He wasn't so sure about Toonsang.

He laid the M-16 across the packs, within easy reach. Suong scuttled to a corner to wait. As a female she had no place at the table. Toonsang, an impudent grin on his face, came over and sat at the table with his back to the open porch, as if to show that he hadn't an enemy in the world. A Hmong woman brought them bowls of rice, but Sawyer motioned her to wait.

"Later, with your permission, uncle," to the headman. "I owe this man," indicating Toonsang, "six chi of gold and would first pay my debts."

The headman nodded as though appreciative of such prudence. He had a good face, lined with age, but alight with curiosity at the unexpected appearance of a European in his village. They weighed out the gold, and afterward Sawyer added an extra chi for the headman. Toonsang's eyes narrowed as he watched the headman take his gold.

"For rice beer for all, and also rice cakes to take," Sawyer explained.

"Younger brother is most generous," Toonsang growled.

"I like to make friends." Sawyer smiled.

"Any man who seeks Bhun Sa needs all the friends he can find," Toonsang said loudly, and Sawyer couldn't tell if he were bragging or simply announcing Sawyer's obituary. At the mention of Bhun Sa's name, the hut grew very quiet.

"Has the honorable stranger met Bhun Sa?" the headman asked.

Sawyer shook his head.

"Ah!" the headman clicked his tongue and said no more. It reminded Sawyer of when Brother Rap had asked a gung-ho captain straight from Fort Benning if he'd been in Nam before. When the captain had said no, and he didn't see that it made a goddamn bit of difference, Brother Rap had said "Yeah!" in exactly that same tone, meaning this one won't be around long enough to worry about. And sure enough, on the captain's first patrol his backpack caught on a twig. The captain twisted around to free it, and the grenade it was attached to blew his head off.

The Hmong women brought them bowls brimming with rice beer, and as the other men were served, the silence that had been there since Bhun Sa's name had been mentioned was broken by the low hum of conversation.

"Wealth and long life," the headman toasted, and they drank.

"Bhun Sa, eh?" Toonsang grinned. He wiped his mouth on the back of his sleeve and watched them both, an amused glint in his eyes.

"What manner of man is he?" Sawyer asked.

"A friendly man. He has only friends, hey?" Toonsang called out, looking over at his men and was answered by coarse laughter. "Know why he has only friends, younger brother?" Toonsang's eyes dancing. "Because"—not waiting for Sawyer to respond—"he kills all his enemies!"

Toonsang guffawed so hard at his own joke he almost fell down. Sawyer and the headman looked at each other.

"Have you met Bhun Sa?" he asked the headman.

"To know the servant of the prince is to know the prince," the headman said, glancing over toward Toonsang, who finished his beer and clapped his hands for another bowl.

The women brought beer and rice with chicken, the head going to Toonsang and the comb to Sawyer, as honored guests. As custom dictated, Toonsang loudly crunched the head as a sign for them to proceed. Toonsang drank the strong beer steadily, and by the time they finished, his small round eyes were swimming. Sawyer gave a long polite belch and the headman smiled.

"Perhaps a pipe later," the headman offered.

"A ten thousand of thanks, no, uncle."

"A vow?" the headman inquired delicately.

"Not even, uncle. Only prudence. A trader who is his own customer will see his profit go up in smoke."

"By the phi, there is truth," Toonsang said thickly, slapping his thigh with a blow that cracked like a whip.

"You trade the opium, then?" the headman asked.

Sawyer shook his head.

"I buy the bricks of white powder that come from the opium, uncle. Only bricks and only large quantities from such as Bhun Sa," Sawyer said hurriedly to forestall their own interest in doing business.

The headman looked at Sawyer with sharp curiosity.

"There are whispers in the hills that Bhun Sa has amassed a mountain of opium. Much of the second and the third cuttings of the Three Lands. It is said he has melted these into the white bricks of which our honored guest speaks and has hidden them away. Though there are those who do not believe of the tale," he cautioned.

"Do the whispers tell where the white bricks are hidden?" Sawyer asked.

The headman sat still, the only movement the blinking of his eyes.

"This no living man can say."

Toonsang rubbed his hand across his mouth.

"This of a mountain of white bricks is women's chatter. It would take more gold than our younger brother's twelve of chi to buy so much," he growled, glancing over at Sawyer's pack.

Sawyer's smile was deliberate.

"Gold can be stolen. Prudent men can find other things of value to trade."

"What things? Your woman?" Toonsang demanded, a snigger in his voice.

For an instant, all eyes turned toward the corner where Suong squatted, motionless as a statue. The headman frowned but said nothing. This was a place of business, and anyone may make an offer for goods on display.

"What say, younger brother? I make you fair trade for the woman. I give you back the six chi plus ten joi of opium and a good Kachin pony. All this and you are saved the expense of the trip to Bhun Sa," Toonsang offered, a lopsided grin splitting his face like an overripe fruit.

"The woman is not for sale," Sawyer replied, a sickly feeling in the pit of his stomach.

The room was very still. Sawyer could hear the creak of wood as someone shifted their weight, but he couldn't see who it was because he couldn't afford to take his eyes off Toonsang. He could hear the sound of breathing and the whisper of wind in the pines outside. His hand edged down toward the M-16. He was thankful he had kept the safety off.

"Yah, and friends should not haggle. Say twenty joi and be damned." Toonsang smiled, staring at Sawyer with eyes that had no drunkenness in them.

Sawyer's hand closed on the grip of the carbine.

"To the ghoul spirits with your twenty joi. The woman is not for sale," Sawyer said, his voice tight. All around him he could sense men reaching for their weapons. As if only just now realizing what was happening, Toonsang shook his head as though to clear it.

"Nay, nay, younger brother. I meant no dishonor, only a fair offer," Toonsang whined, raising both hands, the fingers splayed apart, to show he held no weapon.

"Take your offer to the clapped-up night chickens of Mae Lai," Sawyer snapped, naming the border town whose ramshackle brothels were frequented by smugglers and soldiers from all over the Golden Triangle.

"We will, we will! Clap and all!" Toonsang cackled and a burst of coarse laughter eased the tension. The room once more sounded to conversation.

As a peace offering, Toonsang held out a chew of betel mixed with ground lime and wrapped in a leaf, and when Sawyer declined, shrugged and took a bite.

"Women on a trip are a cause of much difficulty," the headman observed, accepting a chew from Toonsang now that it was over.

"Women are a cause of difficulty anywhere." Toonsang turned and spat. The headman nodded sagely.

"How long will it take us to reach Bhun Sa?" Sawyer asked, wanting to get off the subject of women. The effect Suong had on men was scary, and it was throwing a monkey wrench into the mission like nothing he had ever seen.

"Who can say? He is maybe Burma-side? Maybe Lao-side? Where does the tiger sleep?" Toonsang grinned oafishly, and this time Sawyer was sure he wasn't the fool he pretended to be. Knowing how long it would take to reach Bhun Sa might be an indication of where he was.

"Wherever he likes," Sawyer replied.

Toonsang guffawed and the Hmong tittered among themselves. At least that was better than the first time he had heard the joke, Sawyer remembered. Brother Rap had told it at the Continental Shelf terrace bar in Saigon, only then the question had been, "Where does a six-hundred pound gorilla sit?" They had all laughed until a REMF captain at the next table had said with a drawl that stretched all the way back to Alabama, "If Ah was a nigger Ah wouldn't be telling no jokes about no big black gorillas, boy," and Sawyer had to grab Rap to keep him from taking the captain out then and there. "He's an officer, man. That's just what he wants you to do," Sawyer had breathed in Rap's ear. Later, they stalked the captain through the streets back to his apartment, Rap getting close enough to drop a "frag" in the captain's bedroom before Sawyer managed to talk him out of it.

"Make it count," he had told Rap, who wound up spending the remainder of his R 'n' R in Soul Alley, a tawdry neon ghetto near the Tan Son Nhut airbase, eating fried chicken, flying high on Buddha grass, and taking trips in back with the disease-ravaged Vietnamese girls who weren't pretty enough to make it on Tu Do Street. Sawyer finally came to collect him at Mama Jo's, where they used to hang the red, black, and green striped flag of the Black Liberation Front behind the bar and where the MPs never came, because the last time they had tried to move in, Mama Jo, a six-foot-four former linebacker, now a permanent AWOL, had greeted them with a blast from a twelve-gauge shotgun.

"Ain't going back, man. It's a fucking white man's war," Rap had said.

"I'm a white man," Sawyer had said.

"Then fuck you too."

"Okay," Sawyer had said and started to go, and then Rap had sighed and slid off the bar stool.

"Fuck it, I'm coming."

And Mama Jo, light gleaming through the bluish haze of marijuana smoke from the gold ring in his nostril, had simply shrugged and muttered, "Dumb nigger."

Sawyer remembered how, even when they were back in Indian country, Brother Rap always talked about looking the captain up when they got back to the World. He concocted all sorts of ingenious revenges, but it never came to anything because Rap never did make it back.

The headman smiled at the success of Sawyer's joke.

"Even so, honored guest. Only enter the land of Bhun Sa, and if you do not find him, he will find you."

"And pay him with what, younger brother?" Toonsang wanted to know. "By the phi, I will bring you safely to Bhun Sa, but be warned against playing these European tricks as the reaching for your rifle with Bhun Sa. You have already lost the one eye."

So he had caught that, Sawyer thought. Well, perhaps it was for the best that they knew he didn't trust them.

"I still have two of something else," Sawyer said quietly.

"So speaks a man!" exclaimed the headman, and there was a murmur of approval from the Hmong.

"Even so. It will be good to have our younger brother's rifle with us on our journey," Toonsang agreed. "But it is more than idle curiosity that prompts my question. If what you bring to Bhun Sa arouses his displeasure, all our lives may be forfeit," he argued.

"This is truth," the headman agreed, unable to suppress the curiosity in his own eyes.

Sawyer sighed as if conceding the justice of their request. If he couldn't convince Toonsang that what he had in his pack wasn't worth stealing, the mission was over.

"I have arms to trade for the bricks of the morphine. In these packs is not gold, but books with pictures of different kinds of weapons and papers for the trading."

"Pah! Only pictures." Toonsang turned and spat a stream of juice red as blood.

"Have you no guns with you? This would be of interest to us," the headman said. The young Hmong began to speak among themselves.

"Only a few piddling things for personal use. Of little value." Sawyer shrugged.

"And if we wanted to buy?" the headman persisted, sensing the restlessness of his young men.

"And I too, by the phi!" Toonsang objected.

Sawyer smiled. It was what he had been waiting for.

"It would be my honor and pleasure to trade with you— upon my safe return," he said.

"Then it is as a thing that is well and done," Toonsang declared heartily, slapping the table like a judge with a gavel.

There was a stir as everyone got up to leave. Although the clouds were low and threatening, there were still at least three hours of daylight left for travel. Sawyer grabbed his M-16 and one of the packs and gave the other to the woman.

"Tu comprends ce qu'il faut faire," she whispered as he handed her the pack, her disconcerting eyes looking through him. And as if he could read her mind—no, as if they were one mind—he knew not only what she meant but that he thought the same.

As they loaded the mules, Toonsang cast a rueful eye at the pack Sawyer was tying on to his pony.

"Only pictures after all, eh, younger brother?" as if the joke was on him.

"See for yourself," Sawyer shrugged, knowing they didn't believe him. Anyone seeking to buy a mountain of morphine, if such a thing was possible, would have to be carrying something of great value in his pack. Without saying it, the woman had told him quite explicitly what had to be done.

At the first opportunity, he would have to kill Toonsang.

9

Fire above heaven.
The wealthy man represses evil
and honors good.
The large wagon
has a full load.

THE moon wore a ghostly halo as it broke through the haze. The silvery light revealed the giant carved head atop the stone gateway, the face of the god a hazy white as if it were on a negative. A tendril of vegetation made a diagonal scar from the forehead to the chin, dividing the face into two unequal parts. Without a word, the soldiers took up positions by the gateway, joining the long columns of stone gods on either side of the road guarding the way into the ancient city.

Only then, when the soldiers had disappeared into the shadows, did a single dark figure emerge to stand alone in the center of the road that was white as snow in the pale light. By some trick of the light, the figure's face was almost a mirror image of the god's face, though few saw it. For rarely, even among his own soldiers, did any dare look directly upon the face of Son Lot.

Yet conscious of their eyes, he strode like a conqueror through the deep shadows of the vaulting gateway into the empty city. He walked down the great roadway, the paving stones long since crumpled and broken. Once, he heard something and turned, but it was only the flutter of the bats coming out to hunt. No one had followed him into the city. He was alone.

He walked through the empty streets, intricately carved galleries and towers looming on all sides. He found a high place and looked around at the shadowy ruins. A thousand years ago this place had been the center of the universe. "And will be again," the voice of his other self whispered to him, and he shivered.

"But there are so many imponderables," he told the voice.

"You have a prisoner," the voice insinuated.

"Parker has told us all he knows. We have opened his head like a can of sardines," thinking of Parker's screams.

Pranh! We were friends for God's sake! Parker had begged.

What children you white men are. Is the fact that we knew each other once supposed to make me betray the revolution? he had said.

"Parker has not told you all he knows, merely all he thinks he knows. Surely you can persuade him," the voice mocked. It held an echo, like the lonely sound of his footsteps in the darkness.

He came down an old stone stairway and walked on until he came to the place he sought. A temple ruin among a thousand other temples in the city, overgrown with vegetation. The temple was smaller than most and very old. He climbed the broken steps, the centers worn smooth and concave from centuries of bare feet, and came to where an ancient altar had once stood under a soaring dome, the roof now broken and open to the sky.

The wind whistled through the chinks and around the ancient stone corners. It spoke in voices a thousand years old. The intricately carved stone walls were hidden by the darkness, and statues of gods far older than the Buddha stood in the silent dust of centuries like an army of shadows.

Then one of the shadows moved.

"Where is it?" Son Lot demanded, his voice sounding harsh even in his own ears.

"This way," the figure said, and led Son Lot down a passageway behind the altar. The way was narrow and dark and they had to feel their way. The air was stale, lifeless. It smelled like a tomb. There were a number of turnings down side passages, and if Son Lot had not been following, he would have lost his way. Then he saw the light from a single candle gleaming from a subterranean passage at the bottom of a stone staircase.

They went down the stairs and into a large stone storeroom packed floor to ceiling with thousands of wooden cases. The air had a medicinal smell. A squad of heavily armed soldiers lounged around the room, their eyes on the two who had just come in, one of whom grabbed a wooden case at random, took out a knife and pried it open. Inside was a single large white brick imprinted with the number "999," the raised numbers obviously done in a hand press. The man broke off a corner of the brick with his knife. He crumpled it to white powder with his fingers and held it out to Son Lot.

"This is the morphine base. It makes the heroin of an unbelievable purity. In this room are three thousands and nine hundreds of boxes, each of which contains one kilo. In this room is wealth enough to defeat our enemies a ten of times over," Bhun Sa said.

Son Lot took a pinch of powder in his hand, looking curiously at it for a moment.

"A curious weapon." He smiled. "Lenin was right. The imperialists themselves will sell us the rope with which we will hang them," he said, and blew the powder on his fingers away like a dandelion.

"My men will guard here. Yours outside the city walls."

"It is as agreed."

Bhun Sa looked curiously at Son Lot, his eyes hiding in ambush under his long dark eyebrows.

"Only a most foolish man would think to take the morphine for himself, Comrade General. For such a one would have no one to trade with and worse he would be caught between my displeasure and the fury of the dog-eaters."

"That would be most foolish," Son Lot agreed smoothly. "It is too dangerous for you to keep the morphine powder on your side of the border. Too dangerous for me to take the arms we need on my side where they might fall into the dog-eaters' accursed hands. Like all good agreements, ours is based upon a mutual dislike of the alternatives."

Bhun Sa smiled, a crease deepening along the lines of an old scar on his cheek.

"As it is said, the superior man sees where his own interest lies. But we have lived long enough to see the wheel of karma take many a strange turning, and men are not always wise. While we know that the comrade general is farseeing, yet it may happen that some foolish subordinate who lacks the comrade general's great wisdom may try to take by force what is not his to take."

"A rash and dangerous act," Son Lot said.

"Most rash," Bhun Sa agreed. "To prevent just such a fool-ishness we have planted plastique of a sufficiency to destroy not only the morphine but the very temple around it. An attack would be both suicidal and pointless."

"A prudent measure. The Lord of the Shan is most wise. But could ordinary men be trusted to carry out such an order? For it would mean their own deaths, would it not? Perhaps such men could be corrupted?" Son Lot smiled as he glanced around the room at Bhun Sa's men.

"These are of proven loyalty," Bhun Sa replied airily. "And hardly likely to sell their three khwan upon the word of an armed stranger. Yet the world is a cruel place and even the strongest may falter. Knowing this I have taken hostages of each of these as an added precaution. These hostages would be the first to feel my displeasure." Bhun Sa smiled.

Son Lot could sense a shudder passing through the room like a cold draught. Bhun Sa's cruelty was legend.

"Then it is settled," Son Lot said heartily. "Do you go back shortly?"

"There are matters to which I must attend. Fuk Wa of the Kuomintang has had the impertinence to nibble like a mouse at our opium trade. This has aroused my displeasure."

"Then hurry, for the time is short. Each day the strength of the dog-eaters grows in the hills and along the Mekong," Son Lot said, then slyly, "Where comes a buyer for such a quantity of the white powder?"

Bhun Sa smiled.

"Where there is honey, the flies are sure to gather," he said.

10

Fire over the marsh.
The superior man allows
*   variations within the norm.*
If he meets bad men
he can speak with them.

THEY could hear the crashing of gears from around the bend as the trucks downshifted to take the hill. For an instant, Sawyer's and Toonsang's eyes found each other and then once again they sighted their weapons down at the road. Through the trees Sawyer could see a good stretch of the muddy road as it wound its way through the narrow defile below them.

Toonsang held his M-79 grenade launcher ready. From across the road, the Kachin had signaled four vehicles coming, two jeeps and two trucks with soldiers. With the vehicles having to crawl slowly up the incline and men with automatic weapons on both sides of the defile, it should be like shooting fish in a barrel, Sawyer reasoned, still hoping the soldiers would pass them by. Even with a good ambush, there would be a lot of shooting and an unlucky bullet could do a lot of damage to the mission. Worse, they would have announced their presence here to the world.

The growl of the engines grew louder, and Sawyer held his finger light as breath on the trigger as the first jeep crawled into view. It carried an officer and two men, one a driver and one manning a mounted M-60 machine gun. They wore the dark green camouflage uniforms and black berets of the Thai Rangers. They were anxiously scanning from side to side as the jeep lurched drunkenly through the slimy ruts deep as furrows. The officer looked straight up at Sawyer, who resisted the panicky impulse to duck. The hills were heavily forested with teak and bush, and the officer would have to be Daniel Boone himself to spot anything, Sawyer reassured himself, holding his breath.

As the first jeep went by, the second came into their field of fire. They watched it slipping sideways, wheels spinning in the mud, losing it, and the soldiers getting ready to jump out. The whine of the transmission grew louder. Sawyer's grip tightened, and then it was all right as the four-wheel drive caught and the jeep spurted ahead. Sawyer could see a smile break out on the soldiers' sweaty faces, and shared a quick breath of relief with them as the trucks began to rumble by. Wide-eyed Rangers, their automatic rifles pointed at all angles, peered out from the back of the trucks like frightened monkeys. As they disappeared around the next bend, Sawyer nodded at Toonsang, who grinned back, his betel-stained teeth and upturned eyebrows making him look more devilish than ever.

One for you, you son of a bitch, Sawyer thought irritably, knowing it was going to be a lot harder than he had thought. It was Toonsang who had halted their ponies about half an hour earlier and then, listening intently for a moment, had issued sharp orders in Shan and Isan Thai to set up the ambush. When Sawyer had looked at him questioningly, Toonsang had pointed up the road.

"Soldiers coming. Thai patrol, maybe."

"How do you know?" Sawyer asked. He had heard nothing.

"Petrol." Toonsang grinned, tapping his nose.

And now that he had mentioned it, Sawyer too was suddenly conscious of the faint whiff of gasoline fumes. He cursed himself for an idiot, all at once remembering how the VC used to spot the coming of American patrols in the dense jungle by the smell of the Americans' after-shave lotion. He would have to do better, he warned himself. It had been a long time since Nam and he was older and rusty, and if he wanted to survive the next twenty-four hours, he was going to have to do a lot better.

As the sound of the trucks faded in the distance, Toonsang's head popped from behind a mound of earth like a groundhog. He looked and listened and then got to his feet.

"We go now, yes," Toonsang said, slinging the M-79 across his back and politely motioning Sawyer ahead of him. Sawyer complied, scrambling up the steep hill. Not to have done so would have been bad kreng chai, but he could feel Toonsang behind him every step as he went up to where the ponies were tethered.

Suong was waiting with the animals. They began loading up with the relieved, yet vaguely disappointed cursing of men who have avoided an expected combat. Toonsang insisted on helping Suong mount her pony. She told him she needed no help, but he managed to slide his hand between her legs as he pushed her up. She angrily kicked the pony away, her dark eyes flashing. Toonsang laughed.

It wasn't normal behavior for an Asian, for whom public touching is offensive. Toonsang was only doing it to provoke him, and maybe now was as good a time as any, Sawyer thought, anger rising. He already had the safety clicked off when he realized that the Thai patrol was still close enough to hear a shot. As he slung his M-16 over his shoulder, he felt a prickling along his spine, a warning from the Reptile. Turning, he caught a nasty grin from the Kachin coming up from below and lowering his weapon, as though he too had remembered the Thai patrol just in time.

Tough luck, you son of a bitch, Sawyer thought, as he checked his pony. Another second and both Toonsang and he would have been dead and the Kachin would have had Toonsang's opium and the girl. Sawyer tightened the bed roll and saddlebags carried mountain-style, in front of the rider, and mounted.

That was the problem, Sawyer thought. There was always at least one of them behind him and they were too spread out. He couldn't hope to get them all at once. Especially now, going single file along the narrow trail that roughly paralleled the road but was about halfway up the hill.

It wasn't going to be easy, he thought, looking back over his shoulder at the Kachin, who grinned as though they both shared the same joke. Ahead, the trail was a tunnel of hanging vines and leaves a thousand different shades of green. Wind hissed in the treetops high above. A twig fluttered, and at the same instant both

Sawyer and the Kachin started to swing their weapons around, then relaxed as a parakeet flitted, a blue spark between the branches.

The hooves of the ponies and the mules made soft padding sounds on the trail, sodden with wet leaves. All around, the teak trees towered straight and brown or slanted one against another. Higher up, the branches intertwined to form a latticework through which the colorless light filtered, forming intricate shadows. Always there was the sound of water dripping from above and the smell of wet vegetation. Now and then they would come across a grove of dark Yang trees, the kind that are tapped for the lacquer, and across a fallen trunk, a profusion of wildly colored orchids, startling as a neon sign.

Ahead, Sawyer could hear the sound of rushing water. It grew louder and they came to a tiny stream splashing down the rocks and across the trail. A brightly colored kingfisher flew up the stream. As he guided his pony through the rushing water, Sawyer noticed the tracks and leavings of a Lyre deer on the muddy bank.

The wind came up. The tall trees began to creak, and Sawyer felt a sense of foreboding. The forest seemed ancient, and he remembered Vasnasong's curious remark that "sex was older than mankind." Well, there were a lot of things older than mankind, dark things buried deep in the makeup of man from the time before we were human, and it was as if the forest was calling them up. He didn't want to go any further. He couldn't shake the feeling that going up the trail was like going back in time. To a dark time when only force ruled and anything was permitted. But anything *is* permitted if only you allow yourself, came a secret voice from his subconscious. *Anything*.

The voice had the sound of the branches swaying in the wind. The skin at the back of his neck tightened and he let it. He would need all of the Reptile's cunning if he were to survive, remembering the quick whispers with Suong by the ponies before they set up the ambush.

"I can't get at him. He is cunning," he had whispered.

"Yes, but only cunning. You will need cleverness," she had whispered back.

"But how? . . ." he began, but it was too late. Toonsang had come up and was grinning at them both. His yellowish skin, the gaps between his teeth, and the crushed porkpie hat combined to give him the appearance of a vaguely demented jack-o'-lantern.

He could see Toonsang's broad back up at the head of the column. Even from the back, there was something brutish about him. Sawyer's fingers itched for the gun. Not yet, he told himself. She's right. It needs more than brute cunning. The son of a bitch won't give you a shot at him unless he's already got you covered.

The trail began to dip down toward the road. The pony started to move too quickly and Sawyer had to rein him back. The mules perked up their ears and Toonsang halted. They listened to the wind in the leaves, the breathing and stamping of the mules, and always, the drip of water. Sawyer could see Toonsang's nostrils widening and shrinking as he sniffed deeply of the forest air. Then Toonsang dismounted and began to probe the trail for booby traps and mines, his pony following slowly behind.

Suddenly Toonsang stopped. He looked up and sniffed again, and then Sawyer smelt it too. Smoke from a campfire. Either a very big party, or fools, Sawyer thought.

They were fools. Two of them were roasting chunks of meat over a small fire while a third soldier bent a village girl facedown over a log. Sawyer could see her white buttocks gleaming as he plunged in and out of her anus. The two reached for their rifles, but Toonsang, the Karen, the Shan, and Sawyer had them covered. The two looked white in the face, but the third turned from the girl and faced them boldly, a Colt .45 in his hand, his penis still red and impudently pointed up at the sky.

"A thousand of greetings," the soldier called loudly in Isan Thai. He had a broad Chinese face with ears that stuck out like jug handles.

"I fear we interfere with your pleasure," Toonsang replied, grinning hugely.

"Pah! Little enough pleasure from a Lisu bitch! Take her yourself and good riddance," Jug-Ears said, grabbing his penis and shaking himself elaborately. But he kept the pistol pointed at Toonsang.

"We will, we will—and everything else, even your pants!" Toonsang declared, and even Jug-Ears joined in the harsh laughter. But the two soldiers could only manage sickly grins. The Lisu girl grabbed her clothes and squatted on the ground, not daring to look at any of them.

"Enough talk! Let us kill them and go," the Kachin said, coming up. He swung his Chinese SKS carbine into position. Jug-

Ears' eyes narrowed as he took in the new factor of the Kachin. The other two were frozen like rabbits caught by headlights at the side of a road.

"So be it! This one is ready for the long night. I take you" —Jug-Ears gestured with the pistol at Toonsang—"and with joss, maybe one other with me"—scanning them. Then his eyes widened.

"By the phi, a white man!"

"A trader, he says," Toonsang said, elaborately picking his nose with one hand to cover his other dropping down to a Tokorev pistol he had gotten from God knows where.

"What you trade?" Jug-Ears wanted to know, his forehead furrowed as if debating Sawyer as a potential target. Sawyer felt all their eyes burning on him and wondered whether he had more to fear from a shot from the front or the back.

"Life and death," Sawyer replied.

Jug-Ears' face brightened.

"Then we are all in same business, neh?"

"What is this stupidity? It is a dead man who speaks," complained the Kachin, urging his pony a few steps forward.

"But still more of a man than you," Jug-Ears retorted, grabbing his penis. But this time it didn't cooperate, and as it shriveled, so too they could see Jug-Ears visibly deflate.

They would kill him now, Sawyer thought, and he decided to take a chance, because once they started shooting, they might decide to take care of him at the same time.

"What is the Kuomintang doing so far Thai-side?"

"Retreating," Toonsang sneered, and their guffaws echoed in the woods. Only the two soldiers and Jug-Ears didn't laugh.

"They've been doing that since Yunnan." Sawyer smiled. "Who's chasing you this time?"

Jug-Ears looked suspiciously up at Sawyer.

"How you know we are KMT?"

"Who else would stoop so low as to raid a Lisu village?" Sawyer shrugged, and this time Toonsang laughed so hard he had to wipe the tears from his eyes.

Jug-Ears flushed. He looked up at Sawyer with hatred. Sawyer tensed to start shooting. Then the look faded. Jug-Ears had found the opening Sawyer had left him.

"We took the village to remind Bhun Sa we can come Thai-side too. Now, we leave." He shrugged. "If this one is permitted, better to die with pants on"—and when Toonsang nodded, he began to pull on his clothes.

"Stupid! These not KMT. These are deserters!" the Kachin insisted.

Toonsang shrugged.

"Where there are three of the KMT, there may be more," the Karen said, reining his pony tighter. It was a Yunnan pony, sandier in color and less shaggy than the Kachin ponies. At this, Jug-Ears looked up sharply.

"Truth," he growled.

"Lie! He makes the pretend only to stay alive," the Kachin spat disgustedly.

"Truth," Jug-Ears repeated.

"Truth, lie. What we do now? Shoot or eat? You say," the Shan declared to Toonsang, speaking for the first time. He aimed his rifle at Jug-Ears, his elbow out to the side as though he were holding a crossbow.

"We have no quarrel with KMT—" Toonsang began.

"Stupid! You not see what he trying—" the Kachin hissed. The two soldiers blanched at the sound. The girl covered her head with the colorful blue and red scarf of the Lisu and rocked silently back and forth on her heels.

"Be still!" Toonsang snapped.

"But is lie—"

"I command here. Does any dispute this?" Toonsang roared, aiming the pistol at the Kachin. There was a murderous look in Toonsang's wide-set eyes, and the Kachin looked away disgustedly.

"Better not to kill us," Jug-Ears said carefully, looking from the Kachin to Toonsang, pursing his lips with the effort of judging such a weighty matter.

Finally, Toonsang leaned forward over the pony's neck and pointed the Tokorev at Jug-Ears. "You may leave with your lives. But your ponies and goods we take. Also the female," Toonsang pronounced.

At this the two soldiers looked up in disbelief, not daring to believe their good joss. Jug-Ears eyed Toonsang warily.

"What of our weapons?" he asked.

"We take."

Jug-Ears shrugged and pointed the Colt back at Toonsang in a kind of Mexican standoff.

"Then shoot us now. Without guns we are dead men."

Toonsang considered this for a moment. No one breathed. A bird chirped somewhere, and it seemed to Sawyer that time had stood still and that a scene such as this had been played and replayed for eternity.

"By the phi, you have a prick and balls. Take your guns and go, but quickly," Toonsang declared magnanimously, waving them away with the pistol.

"Bad business," the Kachin growled, but Toonsang was enjoying his moment too much to bother squashing him. Still, Jug-Ears looked distrustfully up at them.

"Truth?" he murmured.

"You have a distrustful nature." Toonsang laughed and ostentatiously clicked on the safety and stuck the pistol into his waist sash.

At this, Jug-Ears growled something to the other two and they hurriedly grabbed their rifles by the slings and made ready to go. Jug-Ears smiled up at Sawyer.

"May fortune follow you, One-Round-Eye."

"And you." Sawyer smiled.

With a last wary look at Toonsang, Jug-Ears turned to join the two soldiers who'd begun to walk hurriedly toward the far side of the clearing. Jug-Ears muttered something and they tried to make a show of it, but their movements were stiff and unnatural as marionettes.

They hadn't gone ten meters before a burst of automatic fire cut them down like toy soldiers at the hand of a bored child. Toonsang had pulled an AK-47 from a sheath hidden under his saddle blanket. The Kachin was firing too. Jug-Ears almost succeeded in turning around, rifle coming into line before a piece of his head flew off and he toppled forward spilling blood. The others joined in firing long bursts at the bodies. The Lisu girl began to run in circles, screaming all the while until a short burst from the Kachin knocked her off her feet. The Kachin turned toward Sawyer, only to find the M-16 covering him and Toonsang, who shrugged and sheathed the AK-47.

The Shan and the Karen slid off their ponies and ran to strip the bodies and gather their ponies and booty, as the Akha and the Thai came up with the mules. Suong was with them. Toonsang kneed his pony and came between Sawyer and the Kachin.

"Better this way, younger brother. More easy. If we let them live, they maybe sell us to KMT, maybe Birman army. That one have big prick and balls. If we shoot face-to-face, he make somebody die. Maybe you. Maybe me." He grinned.

"Better to shoot him in the back."

"Ah yes, much," Toonsang agreed cheerfully. He glanced back at the Kachin and they both began to laugh, their betel-blackened teeth giving them the appearance of demons.

Sawyer looked over at Suong. Her face was calm, but there was a faint moustache of perspiration on her upper lip. He wanted to talk to her, but it was too dangerous. Toonsang drew his pony alongside Sawyer and they rode across the clearing side by side.

"Then the feud with the Kachin was a thing of shadows, like the play-acting of the nang?" Sawyer asked.

"Of a certainty. That one with prick in air was a fool to believe."

"Brave, though."

"Ah yes. Big prick and no wits." Toonsang sniggered.

"A fool, you say?"

Toonsang looked at him blankly.

"Who else would trust his life to a stranger?"

By the time they reached the pass, the shadows were long across the road. It had rained earlier and gray clouds still shrouded the holy mountain Doi Tung; the pagoda near the peak could not be seen. Although they remained watchful, they had relaxed enough to come down to the road. Ambushes were unlikely here, for this was sacred ground. It was said that a band of Communist insurgents had once passed a column of Thai Rangers on the opposite side of the road with nothing more deadly exchanged between them than wary looks.

The road was a brown gash between the hills. It wound upward through the pass, tiny rivulets of runoff water snaking down from the muddy slope. Somewhere between here and the Salween, though no one, not even the mapmakers in Bangkok and Rangoon could say where, was the Burmese border.

The green of the hills was very deep, mostly from pine because of the altitude, with an occasional oak, and the road was bordered by a fringe of brown pine needles. The mules were strung in a long line and they moved with shortened steps to take the incline, the sound of their hooves muffled by the pine needles. Toonsang's men, mounted on ponies, were spaced at intervals, each man leading a string of four mules, so that if they came under attack they could disperse quickly without losing all the animals. Birds chattered in the trees, a comforting sound. If they grew silent, it would be a warning of an ambush.

Sawyer and Suong rode side by side, not far behind Toonsang. Since the shooting, she had said little. Not far behind them rode the Kachin, the SKS held across his thighs for quick access. From the way she held herself, Sawyer knew she could feel the Kachin behind her.

"He means to kill you," she said.

Her voice was soft, so soft he might not have heard, and despite the words, so sensual it was as if she had stroked him with soft fur. She couldn't help it if she wanted to, Sawyer thought. It's how she is. There was no part of her that didn't set a man to thinking dangerous thoughts.

"I know."

"That one wants me"—a jerk of her chin indicating Toonsang's broad back, the porkpie hat perched absurdly on the top of his round head as on a snowman. "Always I feel his eyes on me. He will come tonight."

"Let him come," Sawyer said.

She looked at him, only darkness in her eyes.

"You wish this?"

"Let him come," Sawyer said. "I'll be waiting."

She didn't say any more and he was grateful for that. Because he was starting not to trust himself where she was concerned. His feelings were all tangled up. He let her move ahead a bit so he could watch her tight little behind sway with the pony's stride. He felt himself harden, and at that moment he wanted her so badly he could barely keep from throwing himself upon her right then and there in front of all of them. Why lie to himself? he thought. Seeing the rape of the Lisu girl and its deadly aftermath had in some dark way fired his blood. But what he felt for Suong wasn't just sex. It was more than that. But it wasn't love either. Because they were using each other. Tonight he would use her in the vilest way a man can use a woman, he thought. As a pimp for his own purposes, so he could get at Toonsang. That wasn't any kind of love, unless Vasnasong was right and love wasn't the selfless bullshit we were always taught, but something far more ancient, with selfishness and using as much a part of it as anything else.

Because he was so absorbed in his thoughts, he was slower than the others to react, and when he did, at first he missed it. Because the figure up ahead was so utterly motionless he assumed it was just a roadside Buddha, one of the crude little shrines one would come across now and again in these hills.

As first Toonsang and then Suong came abreast of the figure, each in turn made the wai sign to the forehead, which is reserved for holy monks and the Lord Buddha himself. The figure was draped in a ragged monk's robe, the orange color sun-faded pale yellow, the right shoulder left bare as is the custom. It was seated in the lotus position and like a statue was utterly oblivious of them. As Sawyer rode up, he could see that it was an old monk, though how old it was impossible to say. The face was gaunt, yet barely creased by time, and burnt the color of teak by the sun. The head was utterly bald, so that it was easy to see the death skull it would someday become. But its appearance was not forbidding. The face wore the half-lidded smile of the Buddha, and the dark eyes were fixed upon eternity. So when Sawyer too wai'd, he was utterly startled when the statue suddenly came to life and wai'd back at him.

The pony shied at the sudden movement, and with a curse, Sawyer yanked at the rein and stopped it, facing the monk.

"Blessings and greetings, holy one."

"Greetings and blessings, brother. This humble one fears he has startled your pony," the old monk said. His eyes were younger than his face. They sparkled with intelligence.

"And not only my pony, by the phi. I nearly shot you— or worse, this fornication of a pony," Sawyer said, yanking the pony's head around.

The monk smiled.

"Like most shootings, that would have been of benefit to no one. As for your pony, the sight in his right eye is imperfect, hence he has fear on that side. Only let him turn his head to smell the man smell and see that this humble one poses no danger and he will stand easily."

Sawyer turned the pony's head. The pony quieted. He leaned over and patted the pony's neck. As he did so, he checked the positions of Toonsang and the Kachin. And Suong. They had all stopped to watch.

"You know ponies, then?" Sawyer asked.

"Animals are simple. Men less so," the monk said in a way that indicated he had seen Sawyer's action.

Sawyer squinted up the empty road. Except for the hoofprints of Toonsang's ponies and mules, there were no recent tracks. The sky was a slate gray ceiling over the hills, and when he looked back down at the old monk, he smelled the wet pine needles and earth, as though the monk was indeed a crude village ikon made of mud and straw.

"A lonely road to beg rice," Sawyer observed.

"And yet you have come," the monk replied, his eyes twinkling. Then Sawyer noticed that his begging bowl was turned facedown on the ground. A sign he sought no alms.

"That cannot be denied, holy one." Sawyer smiled. "But this one meant only that this is a most dangerous place. Have you no fear of bandits?"

"A monk's poverty is his safety. Is this not true?"

"Here, perhaps. In my land, even poverty is no protection against bandits."

"That is a hard land that breeds such desperate men. And are the rich safe, then?"

"Not even." Sawyer shook his head.

"Then you too live in a most dangerous place, brother."

"Every place is dangerous, holy one."

"That is truth—for we carry the most dangerous place of all with us always," the monk replied, glancing down at his own chest as a way of avoiding pointing at his head, which would have been bad kreng chai.

"I have more danger than that with me, holy one," Sawyer said, glancing back at Toonsang out of the corner of his eye.

"Yes, that is plain," the monk said, following his glance. "The men of the opium trade are desperate men. But perhaps you are such a one yourself, brother"—eyeing Sawyer's M-16.

"I must do business with these men. But I am not of these men, holy one," Sawyer said, unable to keep the disgust out of his voice.

The old man got stiffly to his feet and peered intently into Sawyer's good eye as if to read his thoughts.

"Truly, you believe this, brother. But if you do business with them, are you not one of them?"

Sawyer felt as though he had walked into a wall. The old man's eyes seemed to see into his very soul. For some reason, he knew his answer mattered. He didn't know why, but it mattered.

"I don't know," he said.

The old monk smiled. His face creased deeply along ancient laugh lines.

"That is good. Not to know is a much higher state than knowing for a certainty that which is not so," he said, gathering up his bowl. "I will come with you as far as the road to Doi Tung," he said loudly so that all might hear. Then softly to Sawyer, "There will be no killing while I am with you. Even for desperate men, to kill before a monk's eyes is most terrible bad karma that a hundred lifetimes could not redeem."

Under Toonsang's watchful eyes, Sawyer readied a mule for the monk to ride. Toonsang made no effort to stop him, and Sawyer wondered at that until he realized that the monk's presence was a safe conduct for all of them in these hills. Despite his years, the monk scrambled up on the mule as agilely as a monkey.

Once more, Toonsang led them up the road, now completely in shadow. The monk and Sawyer rode side by side.

"Is Doi Tung your home?" Sawyer asked.

"A monk is always at home everywhere. The bot atop Doi Tung is a place I sometimes stay. And you, brother," glancing sideways at Sawyer, "where is your home?"

"The village of the Angels in the land of America."

"The Angels, as in Krung Thep?"—giving the Thai name for Bangkok.

"The very same."

"A big village?"

"Ah yes. A thousand of huts and more."

"What a terrible liar you are, brother! Worse than any 'guest,' " the old monk cackled, referring to the common belief that all Indians were unscrupulous liars who, even if born in Thailand, were always contemptuously referred to as "guests," "for I have seen a photograph of your village of the Angels in the newspaper. It is a great city, like Krung Thep. Only the people must hide in automobiles, for there were thousands in the picture on big roads intertwined like vines on the teakwood. But no people. Truly, the American is most strange."

"Why strange, holy one?"

The monk looked curiously at Sawyer.

"Do you not think that to build a city for machines and not people is most strange?"

"That is truth." Sawyer smiled, but his mind was elsewhere. He had caught a whiff of smoke on the wind. He could sense the nervousness in the ponies and mules, and up ahead, Toonsang was anxiously scanning the darkening hills.

"Soon now," the monk said.

Sawyer turned sharply, hand moving to the M-16.

"Soon for what?"

But the monk's smile was the imperturbable calm of the Buddha. Although his lips moved, his words seemed to come from somewhere else, like a ventriloquist's trick.

"That which you seek, brother. The war without only mirrors the war within."

Suong looked anxiously over her shoulder at Sawyer. Tightening the grip on his M-16, he spurred his pony forward, flicking off the safety as he came abreast of her. Toonsang had already gone around the far bend in the road to scout ahead.

Suong and Sawyer looked at each other. Her hands were clenched tight in her lap, and then he saw that she was clutching a hand grenade.

The sky had turned a deep violet. Soon it would be night. Sawyer looked back, and the Kachin grinned at him. He was cradling the SKS in his arms, but as long as the monk was there, Sawyer thought he wouldn't shoot.

They saw it as soon as they came around the bend. The entrance to the Lisu village was a gap in a split-rail and bamboo fence about a hundred meters off the road. The entrance was lit by a towering bonfire, deliberately set to illuminate the scene before them. The flickering yellow light brought the shadow to life. The roar and crackle of the fire was all they could hear. Beyond the entrance, Sawyer could see a body lying in the mud. From here he couldn't tell if it was male or female. But there was no mistaking the things lined up like telephone poles along the trail to the village entrance.

There were six of them. They looked very young. Mostly recruits, no doubt. All in the uniform of the Kuomintang. Each of them had been impaled on a sharpened bamboo stake between their legs. Their hands were tied by a cord looped over the long crossbeam of the crude scaffold. They hung from the crossbeam like chickens, the height carefully set so that they would have had to strain up on their toes to keep the point from penetrating deeper, but just high enough so they couldn't sink down and end their appalling agony too quickly. Their pants were wet with dark stains, and at their feet were black pools swarming with crawling things. From the expression on their faces, they must have taken many hours to die.

Toonsang sat on his pony, a cheroot glowing in his mouth. As Sawyer came up, he spat.

"Welcome, younger brother," Toonsang called out. He was smiling. In the flickering light his betel-stained teeth seemed to drip with blood.

"Welcome to the land of Bhun Sa."

11

The marsh drains into the deep.
Confined by a rock,
the man grasps at briars.
In his palace,
he does not see his wife.

PARKER sat in the darkness of the pit, his hands tied behind him, and prayed to die. Not that he believed in God. Or in anything anymore, except the pain in his feet that was more terrible than he had ever conceived pain could be. Christ, let me die. Please, sweet Jesus. Please please please let me die, he prayed.

He would do anything. Sell his soul. Betray his country. Anything. He had begged them to let him confess. They could name the crime and he would swear to it. Did they want CIA secrets? He'd give them the whole ball of wax. But they didn't care. They just smiled and kept asking him the same questions over and over again.

Would the CIA deal with them directly? Would they betray Bhun Sa? Did they have secret contacts with the dog-eaters? Would they send another? One who was empowered to negotiate? He had told them everything he knew over and over. Why wouldn't they believe him? Or just kill him, please God?

He had been one of the proud ones, he remembered. One who had always refused the standard issue cyanide pill and who had looked a little contemptuously at those who took them. The pill just tells the Opposition that you know something that makes your head worth opening, he used to say. Without it you might bluff your way out, or disinform them, snatching a kind of victory from the pain. There's a limit to the pain, and besides, you're worth more alive than dead to them, maybe as part of a swap, and once you know that they won't kill you and that there's an end to it somewhere, you can stand any pain, he would argue.

Besides, if you want to run with the big dogs, you've got to be willing to piss up tall trees, he'd say, implying that those who took the cyanide pills with them didn't really have what it took.

Except he was a fraud. His whole life was a fraud, because he didn't have what it took at all. Only now he couldn't lie about it anymore. Not to himself. Not to those grinning fucking monkeys who would do things to his feet. Not to anybody.

He'd lied about it all the time. Bullshit. That's all he was was bullshit, like the time he'd sworn on his mother's life that on his first time out as an LRRP, he had taken out a VC with a bicycle chain only inches from a whole fucking NVA squad. He had originally heard it from some Aussie Ranger, who used to carry VC ears in a tobacco pouch and trade them as though they were stamps, and took the story for his own. The Aussie had said that he had cut fourteen ears off of VC he had personally killed, but Parker didn't believe him any more than he believed himself the first time he told the bicycle chain story. The truth was that he had spent the whole night cowering in the bush, jumping at every sound. In the morning on his way in, he had found a dead VC near the trail and those were the ears he took, trying not to look at the bottom half of the body, mangled from a B-52 strike and swarming with insects, as he did it. Then he threw up.

And yet, incredibly, everyone believed him. Parker was a tough motherfucker, they said. When he transferred from Special Forces to the Company, the stories followed him. The Company execs loved that shit as much as the guys in Nam did. They gave him a promotion. They used to point him out to CTP trainees, who wouldn't dare approach him. After a while, he almost believed it himself. In his mind's eye, the image of himself wielding the black-taped bicycle chain, the VC's face as he went down, was as real as any memory.

Only once had he ever let the mask slip. The night Brother Rap died. The night they had sworn never to speak about. But he'd tell them now, all right. He'd tell anybody anything if they'd only make the pain in his feet go away. Christ, give him an ax and he'd chop his own feet off himself! Anything, please, he moaned, staring up into the blackness, not knowing if it was day or night.

The pit was dark as a grave. Then he saw a star through the bamboo lattice above and realized it was night. He began to struggle against the ropes tying him down, but all his movements did was send the pain shooting up his legs. He screamed. And screamed.

He must have passed out, because he awakened to a scraping sound. They were opening the lattice on the top of the pit. "Oh, God," he mumbled. They had been right. Brother Rap had been right. Sometimes death is better. He wondered if they had sent someone after him. They must have, except he no longer wanted to be found. He wanted to die before they ever found him. Where were they? Who was coming after him? That's what they wanted to know, only he didn't know who was coming. Except . . .

Oh, Jesus! They wouldn't send that one-eyed son of a—

The pit flooded with light from a flashlight. It hurt his eyes and he turned his head away like a thing that prefers to cower in the dark. A high-pitched voice barked a command, and he obediently raised his head and tried to force his eyes open. He squinted up at the opening. It was a rectangle of gray dawn light. A teenage face wearing a KR cap peered down at him.

"Please, don't," Parker whimpered.

"To dah dei oun. It is time to wake the earth," the boy said.

12

The marsh above the trees.
The beam is weak;
it will collapse.
The man places mats of white grass
beneath objects set on the ground.

OME say the gods made the world to give them a place to fight," said Chaw Wah, the phu yai ban of the village. He was a thin man, not old, with a narrow triangular face and a long nose with a sideways bend that made him at once ugly and interesting to look at. At his words there were murmurs of agreement.

"The Chinamen say the gods created the world to give the bureaucrats something to do," Sawyer remarked. It was an old joke but still successful and the others laughed over their cups.

"That is truth," Chaw Wah agreed sagely. "It is said the neak ta spirits complain that even in the Other World there is too much bureaucracy." And the betel chewers among them turned and spat in delight at the saying.

They had finished eating and were seated around the fire in a crude hut made to shelter villagers during the long nights in the fields during the time of planting. The hut was of pine and stood on stilts in a terraced poppy field several hundred meters from the village. The forest pressed close around. As they ate, they held their weapons as unselfconsciously in their laps as Westerners might wear napkins.

It had been a poor meal. A single grilled plat taw fish. A dab of fish paste. Rice. The only fruit a few papayas and rambutans. But after the fighting the village could offer no better, and as a consolation, they warmed their bellies with the potent corn liquor brewed by the local spirit doctor. Night had fallen. Rain dripped steady as time from the thatched eaves of the hut.

Only the old monk sat apart. He had eaten of the rice only, for the monsoon season was also vossa, the time of purification. And the woman, of course. Earlier, she had taken a portion of food to the Akha, who was keeping the first watch over their animals and goods. When she came back, they all turned. The rain had soaked her peasant clothes, molding them wetly to her body. Their eyes were on the smooth swell of her breasts and belly, the dark depression between her thighs. Only the monk looked away; the sight of such as she was a detour on the Eightfold Path. Toonsang had stared at her like a man in a fever. His fingers curled into claws. As she passed, her thigh brushed Toonsang's hand, and Sawyer, who suspected that she had done it deliberately, curtly motioned her away. That was his part and he played it, feeling like the cuckold in a French farce. Since then, she had sat in a corner, keeping tight-lipped guard over Sawyer's pack and hers like a bitch over a new litter. In the shadows, only her eyes could be seen.

But though none looked at her, they could all feel her presence. Toonsang busied himself lighting a black cheroot. He avoided Sawyer's gaze because the sickness for her was burning in his own, and if their eyes were to meet, it would end with killing then and there. The Kachin smiled. But Toonsang, ever wary, found his voice as he passed the lit cheroot to Chaw Wah.

"May the phi bop take this talk of bureaucrats. What of Bhun Sa and this pestilential Fuk Wa of the Kuomintang?" Toonsang growled.

"With those two is battle unending, as that between the noble Rama and Thosakanth," Chaw Wah replied. Rama was the hero and Thosakanth the villainous monkey general of the *Ramakien* tales. Chaw Wah's cheeks hollowed as he drew deeply on the cheroot.

"Ah, but which is Rama and which is Thosakanth?" the Kachin said, holding up his hand, the thumb and forefinger outstretched. Everyone laughed. The sound was harsh and male. The

Kachin turned his hand so the two fingers switched positions, and they laughed again.

"That depends on who occupies the village!" Toonsang called out, and there were more guffaws and the slapping of thighs. The Kachin, grinning like a street urchin with a new trick, turned his hand back again to still more laughter. Toonsang crumpled his porkpie hat in his hand and dabbed at his eyes with it, as the laughing subsided. The tension had eased, and when Chaw Wah, himself smiling broadly, grunted, a girl in the red-sleeved blouse, colored phanung and apron, striped shawl, and multicolored turban of the Lisu women poured them another round of the dark brown liquor. It burned like acid going down and there was much lip-smacking and belching as they drank.

"That is truth," Chaw Wah agreed. "Always before, we sold the opium to any who would pay. There were raids and stealings, but with prudence, the water did not overflow the banks of the river, as it is said. The road itself was safe for those of prudence and the village also, for it lies in the holy shadow of Doi Tung. But for Fuk Wa and Bhun Sa, not Mount Meru or the world itself is of a sufficient bigness. Each will have the opium trade for his own. Thus when the Koumintang came this time, it was not to trade but to stay. They left those you see now hanging at the village gate to hold the village for them.

"At first we gave them, of food and some few baht and kyat as we had, hoping they would go away. For we are a poor village," Chaw Wah added, glancing sideways at Toonsang's men and their guns.

Toonsang grunted. Message delivered, Chaw Wah went on.

"But they wanted all, even the scrapings of the fourth cutting of the opium. They drank and ate, and when there was no more of the corn liquor, they slapped the face of Ah Chaw, the spirit doctor, and threatened to cut off his manhood if he did not find another jug. And they took the women as they pleased, anywhere, even in the middle of the village, like dogs. Any woman. Even those who were married and those at the time of their bleeding. And when finished, would leave them with their skirts over their heads, though from the women's pleading they knew that the husbands would have no choice but to put them aside."

"Barbarians!" Toonsang said, and spat into the fire. That was what you said when it was the other side that did it, Sawyer thought. But words meant little. Brother Rap had taught him that.

"What is to become of the women?" Sawyer asked.

Chaw Wah made a vague gesture that might have meant anything.

"What becomes of any woman taken in adultery? Among the American tribe does not the husband also put her aside?"

"That is not the custom, but some do all the same," Sawyer said.

"Ah," Chaw Wah said, meaning he understood, but with exquisite kreng chai did not wish to comment further, because at a deeper level, Sawyer's reply had merely confirmed what they already knew. The ways of the European were beyond rational comprehension.

More liquor was passed around, and as an offering to the protective chao spirits, Chaw Wah spilled a few drops from his cup into the fire. They flared up, briefly burning with a bright blue flame.

"Pah! The most severe punishment for adultery is among the Paduang, they of the long-necked women," Toonsang broke in. His small eyes had begun to blear from the liquor. It made him look more dangerous than ever.

"It is said the women of the Paduang wear so many neck rings that their necks are stretched to three times longer than a normal woman's," Chaw Wah observed.

"That is truth. The rings are of heavy brass, and the wearing of them makes the necks long and slender and the head seem small, which is a mark of beauty among the Paduang. And the punishment for adultery is the removal of these very neck rings. The husband himself must cut them off," Toonsang said.

"Why is that so terrible?" Sawyer asked.

"Most terrible." Toonsang grinned. "After years of rings, the neck is not strong enough to hold up the head. Unless the woman carries her own head in two hands like a basket, it just flops over."

"A terrible punishment," Sawyer agreed, and they drank. Chaw Wah shook his head.

"Not only punishment. Warning, like those the men of Bhun Sa left hanging at our gate when they retook the village. They warned us not to take the bodies down. They said from now on we are to sell only to Bhun Sa."

"Have you not fear of reprisals from Fuk Wa?" Sawyer asked.

The headman made a gesture that somehow suggested all of Asia.

"What is one to do? We are a little village. As it is said, 'When the elephants fight, the grass is trampled.' "

"Some might flee a land of tigers."

Chaw Wah smiled in approval at Sawyer's reference to a famous story of Confucius, who once asked a woman whose family had been devoured by tigers why she stayed in such a terrible place, and she replied: "Because there is no repressive government here."

"Your words have wisdom, honored sir. There are some among us, some of the young, who say this. For we have heard stories. Always there has been fighting, but now the dog-eaters grow very numerous in Laos and in the land of the Khmers, that is already a graveyard. The air smells of thunder and storm clouds gather in the east. Perhaps you are yourself a cloud-bringer, honored sir, for you have the look of a warrior," Chaw Wah said, staring boldly at Sawyer's eye-patch.

To this Sawyer said nothing. Chaw Wah took it for an answer.

"You see how it is. We must stay here and endure where our ancestors are buried. As it is said, 'The boat moves off, the riverbanks remain.' What else can your humble servants do?"

"Pray. We bring you a monk," Toonsang declared rudely. All turned to the monk, still seated in the lotus position. His face was shadowed. His eyes were two flames in the firelight.

"What says the holy one?" Chaw Wah asked.

The old monk picked up his bowl and got stiffly to his feet.

"Only what you already know. Life is dukkha. No prayer will end suffering," the old monk said.

"Even as those poor wretches by the gate," Chaw Wah nodded. "Though we wished them ill, their screams were most barbarous to hear."

"Then it was a good warning. What say, younger brother? Still wish to meet Bhun Sa? Maybe he will welcome you as he does the Kuomintang, neh?" Toonsang said, leering at Sawyer.

"More than ever," Sawyer said.

Toonsang glanced over at the Kachin, and Sawyer saw how it was then. He let his hand fall on his M-16.

"Too dangerous now. Finish trip here," Toonsang declared. "This one will buy the woman so you not lose profit. Better this one than Bhun Sa. For that one will take the woman and give you nothing for your trouble but a sharpened bamboo to sit on."

"Maybe this one take her," said the Kachin, his SKS carbine suddenly pointed at Sawyer.

It was a bad place. They were all too close and there were too many of them. Sawyer had made the classic mistake of letting his enemy pick the time and place of battle, because he had thought they would hold off in the presence of the monk and wait till they could get a clean shot at him, without him being able to get any of them. But this was the place. He tightened his finger on the trigger, knowing he was about to die. They couldn't miss and all he could hope for was to take one or two of them with him.

The old monk stepped between the Kachin's rifle and Sawyer. The Kachin kept the SKS aimed at the monk. His eyes had the killing look. The monk made no move.

Suddenly, Toonsang turned toward the Kachin and spoke furiously in a dialect Sawyer could barely follow. It sounded like a Thai variant of North Shan.

"What manner of foolishness is this? Can you not see the farang's pestilential hand on his pestilential gun. Or the phu yai ban? Or the holy one? And if a bullet should send one of these to the Long Night, who will save us from the wrath of the Lisu? Or Bhun Sa and the SUA? Or the KMT? Or the gods themselves, may the phi bop devour your balls if I do not cut them off with my own hand, for who would not put his hand against us? There will be time enough for the woman and more than the woman, but not for one with the manure of the bullock for wits. Now go to the mules and replace the worthless Akha on guard. Perhaps you can do a thing that does not require more wits than that of the bullock and leave this of the farang to me."

The Kachin didn't move. He glared at Toonsang. But his knuckles were white on the SKS, and Sawyer knew then that he would go stand guard. The Kachin sneered.

"There is too much of talking with such as these. And of

drinking, too much. When the head is dizzy, the man is weak like a woman."

"Is this one a drunkard?" Toonsang demanded dangerously. "Yet even drunk, this one can lead better than one with the wits of the bullock."

The two men glared at each other, Sawyer quite forgotten. The Kachin looked down. He spat into the fire and it hissed back.

"I go. But even the bullock does not forget an injury," the Kachin declared, hefting his rifle.

"More better," Toonsang retorted. "The man wants the bullock to remember the stick."

The Kachin went out into the darkness, his footsteps swallowed by the sound of the rain. Only then was Sawyer able to take his eye from Toonsang. The hut seemed darker, emptier somehow. Suong had gone.

She must have slipped away during the argument, he realized. Her pack was still there, but open, as though she had taken something out of it. Part of him wanted to go after her at once, but he resisted the impulse. There was still unfinished business here.

Toonsang plucked a burning ember from the fire and relit his cheroot. A layer of tobacco smoke hung over their heads like a raincloud.

"Bad kreng chai, that one," Toonsang said in a friendly manner, once more speaking Isan Thai. "It was the drink. Pay no heed. All know the Kachin people have no head for the good corn liquor."

"I have heard this too," Chaw Wah said, anxious to make peace.

"And you, younger brother. Forgive this miserable jesting upon the woman. Such talk is foolishness. Drink talk, no more. This one will take you to Bhun Sa, as agreed. That is of a certainty," Toonsang said.

Watch it, Sawyer told himself. It's when he's at his friendliest that he's most dangerous. Remember what happened at the clearing.

"Mai pen rai. This one never doubted you would," Sawyer replied, raising his cup to his lips.

At this, the old monk made unmistakable signs of leaving. He made the wai to Chaw Wah and then the others, not excluding the little spirit house in the eastern corner.

"Blessings and peace," the monk said.

"Are you leaving, holy one?" Sawyer asked stupidly. He had counted on the monk being there. So long as the monk stayed, there was a chance Toonsang might hold off.

"May you walk the Eightfold Path, brother. This humble one goes now."

"Your humble servant wishes you to stay the night that he might earn merit, holy one," Sawyer said, trying to keep the desperation out of his voice.

The old monk peered nearsightedly into Sawyer's good eye.

"It is better thus, brother. Bad karma if these eyes should see what is to come in this place," he whispered. Sawyer understood. The monk foresaw more killing. For him to witness any of it would be bad for his inner calm and bad karma for Sawyer too, whether in this life or the next.

"But it is dark outside," Sawyer objected.

"The Enlightened One will guide my steps." Then seeing the look on Sawyer's face, he added, "Fear not. There is that which tells this one we shall meet again."

Small consolation, Sawyer thought. He might mean a hundred lifetimes from now. He tried one last time.

"But it is raining, holy one."

"Then this one will get wet."

Gathering his robe around him, the monk stepped outside. Just before he disappeared in the darkness, Sawyer called after him.

"How are you called, holy one?"

The monk stopped and turned. Rain streamed down the creases in his face, gleaming like veins of gold in the flickering light of the fire.

"Utama."

"A fortunate name," Sawyer joked. The monk's name meant "good fortune."

The monk smiled back.

"This humble one's parents were most prudent. And how is my brother called?"

"Sawyer."

"What means this So-yah?"

"A name from a story"—thinking that that was closer to the truth than anyone would ever know.

"May you find peace, So-yah. Though this one does not think you will," the monk added.

"One question more, holy one," Sawyer said, himself stepping out into the rain. "Why were you on that road when there were no begging prospects?"

"Waiting for you, it seems."

The monk smiled and turned away. Sawyer watched him go. He went back to the hut and got his pack, conscious of Toonsang and the others' eyes on his back.

"This one will find the woman and bring her back," Sawyer said.

"We will wait for you, younger brother," Toonsang said. His eyes showed nothing.

Sawyer stepped out, keeping his back straight despite the desire to run. He thought Toonsang would wait till later, but if he was wrong . . . As he walked down the sodden path, he could hear Toonsang questioning Chaw Wah about which way Bhun Sa's men were heading, Burma-side, Thai-side, or Lao-side.

His thoughts were in a turmoil as he moved down the muddy path, going into the silent, groping glide they had used in the jungle trails in Nam. It was too dark to see and it was too dangerous to use a light, so he felt his way, hoping that there were no booby traps so close to the village. The rain soaked his peasant shirt and phanung, worn tucked into his belt hill-style, to make them like breeches. The foliage was wet and he held the branches as he slipped through, to keep them from springing back and making noise. Looking back, he could no longer see the light from the hut. He listened to the rain on the leaves. He held his breath, but he could hear no one coming down the trail behind him.

Where was Suong? he wondered. What was she hiding? And if he could survive Toonsang's treachery, what of Bhun Sa? And Pranh? And somewhere in the back of his mind, Vasnasong still in the game, despite Harris' assurances that he was handling it. And all the while the Vietnamese, with the patience of ants, were carefully moving their men into place. How much time would they give him? And if he didn't get it together soon, they could start quarrying the marble for another damn black wall in Washington and—

He had been thinking so furiously, he almost stumbled over the body lying across the trail. His heart leaped into his throat, but from the bulk of it, he knew at once it wasn't Suong. He felt for the head, hoping to feel the turban of the Kachin—and not finding it, risked turning the body over.

It was the Akha.

He had to have been killed on his way back from guard duty only a few minutes earlier. They had heard nothing in the hut, so it must have been quick and by surprise. Sawyer's pulse began to race. He had to find Suong.

He opened his pack and felt for the stubby Ingram M-10 submachine gun. He snapped in a full clip and stuck an extra in his pocket, though if he ever needed to use more than the first clip, the most likely target would be himself. He screwed on the sound suppressor and switched to full automatic. It would only be good for close work, but at night and in dense terrain, that was the way it would happen. When the time came, he would leave the M-16 with the pack.

Now he had to go carefully. And it all came back, just like that. The imagining of noises and phantom black-clad snipers behind every bush. The sweats at the movement of every leaf. The foliage was dark and damp. It had a slimy feel. Something moved under his hand and he struck at it, hitting nothing but leaves. He cursed himself for making noise and held his breath to listen. His face was wet. He wiped his eyes with the back of his sleeve, not sure if it was rain or sweat. He wondered if he were a coward, because he didn't want to take another step. Something was waiting for him in the darkness.

He had seen it happen to others. Sometimes it was buck fever, the first time out. Sometimes later. And maybe with him, it had come on slowly, the loss of nerve. Maybe people were like machines and courage was a critical part that could wear out like anything else. What did they call it with airplanes? Metal fatigue. That was it. Metal fatigue. And then he thought of Suong and the Kachin and began moving again.

He heard something. It wasn't imagination. He had heard it moving somewhere up ahead. He let the pack slide silently to the ground and laid the M-16 against it. He smeared mud on his face, wiping his hands clean on his phanung. He crept forward, holding the Ingram in front of him with both hands.

At first he thought his eye was playing tricks on him, because there was a tiny light shining in a small clearing. He came to the edge of the clearing. It was a small candle inside a black box set on a tree stump, like a wayside shrine. There were things in the box, but they were deep in shadow and he couldn't make out what they were. Suong was on her knees, head bowed in prayer. He could hear the murmur of her voice, but not the words. He could not see her face from here, but from the way she held her body, he could sense the tension. It was an intensely personal moment and he felt like an interloper.

Then he saw the Kachin.

He was a humped shadow moving up behind Suong, and whatever he had in mind, it wasn't religious. From where Sawyer was, it was a bad angle. He would have to step into the clearing a few steps to be sure of a shot. He hesitated, wondering whether to risk the whole mission right now. Then he thought of the dead Akha and knew he had no choice. The best thing he could do was to cut down the odds, and he had already stepped into the clearing when the Kachin suddenly whirled. Sawyer must have made a sound, because Suong too had started to turn, her startled face white as the moon in the candlelight. For an instant they were frozen, like an image in a strobe light, the Kachin's face a ghostly mask, his SKS carbine already aimed with catlike speed at Sawyer's chest.

Mexican standoff.

The thought flashed into Sawyer's head. No way for either of them to shoot without getting shot themselves. The look in the Kachin's eyes showed that he knew it too and didn't care.

And then it didn't matter, because he was into the sequence they had drilled into them at the Fifth Recondo in Nha Trang, the sudden drop onto his back as he fired. The Ingram jumped in his hands, and the Kachin, unable to react fast enough, looked down in astonishment at the spurting holes in his chest as he toppled backward.

Sawyer got up and went to check the Kachin, though from the way he lay, there was no way he wasn't dead. He started to pick up the SKS and then with a rush Suong was trembling in his arms. She wrapped herself around him, clinging like a child.

"I thought it was you . . ." she began.

"I know."

He held her till the trembling eased, feeling very exposed in the candlelight. The wind stirred the tops of the trees, and it came as a surprise to realize that it wasn't raining. Sawyer tried to peek over her shoulder into the black box but still couldn't make it out.

"We have to go back to the hut."

"Yes," she replied. Her voice was matter-of-fact. She turned, and from the way she stood, he could have sworn she was trying to block him from seeing into the box. But he caught a glimpse of something just before she blew out the candle and closed the box. Except he couldn't understand it.

She started to pick up the Kachin's SKS, and he told her to leave it in a tone that was sharper than he had intended.

"You have reason. Je comprends tout," she said, not looking at him.

"Do you?"

"Your pistolet-mitrailleur is most quiet. You think perhaps they have not heard and will think the Kachin is still on guard with the Akha. You desire that I make the pig-eyed one, Toonsang, to coucher with me."

"Yes," his voice strangled.

She looked searchingly into his eyes. The look on her face made him want to crush her in his arms, but he couldn't.

"If you wish this, I will do this."

He thought of Toonsang, pig eyed, mouth foul with liquor and betel juice, his slimy hands all over her, kissing her, thrusting inside her, and he wanted to tell her not to do it. Give me an out, he thought. Don't do it for me.

"I wish it," he said.

He walked ahead of her till they got back to where he had left his pack and the M-16. He took the clip out and worked the action to make sure it was empty.

"You killed the Akha?" he said.

"Yes."

"How?"

She showed him the knife. It was a tanto-style blade, and he imagined how she must have smiled at the Akha and how he must have been smiling back as she put her arms around him and struck. He held out his hand, and she gave it to him. He put the knife in its sheath and stuck it into his belt.

"Why?"

"You know why," she said.

It was a way of forcing him to act, and despite himself, he knew she had been right. The feeling for her was very strong. He pulled her to him, and they kissed so hard they bruised each other's lips, and the taste mingled with the salt taste of blood.

"Why did you leave the hut? For the Akha?"

She shook her head.

"The Akha was chance. I met him on the path. From the way he smiled at me, I knew what he wanted. Tant mieux, I thought. One less for us to fight."

"Then why did you leave?"

She pressed her face into his shoulder. Her voice was muffled.

"I thought it would be better if I am not there to fight over like a bone pulled between dogs. And the talking of suffering. I could not sit anymore. Men talk. If you want to know what is suffering, you must to ask a woman."

Sawyer caught his breath. He had to ask.

"What is in the black box?"

She shook her head against his shoulder. He pushed her away, forcing her to look at him. She tried to pull away, her eyes shiny.

"I cannot tell. Je t'en prie, So-yah," she cried.

"I'm sorry. I have to know."

"That makes nothing. It is nothing for you and for the mission nothing. It is only for me. My khwan, tu comprends. This I will not speak of. If you demand again, it is finished with us. It is all finished," she said, her voice surprising him by its firmness.

It must be a religious thing, he thought. He had asked because he was an agent and because you never knew what might ultimately be critical to a mission. And it was astonishing the things people would sometimes tell you in response to a straightforward question. But he couldn't risk pushing her on it. She was vital to the mission and maybe to more than the mission. And if she had a secret, he asked himself, well, what woman didn't?

He handed her the empty M-16 and the pack to take back to the hut. If Toonsang asked, she was to tell him that she had found it on the trail and that she had seen no one. He hoped that Toonsang would think he was either dead or disarmed. She nodded and started to turn away. Then she came back and gently put her hand to his cheek.

"You are not a believer, So-yah?"

"No. Not in your way."

"The angkar told us that to believe is imperialist treason. But karma requires no belief, my So-yah. Karma is what is."

"Were you praying, is that—"

She put her fingers to his lips.

"Only do not wait too long," she said, and was gone.

He waited till he could no longer hear her moving through the foliage before he struck off the trail. He moved carefully, one limb at a time, so as not to disturb a leaf, remembering how Charley could do it and how they had learned from Charley to let the Reptile, the part of them that was millions of years old, take over, till they could move through the night like stalking cats. And how to prove it, Parker had once taken out a VC on a night LRRP patrol with a bicycle chain wrapped in black tape and then got away without the rest of the VC squad, only inches away, ever knowing that he was there.

He moved away from the path in a wide circle to approach the hut from the opposite side. From the shadow of the bamboo fence, he could just see the fire and Suong from the side. She was leaning over Toonsang, putting something on the table. She had unhooked the top two eyelets of her shirt and her breasts swung tantalizingly close to his face. He had only to raise his hands to cup them. The Shan and the Karen stared transfixed. Suong smiled. Toonsang licked his lips like a beast.

They were talking, but Sawyer couldn't hear what they were saying. Probably about him, he thought. Whatever it was, Toonsang seemed to be buying it, because he was smiling like the cat in the cream. Chaw Wah and the Lisu woman had gone. Sawyer wanted to watch it all, but he had to go around to get into position. He started moving again. The side of the hut blocked his view as he came around. He moved from shadow to shadow, his ears straining for any sound. Whatever else happened, if he was spotted now, it was all over.

A village dog started barking. He froze. The dog wouldn't stop barking. It was coming closer. Shut up, shut up, he thought. The barking got louder. The dog was moving fast. It had almost reached the last huts on the outskirts of the village nearest the field. Sawyer pulled the knife. Suddenly there was a muffled curse and the sharp yelp. The dog barked again, only now the sound was moving away. Another curse, and he could hear the dog growl as it slunk away.

The village was quiet. Sawyer crouched in the shadows under the hut by the outer stilts. The ground was dank and muddy enough to make him worry about his footing. He cautiously peeked over the edge. His heart almost stopped.

He was only a foot or two from Toonsang. Luckily, Toonsang was looking the other way, watching Suong prepare the bed matting. Sawyer ducked his head back down.

Now there was only the waiting. "Only do not wait too long," she had said. He readied his knife. The Ingram hung from a strap around his neck. He had to keep blinking the sweat from his good eye. He could hear Suong lie down on the matting and the swish of clothing. He tried not to think of what was happening, but it was impossible. Think of something else, he told himself. Why wouldn't she tell him about the box? Was it some kind of portable shrine that she took everywhere? But it made no sense. Because unless his eye had deceived him, the only thing in the box was a pair of shoes.

He heard muttered talk and sounds of movement on the wooden floor of the hut. He tightened his grip on the knife. He tried to swallow and couldn't. Heart pounding, he waited in the dark for Toonsang to mount his woman.

13

The pond is cradled by the
* mountain.*
The superior man feels calm and
* chivalrous.*
The man wiggles the big toe.

IT was crowded on the train to Sheng Shui. That was because it was race day at the Shatin track. This showed good planning in Lan Fong's opinion, and he approved. Luckily, he had boarded in Hung Hom and was able to find a seat. He looked at the crowd packed around him, swaying to the movement of the train, but his instructions were not to make a study of it. At this point he could be watched by a ten of ten men and not know it.

He pulled a popular racing sheet from the bag on his lap. Only two weeks ago, the paper's tout had, with great joss, predicted three winners in one day, and Lan Fong noticed that there were more than a few in the crowd going over the same paper. The bag was from Yue Hwa department store and contained only underwear and a new shirt he would not be keeping. He pretended to concentrate on the paper, glancing up only when the train slowed to pull into a station.

As the train pulled out of Tai Wai station, Lan Fong could sense a growing tension in the crowd. The racetrack was the next stop. Even before the train pulled into Shatin station, the crowd was already surging for the door. Lan Fong got up and pushed his way into the crowd, shoving the paper back into the bag.

The doors opened and the crowd spilled onto the platform. Lan Fong was jostled as he hurried toward the gate, and felt a slight tug as something was stuffed into the bag. He didn't turn around to see who had done it. He didn't want to know.

He followed the crowd into the street all the way to the racetrack. There was a logjam at the general admission gate, and he held on tightly to the bag. Once inside, he waited for the incoming rush to ease, then darted out one of the exit gates and headed for the taxi stand.

If there was a watcher on him, this is where he would reveal himself, Lan Fong thought. Because he would have to commit himself in order to follow.

There was one. A tall Chinese in a dark blue short-sleeve shirt and sunglasses. Whoever he was, he hadn't been at it long, because he had made the novice's mistake of standing in front of a billboard with a white background. As soon as he saw Lan Fong move toward the first taxi, Sunglasses broke for a rank of parked motor scooters.

"MTR. Fie dee!" Lan Fong told the driver. As they swung out into traffic, he looked over his shoulder at the rear window. Sunglasses was jumping on the scooter's starter.

As the driver maneuvered through the traffic, Lan Fong glanced down at the bag. There were now two identical newspapers jammed into the bag. Lan Fong took out his original paper, marked by a small tear near the corner of the front page, and carefully dropped it in the corner of the backseat, out of the driver's line of sight, as though it had been left by a careless passenger. He left the second paper in the bag. Glancing out of the back window, he saw that Sunglasses had almost caught up.

Lan Fong's heart pounded. He wondered who Sunglasses was working for and how he had learned of Lan Fong. Many times he had been a courier, and this was the first time he had ever been followed. Either he had been betrayed—an unthinkable notion, for he was known only to Wong, his father's sister's son, who had told him that all the couriers were Hakka like himself—or the message he was carrying was of an indescribable importance.

Lan Fong's chest swelled with pride that he was thought

worthy to carry a message of such importance. And had not his estimable cousin Wong hinted that the payment might be greater this time? Lan Fong was overcome with curiosity. What could the message be? Always before he had obeyed Wong's injunction never to examine what he was carrying. "That is the courier's duty. Also less baggage to carry if captured by those who wish us ill," Wong had said. But this time, Lan Fong couldn't resist a peek. There was time, he knew. Sunglasses would stay in their rear window, and nothing would happen till they got to the metro station.

He found the little pencil notations on the fourth page of the paper, next to the lineups. Numbers. Gau. Chut. Ng. Baht. And so on. Obviously, selections to bet on for each race. Mm gon yo, Lan Fong told himself as he refolded the paper and put it back into the bag. If there was a code there, he had no way of understanding what it was.

In fact, the numbers had nothing to do with the numbers assigned to the horses, but after a complex series of calculations, were used to count backward the letters of the horses' English names to arrive at a meaningless sequence of letters. These letters referred to a one-time pad, where each letter indicated a specific word or phrase on a single page. The only copies of the pad were held by the ultimate sender and receiver, each of whom would destroy that page after this one-time use.

The taxi was caught in a traffic jam near the station. Slapping the fare and a twenty–Hong Kong–dollar tip—thinking he would tell his cousin Wong he had given fifty—into the driver's hand, Lan Fong suddenly jumped out of the taxi and began weaving through the stalled traffic. Only when he reached the safety of the sidewalk, did he glance back out of the corner of his eye at Sunglasses, who had abandoned his motor scooter to loud honks and curses and was desperately trying to follow.

Lan Fong raced into the station and headed for the Kowloon platform. He joined a number of Chinese men, most of whom were wearing white shirts similar to his, and stood next to a gray-haired grandfather in wire-rimmed glasses, tall for a Chinese, so he could observe new arrivals while staying partially obscured. He could hear the rumble of the approaching train. Fie dee, fie dee, oh, pestilential train, he thought. He felt the rush of air pushed ahead by the train just as Sunglasses ran onto the platform.

The train whizzed by, the faces a blur. It came to a halt with a loud screech, and Lan Fong felt himself being pulled by the crowd onto the train. But he resisted, standing by the open door until he saw Sunglasses hesitating by the door of the next car down. He heard the sound of air as the doors started to close, then leaped aboard. Sunglasses dived for the doors. Just as they closed, Lan Fong jumped back out onto the platform.

He was alone on the platform. The train began to roll. He watched the windows as an agonized Sunglasses was swept by. Allowing himself a small smile, Lan Fong crossed over and took the next New Territories train to Taipo Market, where he boarded a Kowloon–Canton line train back to Mongkuk station in Kowloon. During the trip he changed cars back and forth but could spot no one. In Kowloon, he caught another taxi to the Star Ferry landing and waited until after they had docked on the Hong Kong side and were on their way back to Kowloon before he went to the lavatory, having made sure no one else in the big passenger cabin was also making the trip back, except for the dreamy-eyed girl student in braids who had looked around in confusion when the ferry had pulled in at the Queen's Pier Landing, and the tourist couple, obviously American, the wife wearing heavier makeup than a Tsimshatsui girl, chattering without pausing for breath at the husband, belly sagging over his belt, wearing a curious shapeless hat and a camera strap diagonally across his chest like a Sam Browne belt.

The lavatory stank of years of urine and disinfectant. The third cubicle had an "Out of Order" sign, crudely lettered in Cantonese and English, taped on the post. That was the one Lan Fong chose, tearing off the sign as he entered. Propped next to the toilet was a Yue Hwa bag identical to the one he was carrying. As he bent down, he could see the shoes and Western trousers of someone in the next cubicle. In a moment he had made the switch, flushed the toilet and left, feeling very pleased with himself. The sound of flushing covered the retrieval of the bag by a hand under the partition from the next cubicle.

Within the hour, the coded racing paper was on the desk of the local MI6 station chief. Next to it was the page of the one-time pad. Working slowly, methodically, because he was a careful man, he translated the code. After checking it for any possibility of mistake, he destroyed the pad page.

He whistled to himself as he studied the message. London would have to be told at once, he thought. Because the message confirmed that the Vietnamese had just sent another fifty-five thousand troops into Cambodia. Before the monsoon season ended, they would be completely mobilized for war.

14

 The stranger kindles his fire with
a bird's nest.
This gives joy to the fire
but undermines the man.
Ominous.

THE flare floated down over the village, opening a seam of white light in the night. A machine gun opened up near the village gate, and small arms fire flickered along the tree line. Sawyer watched the aquamarine trails of tracer bullets spin toward the village with dreamlike slowness. Suong! he thought, his stomach giving a sickening lurch. He ducked out from under the flooring of the hut and smashed through the bamboo side-screen just in time to see the shadows of Toonsang and his men leaping from the hut, packs and weapons in hand.

Suong was sitting bolt upright, her face white and strange in the harsh flare light. It didn't look like her and for an instant he recoiled. It was as if he could see the skull, hollow-eyed beneath the skin. A memory stirred. Something Pranh had told him once, some Cambodian superstition about how death is a pale woman in white. Through the open side of the hut he could see the villagers firing back, red and aquamarine tracers crisscrossing in a spider web of color. For a moment, the scene was so like his memories of Nam, that he just watched, spellbound.

Then the fear hit him. It was like waking up. Suong's face was hers. It was just that her eyes were round with fear, and he shoved her down, hissing in her ear to be still. He leaned over her, the Ingram ready, but they were alone in the hut. The flare went down somewhere beyond the trees and the night returned, darker than ever. He had seen no sign of Toonsang and the others.

He could feel Suong breathing under him. She was trying to catch her breath. He squinted, trying to clear the imprint of the flare from his eye and make his night vision return faster.

"So-yah?" raising her voice to be heard over the sound of firing.

Somewhere off to the right came the unmistakable stutter of an RPD machine gun opening up. It was a sound you could never forget.

"We have to go," he said, pressing his lips to her ear.

"What is happening?"

Who was attacking the village? Sawyer wondered. Bhun Sa? The KMT. The Thai Rangers? Not that it mattered at that instant. As Brother Rap once said, on that patrol when the ARVN dug up some previously buried VC bodies so they could up the body count for an extra beer ration, "It don't matter who pulls the trigger and it don't matter when. You is dead just the same, bro'."

"They're attacking the village."

He felt her squirming, trying to get up. Suddenly he was enjoying the feel of her moving under him. Of all times! You crazy son of a bitch, he thought, feeling himself harden against her belly. He began to move, pressing himself into her.

"Please, So-yah. This is bad time. We must go now."

"Yes," he said, not stopping.

Suddenly there was a sound of firing from further away and the shooting began to intensify. But their hut was well away from the village; the firing was not directed at them. They could see lights flashing like a son et lumière. They had a ringside seat. Aquamarine tracers were now firing in two directions, toward the village and away from it. It made no sense. If someone was attacking the village from the trees, why would they also be firing away from the village. Unless . . .

All at once, his excitement growing, Sawyer realized what was happening.

That sly son of a bitch, Bhun Sa. He had left the bodies by the gate as bait, knowing the KMT would attack the village for retribution. Only he must have left the Lisu some arms and a spy among them to let him know when they came back. That's why the phu yai ban had insisted on them staying in the field hut, instead of the village guesthouse. At the time, Sawyer had thought it was because Chaw Wah didn't trust Toonsang, but it wasn't that at all. Chaw Wah had been in on it all along. It was a trap for the KMT, who were now caught between the village and Bhun Sa.

Although he didn't think it was deliberate, she was moving wonderfully under him. His breathing grew short. He forced his leg between her thighs. But he kept one hand on the Ingram.

"Not now, So-yah. We go now, yes?"

"Better later, when the shooting dies down," he said. He felt her tense under him, her thighs pressing tight against his between them.

"Please, So-yah," she whispered, biting her lip.

Then he knew. She felt it too. With a tug, he opened her phasin, her thighs creamy white in the flickering light. He glanced down at her naked body, at the long legs, firm young breasts, strong hips and thighs, long hair black as ink spread beneath her head and shoulders like a shawl, the haunting Eurasian beauty of her face, the sheer perfection of her, and he felt the tingle growing, knowing that she was his and he could do anything with her. Anything! He bent over her, pinning her down.

The rattle of gunfire grew louder, more deadly.

And then she was no longer fighting him, but moving with him, the danger taking them quickly to the edge, making it all the more intense.

He had never felt anything like it. He was like a god, inviolable, floating, the sensation exquisite and the nearby battle merely a play of shadows like the nang. He could feel himself being pulled into her like iron to a magnet as he watched shadows break desperately from the trees toward the village gate. A hidden M-60 suddenly opened up, cutting them down, and then he couldn't watch anymore because there was only her mouth, urgent, hungry, and they were like beings possessed, making love as if fighting for their lives against the surrounding shadow of death all around them. And then they were together, man and woman, each of them invading the other, completely filling the universe, obliterating everything else.

A mortar explosion in the trees lit the sky with a red glare.

They could see the trees burning. The thick perfume of cordite washed over them and they were still. They lay in each other's arms, still locked together, and listened to the sound of fighting.

She rubbed her cheek catlike on the stubble along his jaw, sniffing at him like an animal. Her long hair brushed his face, silky, black, the smell of sex mingling with the scents of cordite and the dank earth into something that stirred in the dark recesses of his mind, something very ancient.

He didn't say anything. He didn't understand what had come over him. Somehow the lovemaking had gotten all twisted up with the killing and the danger. And yet it was as exciting as anything he had ever experienced. It was crazy and yet—he knew he had touched something at the very core. Something utterly primitive. And he could almost hear Vasnasong's voice whispering in his mind: "One thing you must to remember, Sawyer-khrap. Sex is older than mankind."

The sound of the firing began to die down. He listened, hardly breathing. Short bursts of submachine fire came from the direction of the trees. It sounded like Bhun Sa's men were mopping up. Now might be their only chance.

"We have to go," he whispered.

"I know." She sighed, but made no move to leave.

He understood her reluctance. Somehow their passion had made the hut a kind of refuge.

The renewed rattle of gunfire came like a splash of cold water. A stray tracer seemed to fall from the sky like a shooting star. It plunked into the mud within a few feet of the hut. Someone in the trees was screaming. Sawyer couldn't make out the words, but it didn't need a translation. All at once, they heard a short burst from a submachine gun and the screaming was cut short. But the scream seemed to leave a space in the sudden silence.

The firing had stopped.

They had to go. To stay in the village any longer would be suicidal. Keeping low and moving quietly, he pulled on his clothes and reached for his pack. She started to say something and he put his finger to her lip. She froze.

They could hear the cautious tread and faint jingle of soldiers coming down the path toward the hut.

Still naked from the waist down, she grabbed her things. They slid silently through the gap in the bamboo screen down to the murky darkness beneath the hut. Sawyer, followed by Suong, crawled on all fours into the poppy field on the side away from the soldiers. Suddenly there were lights behind them and the sound of soldiers ransacking the hut. They scampered into the woods. In the mossy darkness behind a large fallen tree, Suong stopped and fastened her phasin around her waist once more. She hurried to catch up with Sawyer, already moving soundlessly through the dense forest as if he knew the way.

Later that night, she prayed again at the little wooden shrine, despite his misgivings about her lighting the candle so near to the road. But the look on her face had told him there was no point in arguing.

They were in the small clearing near the dead sentry. It was hard to say on whose side he had been. At first, Sawyer had thought the sentry had them dead to rights. He had already started to raise his hands and think of ploys, when he noticed the unnatural stillness of the man's head. He was holding what looked like a brand-new M-16 in his lap. Suong had already begun to reach for it, when Sawyer grabbed her arm and pointed at the almost invisible black wire attached to the trigger guard. By this time, they were both punchy from fatigue, and as soon as they came upon the clearing, they dropped their packs. She told him she would take the first watch, but he fought off his desperate need to sleep. There were still too many unanswered questions he had to sort out.

"Why didn't Toonsang try to rape you?" he asked, coloring slightly. What he himself had done wasn't that far from rape either, he thought.

She wiped her face on her skirt.

"He is crafty, that one. Perhaps he know you lie in waiting. I think he comes, but still he waits. In the darkness, I felt him watching, always watching, and I thought, now he will come. Then came the brightness in the sky and they are gone like thieves."

"It's curious he didn't try to steal my pack."

"Maybe they fear Bhun Sa. They ran as if the phi bop chases them. Sauve qui peut. Maybe they still running," her voice contemptuous.

"Maybe," he muttered.

He felt her hand, cool on his forehead.

"You sleep now, So-yah. I pray and watch."

He tried to talk her out of it, but the more he talked, the stupider he felt. If he could just close his good eye for a minute, maybe he could think it all out. Just one lousy minute, then he would go down near the road and stand watch.

A sudden sharp pain in his ribs woke him up. The boot kicked him again. He reached out to grab the foot and became aware of the rifle muzzle pressed between his eyes. He looked over and saw Suong, already captive, her hands tied behind her. Her eyes were frightened and there was a look of pleading in them. Or maybe it was guilt. That fucking candle! he swore to himself. It must have drawn them like moths. One of them kicked him again and Sawyer stumbled to his feet.

There were eight of them. Shan, by their tattoos, and heavily armed. They were thin and savage looking, their hill clothes ragged. VC dragged out of tunnels after weeks underground never looked that scruffy. Their eyes had the blank stare that in Asia means a captive's life is hanging by the barest thread.

Take the initiative, went Langley doctrine. Sure, Sawyer thought, wishing the skinny prick in Langley who thought that one up were here to do it instead of him. But he had nothing else.

He started to say something and one of them, tall, with long greasy hair down to his shoulders and the look of a starving timber wolf, slammed him in the mouth with the butt of what looked like a World War II–vintage M-1. Sawyer staggered to his knees. Blood dripped down his chin. He felt gingerly with the tip of his tongue. His two bottom front teeth were loose and his lip was split. It hurt like hell.

A sharp pain from a hard poke to his kidneys brought him back up to his feet. Someone grabbed his wrists and roughly tied his hands behind him. Another whack in the kidneys got him moving.

An M-1, Sawyer thought stupidly, as they prodded him along the trail. An M-1, for Chrissakes. Up ahead he could see Suong look back despairingly at him over her shoulder. Timber Wolf shouted something and another blow slammed into his kidney. Sawyer stumbled forward.

By the time they reached the road, a misty rain was falling from a leaden sky. A mud-splattered Land Rover was waiting in the middle of the road, its engine running. At the sight of it, the Shan went rigid, and even Timber Wolf stiffened and made something resembling a salute. Timber Wolf proudly pointed out their booty and captives to a large swarthy Asian in the backseat.

The Asian wore a dark green officer's uniform, though Sawyer could not identify the insignia with any army he had ever heard of. An old scar ran down into the corner of the Asian's mouth. It gave him the mean look of a veteran brawler. His eyes were dark brown and deep set under long dark brows. There was a ruthless intelligence in them and something else. Something Sawyer had seen only once before, on the face of General Easterbrook when he had visited them in the hospital in Zama. It was the glint of raw power. Looking at him, Sawyer had no doubt whatever that it was Bhun Sa.

Ordinarily he would have studied Bhun Sa's face with great interest, except that he couldn't help staring at the other apparition in the Land Rover. Because there, seated next to Bhun Sa and grinning like a banshee, was Toonsang.

15

The deep has been contained with
wood and made into a well.
The plan of a town may change
but the location of its wells
   remains.
There is a leak in the well.
The insects and worms are refreshed.

THE two men, one bulky in the uniform of a Vietnamese officer, the other a short civilian wearing the gold sunburst badge of the RPK on his shirt pocket, watched the interrogation through the one-way glass. In the room beyond the glass, they saw the prisoner try to say something and the interrogator scream and slap him viciously across the face three or four times. The interrogator pointed at the primitive electrical apparatus on the wooden table and then at the prisoner's penis, then grabbed the black cables, their serrated metal clamps making them look almost exactly like snakes, and shook them in the prisoner's face to emphasize his point.

The prisoner looked desperately around the room as though there might be an escape somewhere, but except for the table and the chair he was bound to with heavy leather straps, the room was utterly empty. The walls were whitewashed and the concrete floor dipped to a drain in the center of the floor, but all the hosing in the world could not eradicate the dark stains that spotted the floor and walls, almost to the ceiling. A set of security regulations were taped to the locked door.

In addition to the interrogator, two guards stood on either

side of the prisoner, their faces blank with boredom. They toyed with their heavy rubber truncheons in the monotonous manner of men anxious to use them.

Watching the interrogation in silence through the glass gave it an air of make-believe. It was like watching a movie on TV with the sound turned off. There was a speaker on the wall that could be turned on at any time, but the two men preferred to keep it off. There was nothing that either the interrogator or the prisoner had to say that was of any interest to them.

There was a knock at the door, and a young RPK lieutenant came in. He saluted the general, who merely nodded and turned back to the glass, and then, after a moment's hesitation, the civilian, who beckoned him forward. The lieutenant whispered something in Khmer to the civilian.

"They want to know whether to use the electrics," Heng Ry said in perfect Vietnamese.

"Of course they do, the idiots," General Lu made a face. "Mon Dieu, the stench of this place," he added, as though the thoughts were somehow connected.

Heng Ry nodded. The very walls reeked of urine and carbolic acid and something that in an open field would have drawn vultures from a hundred kilometers around.

"No electrics," Heng Ry told the lieutenant in Vietnamese, as a signal for him to speak in that language in the general's presence.

"But, Comrade General, the prisoner tells us nothing," the lieutenant protested.

"A good thing, too. Otherwise we might have to do something about it," General Lu observed.

The lieutenant stood there gaping.

"A thousand pardons, Comrade General. This foolish one does not understand," the lieutenant said.

"That too is a good thing. If mere lieutenants can understand a general's plans, so can the enemy." General Lu smiled, obviously enjoying himself.

"The comrade general already knows the prisoner's secrets!" the lieutenant exclaimed, then clapped his hand over his mouth in embarrassment.

General Lu roared, and even the normally stone-faced Heng Ry had to smile.

"By the Lord Buddha! A thinker, this one. Your RPK begins to show progress, Comrade Heng," General Lu remarked.

Emboldened by the general's good humor, the lieutenant dared to speak again.

"Our superiors have told us that an officer must learn to use his wits," he declared proudly.

"Not really." General Lu shrugged. "Officers who think for themselves will enjoy very short careers. Only when one has learned not to think at all can one become a general."

Heng Ry smiled at this.

"Surely one of the Comrade General's reputation does not truly believe such a statement."

General Lu's eyebrows rose into his brow like horizontal crescent moons.

"You would be surprised what the Comrade General believes after thirty years of war. Une guerre sans fin. But you are right, Comrade Secretary." He turned to the lieutenant. "Incredible as it may seem, Comrade Lieutenant, the general does indeed have a plan for the prisoner. Or rather, the Politburo itself does."

The lieutenant snapped to attention.

"Much better." General Lu smiled. He glanced back at the one-way glass. The guards were beating the prisoner's stomach with the truncheons. The prisoner was screaming. Bile trickled down his chin. General Lu frowned. He motioned the lieutenant closer.

"About the prisoner," he began.

"Yes, Comrade General."

"I want him intimidated, not damaged. He must be made to understand that he is suspected of crimes against the people. Then you are to go in there and have him released for insufficient proof."

"Released, Comrade General?" the lieutenant asked, blinking stupidly as a bird.

"Comrade Lieutenant, do you know what a captain is? A captain is one who, when he was a lieutenant, did not make his superiors repeat their orders," General Lu snapped.

"Yes, Comrade General." The lieutenant stiffened.

"It is essential that the prisoner understand that he is still under suspicion and his every action watched. I want him to believe that his rearrest is only a matter of days."

"Yes, Comrade General." The Lieutenant saluted smartly and turned to go. Then he turned back and saluted again.

"Begging the Comrade General's pardon, but what is the prisoner suspected of?"

"He is a spy for the Chinese," General Lu remarked off-handedly.

"Is he really?" The lieutenant gaped at the prisoner through the glass. It was the first real spy he had ever seen.

"Of course. The fact that we arrest someone is clear evidence of his guilt. You really must have more faith in our system of revolutionary justice, Comrade Lieutenant." General Lu smiled.

"But if he is an enemy agent, why are we letting him go, Comrade General?"

"Because if one eliminates a spy one knows, the enemy may send another one does not know. It is often more useful to keep the spy where he is."

"If he knows he is under suspicion, he may escape," the lieutenant objected.

"That would be most unfortunate for the men assigned to watch him. Most unfortunate," General Lu said in an abruptly icy tone. It was clearly a dismissal. The lieutenant blanched. His arm shot up in a jerky salute and he scuttled out of the room.

Heng Ry came over.

"Was that wise, telling such a one about the Chinese?" he wanted to know.

General Lu made a resigned Asian gesture as he turned back to watch the one-way glass.

"That imbecile will certainly let it slip out. Better to let the prisoner learn about it accidently in such a manner. Then he will be certain to believe it."

General Lu watched the lieutenant enter the interrogation room and bark an order. The guards put down their truncheons, with some reluctance he thought, and began to unstrap the prisoner. His body sagged and they had to hold him up. They splashed water in his face to revive him.

As they worked on him, General Lu glanced around the tiny cell-like room with an air of distaste. This was an evil place, he thought. He had been in many bad places, and after nearly thirty years of war, he had seen the worst that people can do to each other. But this was an evil place.

He turned his attention to the security regulations taped next to the one-way glass. The crudely typed sheet dated from the time when Tuol Sleng was a Khmer Rouge prison, and was identical to the copy in the interrogation room. He put on a pair of wire-rimmed glasses to read it.

THE SECURITY REGULATIONS

1. You must answer according to my questions. Don't turn them away.

2. Don't try to hide the facts by making pretexts this and that. You are strictly prohibited to contest me.

3. Don't be a fool for you are a chap who dares to thwart the Revolution.

4. You must immediately answer my questions without wasting time to reflect.

5. Don't tell me either about your immoralities or the essence of the Revolution.

6. While getting lashes or electrification you must not cry at all.

7. Do nothing. Sit still and wait for my orders. If there is no order, be quiet. When I ask you to do something, you must do it right away without protesting.

8. Don't make pretexts about Kampuchea Krom in order to hide your jaw of traitor.

9. If you don't follow all of the above rules, you will get many lashes of electric wire.

10. If you disobey any point of my regulations, you will get either ten lashes or five shocks of electric discharge.

"Barbarians," General Lu muttered, folding his glasses and putting them away. He glanced back at the glass. They were taking the prisoner away. He stumbled between them, but apparently was able to walk. "Barbarians," General Lu repeated.

"They were merely following orders," Heng Ry said, having come up behind him. "Besides, we Khmers have no monopoly on cruelty. It was the French who taught us the electric wire. And what of the Americans, preaching of the démocratie while they dropped napalm on babies and took prisoners up in helicopters and forced them to jump without parachutes? Or even our Vietnamese comrades with your 'tiger cages' and 'Hanoi Hilton,' " he added defensively.

"Ah yes. Barbarism is a matter of class and circumstance, not race. We all need someone to do our dirty work," General Lu agreed smoothly. "Now let us exit by another way. I do not want the prisoner to see us."

The two men left the room and were escorted by a pair of guards down long twisting corridors, narrow and dank as a grave, to a side door where a white Mercedes was waiting, its windows tinted so it was impossible to see inside. It was parked in a side alley that gave them a view of the prison's grim main entrance.

"Wait here. I want to see where he goes," General Lu instructed the driver, separated from them by a glass partition, through an intercom phone.

"What makes you so certain he will escape to Bangkok?" Heng Ry wanted to know as the general replaced the phone.

"He knows he's blown. He can't stay in Kampuchea. Where else can he go? It's too risky for him to fade into the mountains and try to find the Khmer Rouge. If we don't kill him, they will. And he certainly won't head for Vietnam or Laos, where he knows no one and which we control. No." General Lu shook his head. "Thailand is the only direction open to him. When he stops panicking he will rendezvous with his Chinese contact, who has been our man all along. His contact will arrange his escape route down Highway Four. Your RPK officers at the checkpoints are to make it look convincing, but no matter how he blunders, we will make sure he gets safely to Kompong Som. From there Khmer Rouge sympathizers will smuggle him aboard a fishing boat up the coast, probably to Trat, across the Thai border. With joss, which as a good Marxist-Leninist I am certain does not exist, but about which as an Asian I know better, he will be in touch with Chinese agents in Bangkok within two days.''

Heng Ry nodded nervously. He began to say something when General Lu leaned forward and tapped the glass partition. The prisoner had emerged into the street. He was blinking as though blinded by the light, despite the gloomy monsoon clouds. They watched him hesitate for a moment, trying to decide which way to go. Then he looked around suspiciously.

"If he heads east, he will be going toward his apartment. West toward Norodom Boulevard will take him toward his contact," General Lu murmured.

All at once, the prisoner seemed to make up his mind. Throwing a last furtive backward glance over his shoulder, he began to walk briskly toward the west.

Heng Ry and the general shared a smile. The driver looked over his shoulder questioningly at General Lu, who picked up the intercom phone.

"Shall I follow him, Comrade General?"

"No." General Lu shook his head. "Take us by way of Monivong Boulevard to the Ministry."

The Mercedes pulled smoothly into the empty street, heading in the opposite direction of that taken by the prisoner.

"When do you leave for the north?" Heng Ry asked.

General Lu stared out his window. Along the side streets were piles of rusting automobiles, stacked like children's blocks for removal to tiny hand forges outside the city. He remembered how the abandoned vehicles had cluttered the streets when they had first conquered Phnom Penh back in '79. He remembered the smell and the corpses in the streets half devoured by dogs that had reverted back to the wild and had to be machine-gunned, the helicopters hovering just above the level of the roofs spraying disinfectant, the weeds sprouting from the cracks in the sidewalk. Now on the main boulevards the palm trees were beginning to flourish again and the intersections were crowded with bicycles and kong dups. Now and then you even came across the occasional curbside stall selling nems or Cha Gio. But most of the stores were still smashed and abandoned. Apartment windows above the stores were shuttered, and in side streets he could still see broken glass and rats squashed by the motorcycle carts.

The driver touched his horn, and the little girl who was directing traffic, in the red scarf and hat of the Revolutionary Youth, waved them through the intersection. They had not seen another moving automobile.

"At dawn," General Lu replied.

He watched the faces turn away as they drove by. There was none of the normal bedlam of an Asian city, the music blasting, the squawling of infants, the shrill voices.

"You can still see it," he remarked.

"What?"

"The fear in their eyes. It's still there, after all these years. They hate us, you know"—gesturing at the pedestrians starting to run as the rain began to fall. Fat wet drops splattered on the Mercedes windshield like translucent insects. "Us, the Russians, all of us. They'd love to see us go."

"And yet we are all that stands between them and the return of Pol Pot and his killing fields, the peal chur chat," Heng Ry objected.

"But we are foreigners all the same. 'Dog-eaters,' n'est-ce pas? Hatred of foreigners is a force that should never be underestimated. It enabled us to drive the Americans out of Vietnam," General Lu said.

"Not 'historical inevitability'?" Heng Ry smiled wryly.

"That too." General Lu smiled back. "Though there were dark times, Comrade Minister, when the Marxist-Leninist 'dialectic of history' did not seem so inevitable at all. The Americans were far more powerful than we. At times their weight was crushing on us, like an anthill upon which an elephant has sat. They were a good enemy."

"A good enemy?" Heng Ry inquired, eyebrows raised.

"Most good." General Lu nodded. "Choose your enemy well, Comrade Minister, for he will be your teacher. In this matter, like you Kampucheans, we Vietnamese were most fortunate in having first the French and then the Americans. They were both good. And strong, especially the Americans."

"Yet they lost."

General Lu stared out at the rain. The driver turned on his lights. The afternoon was dark as night and the rain fell in ropes, as the saying went. Drops danced on the pavement like water flowers. Pedestrians huddled under awnings and overhangs. A motorcycle cart raced by, the driver trying to hold a sheet of clear plastic over his head with one hand as he drove.

"Like in jiu jitsu, it was their own strength that defeated them. They lost because they thought the war was a military matter; that the political solution would come after victory. They never understood that the political issues were all that mattered and the fighting incidental. A Coca-Cola can with explosive would have been enough for us to make an incident and keep the war going forever," General Lu said at last.

"Yet they tried to win the peasants over."

"With words only. 'But if language is not in accord with the truth of things . . .' " General Lu shrugged, quoting Confucius. "They lost because they never saw us. We were invisible. Eh bien, they saw us, we were right in front of them, but they did not truly see us. They thought they were fighting for big things, pour la démocratie and against le communisme, when the war really had to do with who owned the pigs in a village. And because they could not see the world this small, they could not see us. And not seeing us, the only way they could have beaten us was to kill every last Vietnamese. Of this, they were physically, but not morally, capable. As I said, 'a good enemy.' " General Lu grinned.

Heng Ry nodded. Whether he agreed or not, he kept his thoughts to himself. He watched the monotonous slap of the windshield wipers. The Mercedes slowed to go through a deep puddle. The rain was already beginning to turn some of the intersections into muddy lakes. The water was dark as soup. Palm fronds floated on the surface. In the low-lying areas, the Tônlé Sap had already begun to overflow its banks. Along the waterfront the city resembled a Venice of squatters' shacks.

"And now it is we who take the part of the Americans against the Khmer Rouge. This time it is we who are the elephant and they the ants," Heng Ry observed glumly.

"Yes, but we can profit by the example of the Americans. That is why the matter of this agent Pich"—naming the prisoner—"and the opium of Bhun Sa is of such importance," General Lu said.

"But whose is the opium? Bhun Sa or Son Lot?"

General Lu made an open palm gesture as though weighing

something in his hand that in Asia means the answer does not matter.

"Two dogs, one bone. They will not share. The bone belongs to the stronger," General Lu said.

"But will we find it in time? That is the key," Heng Ry said, his mouth pursed with worry.

There was a creaking of leather as General Lu settled back in his seat. He smiled enigmatically. At that moment, Heng Ry thought, he really did look like the Buddha.

"You should have more confidence in the skill of the Americans, Comrade Minister. Have I not said they are a good enemy?" General Lu said.

16

The deep within the deep.
The depths confront him on every
hand.
Everything is dangerous; he is
never at rest.
His struggles will plunge him
into the chasm within the deep.

Y OU owe me six chi of gold, younger brother. Did I not say I would deliver you to Bhun Sa, neh?'' Toonsang declared boisterously.

Sawyer forced a smile.

"For your payment you must ask of Bhun Sa. For all that was mine is now his."

Toonsang's eyes narrowed.

"Younger brother's generosity to the Lord of the Shan shows wisdom. Did I not say Bhun Sa would have all when we were yet in the village of the Hmong? Better to have accepted my offer then," he said, glancing out of the corner of his eye at the woman.

"Ah, but then you would have been richer and the Lord of the Shan poorer," Sawyer offered slyly.

"By the phi, the farang speaks truth. Better with me than in this old thief's hands." Bhun Sa's laugh boomed and the others echoed it nervously. "But among friends there should be no talk of mine and yours. Your pack has been returned and none will dare touch of it," Bhun Sa assured Sawyer, looking keenly into his face. Up close, Sawyer saw that Bhun Sa's eyes were dark and flat as a reptile's. His face was yellow and very Chinese, but Shan tattoos decorated his chest and back and the belly overhanging his waist sash.

"All good friends," Bhun Sa repeated like a car salesman wrapping up a deal. "What you want to drink? Whiskey?" he asked Sawyer, pronouncing it witsake.

"Mountain whiskey or Mae khong?"

"No Mae khong piss. Real Ingrish witsake from Yuessay. See daeng Johnny Warker." Bhun Sa grinned.

He clapped his hands and a Shan woman came out of the cave with a bottle of Johnny Walker Red and clay cups. She handed it to Bhun Sa, who held the bottle up to view like a sommelier. Sawyer squinted to see the label.

"Dee mark," Sawyer said admiringly. "That is the real English whiskey. Where did you get it?"

"We took it from Birman officers near Kengtung. Where they go they are not needing witsake." Bhun Sa laughed in a way that gave Sawyer the creeps.

"Pah, Ingrish witsake!" Toonsang scoffed. "I see Ingrish cinema one time in Chiang Mai. They walk with noses held so, as if there is bad smell in room, and are all the time saying, 'You give me witsake soda, preez, Ho boy,' " Toonsang said, screwing up his face in a striking imitation of monocled aristocratic idiocy.

Even Sawyer had to smile.

"Is truth?"

"I have been in England a ten of times and never have I seen any such as these. Besides, the whiskey comes not from the Yuessay or England, but from the land of the Scotsman."

"Neh! The Ingrish drink the witsake soda all day and night and the women wear longyi that show their bosoms, which are of a monstrous bigness," Toonsang insisted, clownishly holding his hands at arms' length from his chest to demonstrate.

"Who are these of the Scotsman? I have never heard of these," Bhun Sa said to Sawyer.

"They are a hill people. Their land is a part of England, yet they are not English. Once there were wars between them and the English."

"Like the Shan and the Birmans!" Bhun Sa exclaimed delightedly. "Now I know why they make the good witsake!"

Bhun Sa poured the whiskey like water and they drank. It burned like acid on Sawyer's lip and he tried to hide it. His mouth still hurt from the rifle butt, and when he moved, his kidney reminded him it was there.

"Are the hills of the Scotsman like our hills?" Bhun Sa inquired.

Sawyer looked around the camp in the pines. The area was honeycombed with caves and so densely wooded that not many of the Shan could be seen, although Bhun Sa claimed to have over five thousand men in this camp alone.

They were high up in the hills. The air was cooler and wet with mist, and they could hear the rumble of a waterfall less than half a mile down the trail. From the air they were invisible. Sawyer knew this because a few hours earlier a pair of jets, fighters by the sound of them, had flown over, yet there had been no panic.

"Who are they, Thai or Birman?" Suong had asked.

"Neither. Lao air force." Bhun Sa had shrugged.

"What do the Lao want here?"

"They search for me. The Lao government wishes the opium trade for themselves, but we do not allow them." Bhun Sa grinned.

Toonsang spat.

"The Lao are pigs! Food for the dog-eaters!"

"A backward people," one of Bhun Sa's savage-looking Shan chimed in.

Suong's eyes flashed.

"Fool! That is what the Europeans say of us all. I remember when I went to school in Paris I had a friend from Laos. Her father was a wealthy rice merchant in Vientiane. She was most pretty, with soft eyes like the kyi deer, and when we walk in the streets together we make the heads to turn.

"One time we were invited to a party. Very très chi-chi. We were excited to wear our new French dresses, but no, they wanted us to wear our native phasin. We were a nouvelle sensation, you see. Then someone is asking her where she is coming from, and she tell them 'Laos' and they don't know where it is.

" 'Laos is called the Land of a Million Elephants,' she tell them, and someone say, 'You mean Land of a Million Irrelevants,' and because we are good Asian girls our faces show nothing, but back in our room that night she is crying very much."

"What happened to her?"

Suong made an odd gesture of dismissal.

"She fell in love with a French boy and they want to run

away. They are making many plans, all very fou, but her father hear of it and make her come back to Laos, where he marry her to merchant friend, old man of sixty whose wife has died. But of course, that was long ago, before the coming of the Pathet Lao," Suong told them.

That had been earlier, when they were first brought to the camp. Now the light was fading and the shadows were growing longer. Because of the caves and the trees, it was impossible to guess the extent of it, but despite the presence of women, it had the ceaseless activity and air of purpose characteristic of a military base.

Sawyer looked around, admiring how Bhun Sa had done it. There were only two trails in, both well guarded. He could hold off an army, or he could go out the back way and be across any of three borders in a few hours.

"No, the hills of the Scotsmen are colder and there are not so many trees. Instead of wood, they burn old dead plants that have been buried in the ground and which they dry, and it is this smoke that gives the Johnny Walker its taste," Sawyer replied.

"And do they kill the Ingrish as we Shan do the Birmans?" Sawyer shook his head. Bhun Sa made a face.

"This Scotsman place must be a more holy land than I thought. To have someone steal your land and not kill him requires great piety—or perhaps they are cowards," he added provocatively.

"I wouldn't say that to a Scotsman." Sawyer grinned and Bhun Sa laughed.

Bhun Sa poured Sawyer another cupful of whiskey. He made a motion for Sawyer to drink and waited till Sawyer had finished and wiped his mouth with the back of his hand.

"And what would one say to a See-Ah-Ay man?" Bhun Sa asked, watching Sawyer like a snake.

It was a thing Sawyer had been expecting, still it made him weak in the knees to hear it. He remembered the bodies by the gate and knew that if he misspoke now, it was all over.

"Before we speak of business matters, there is the matter of two killings to be settled—that of the Kachin and the Akha. These were necessary for my mission and the protection of the woman, who is here to speak for the army of Mith Yon. But if there is payment due for these, then it is better done now, before enemies share rice and pretend to be friends," Sawyer declared, looking straight at Toonsang and wishing to hell that he had a gun to hand.

Bhun Sa smiled lazily, showing all his teeth like a big yellow cat.

"If these were Shan who died, men of the SUA, you would be begging this one for death even now. But for an Akha, or the Kachin, mai pen rai." He shrugged. "The loss is to this one," indicating Toonsang, "and perhaps no loss since I have purchased his ridiculously priced opium and now there are fewer for him to share with."

Toonsang smiled back, all friendliness.

"The Lord of the Shan is wise. There is no loss, younger brother. The Kachin was becoming presumptuous. The Akha was of no matter. Had I known the Lord of the Shan was desirous of speaking with you, I would have slit their throats myself to safeguard your sleep," he declared impudently.

Bhun Sa turned toward Toonsang.

"Wisely said. To kill one's customers is bad business."

Toonsang flinched under Bhun Sa's unblinking gaze. Sawyer was reminded of the old Cambodian saying that only the gods and the dead never blinked.

"This one never considered an act of such monstrous rashness. By the phi, may the Lord Buddha doom this one to a hundred lifetimes as a castrated pig if this one ever—"

"Do not add blasphemy to your earlier stupidity," Bhun Sa snapped angrily.

Toonsang's smile grew sickly, as if he could already feel the sharpened point of bamboo penetrating his belly.

"Now leave us, before I turn you into a castrated pig in this lifetime," Bhun Sa growled, the scar on his cheek deepening along its uneven crease.

Toonsang hurriedly wai'd and scuttled away. Bhun Sa's own men, recognizing the signs, crept quietly out of earshot, as did Suong, her face an expressionless blank. Only Sawyer and Bhun Sa were left. They watched the sway of her hips as she made her way up the path to the cave.

"She is Mith Yon's woman or yours?" Bhun Sa asked, still watching her.

"Mine—and no one's," Sawyer said, a warning in his voice.

"She has claws and teeth," Bhun Sa agreed. "Any woman is a danger, but that one moves like a tigress."

"Toonsang wanted her. It was the cause of much difficulty," Sawyer admitted.

"Yet you suffered him to live."

"Had the Lord of the Shan not attacked the village when you did, he would even now be with the neak ta."

"By the nats and phi, that is a slippery one. He is like the Hanuman snake, yellow eyed and green as the leaves that hide it till it drops down on its victim from the trees when least suspected, and its bite kills in seconds," Bhun Sa observed, watching Toonsang.

"Yet the Lord of the Shan suffers him to live in this world of dust and sorrow," Sawyer said carefully.

"As the beekeeper suffers the bee to keep his stinger, for without it there is no honey. Does our honored guest wish his death?"

Sawyer spat, but inside, his stomach was turning over. On the road to the camp, Bhun Sa had had the Kuomintang officer who had led the attack on the village tied by his wrists to the Land Rover's rear bumper. After an hour on the road, the officer's hands were the only things still recognizably human. Sawyer wondered if Toonsang was enough of a danger to test Bhun Sa's goodwill.

"Is it offered?"

Bhun Sa considered, thoughtfully rubbing his scar. Then he smiled broadly like a merchant about to quote what he knows is an outrageous price.

"In exchange for additional arms, many things are possible. The Golden Triangle is a dangerous place."

Sawyer shook his head. The water was getting too deep for him. Bhun Sa had let Toonsang ride next to him in the Land Rover. Who could say what their relationship really was? Because someone in that Lisu village had acted as a spy so that the trap could be sprung on the KMT. Toonsang maybe?

"Mai pen rai. Let it be as the Lord of the Shan wishes." Sawyer shrugged. "We have more urgent matters to discuss."

"That is good. And men such as Toonsang have their uses," Bhun Sa declared, offering Sawyer a white Burmese cheroot and lighting one for himself. Although Sawyer no longer smoked, he was too wise not to light up. He considered what Bhun Sa had said. It was as close to admitting that Toonsang was his spy as he was going to get.

"Then the Lord of the Shan must have known of my coming," Sawyer said, trying to contain his excitement and make his voice sound rueful. If true, it meant that not only did the buyer want to buy, but that the seller wanted to sell.

"The Lord of the Shan hears more in the hills than the call of the toktay," Bhun Sa agreed, sending a big puff of smoke to heaven like a signal.

"You have the morphine base, not opium?"

"The white man seeks the 'white powder.' This is known. Also, in these quantities—" He paused. "Does our honored guest know how much of the opium it takes to make the morphine base?"

Sawyer shook his head, although Harris had briefed him. Never show them up was a cardinal rule with Asians.

"It requires two thousands of poppies to produce one kilo of the opium. Ten kilos of the opium make one of the morphine. Who could transport such an amount in opium form?"

"It is said Bhun Sa owns all the opium of the Three Lands," Sawyer said, flattering shamelessly. He remembered something Harris had said a long time ago after coming out of a meeting with a certain secretary of state known for his ego: "You cannot overflatter the really powerful. It cannot be done."

Bhun Sa looked sharply at Sawyer, who could feel a bead of sweat trickle down the length of his spine.

"Not all, honored guest. But enough."

"How much?"

Bhun Sa bent forward and motioned Sawyer to lean closer.

"Three thousands and nine hundreds of kilos of the purest morphine base."

Sawyer whistled to himself. Barnes hadn't been exaggerating. That was worth about a billion dollars wholesale anywhere in the world. Add acetic anhydride and you had an equivalent amount of pure heroin, worth two to three times that in the U.S. or Europe.

"Where is the morphine? Here?"

Bhun Sa smiled.

"Not here."

"But it is ready for delivery?"

"All ready. Is Yuessay government also ready? Long time ago I send word to See-Ah-Ay man, Barnes-khrap. Tell your President Carter the Shan wish to be free peoples. Tell him we trade opium for guns and we kill plenty Birmans, plenty Communists. But the President Carter has no interest. 'The Yuessay government is not in the opium business,' they say. So now I say, is Yuessay ready to do serious business?"

Sawyer shrugged and made a Thai gesture that to Buddhists suggested that the past no longer existed.

"The current president sees things differently. He is not bound by old decisions. My orders come from him through my superiors in the See-Ah-Ay, as you have discovered."

"The See-Ah-Ay has bought the morphine and heroin from us before, in the days of the war in Vietnam."

"Oh yes." Sawyer smiled. "There are those who believe that making money is always in the national interest."

Bhun Sa brought out the big catalog. He tapped the cover with his finger.

"I have looked at these pictures with much interest. Are all here available?"

"We'll trade arms for morphine, as we discussed. M-16 rifles, M-60 machine guns. 'Thumpers'—M-79 grenade launchers, LAW 66-millimeter rockets, claymores. Mortars—60s, 81s. Jeeps, quad-50s, Prick 25 radios. Artillery—105-millimeter howitzers, 175-millimeter self-propelled guns. Slicks—UH-1 Huey helicopters. Stinger missiles. MA's—all kinds of mines, some look like rocks, some to put into streams—all the bullets in the world. Give you any goddamn thing you want. The store is open." Sawyer shrugged.

"Gold?"

"How much gold?"

Bhun Sa pretended to think for a moment.

"Ten millions Yuessay dollars' worth. Five millions deposit in my account in Hong Kong bank. Rest delivered with the arms."

"That's a lot of gold," Sawyer said doubtfully, rubbing the bristle on his cheek. "We'd have to buy it in the open market in London or Zurich. People see such things and questions can be raised."

Bhun Sa looked unblinking at Sawyer.

"Gold is also a weapon," he said finally.

Sawyer nodded.

"What about Kampuchea? We need men to use these arms against the Vietnamese dog-eaters. For guerrilla actions and to lay mines and MA's, booby traps, along the border. Can you do this?"

Bhun Sa puffed thoughtfully on his cheroot.

"We fight the KMT, the Thais, and the Lao army for the opium trade. That is the way of things. But our war is with the Birmans to free the Shan Lands. We have no quarrel with the dog-eaters."

"With the arms we can give you, the KMT will be a memory in the Golden Triangle, even as it is in Yunnan China. You can defeat the Birmans. A pro-Western state on the Thai border would no doubt receive American recognition and with recognition comes much—not the least of which is money." Sawyer grinned.

"What of the gold now?"

Sawyer hesitated like a fly fisherman watching a trout lip at the bait.

"As the Lord of the Shan says, gold is also a weapon," he said carefully.

Bhun Sa studied the ash at the end of his cheroot as if wondering when it would fall off. He blew on it and it fell. He blew on it again and the tip glowed bright red.

"Mines and traps can be laid," he agreed. "That only requires a few hundreds of men and it will be good training for when we use these devices against the Birmans. But for the real fighting against the dog-eaters, we have agreed to supply one-third of all the arms to the Khmer Rouge. They will"—he shrugged—"need little encouragement to use them against the dog-eaters."

"Before the monsoon ends?"

Bhun Sa crushed out his cheroot on the log. He held out his hand, palm up.

"First the arms and gold—here," he said, tapping his palm.

Sawyer nodded.

"You'll get them."

"How will you deliver?"

"By plane to Chiang Rai. Then trucks to any place with paved-road access you designate."

"What of the Thai airport authorities and border patrol checkpoints?"

"They will see only what they have been ordered to see. The

crates will be stamped 'Farm Machinery.' The papers will be in order and the officers will be alerted not to examine further. What of the morphine?"

"By mule from its present location to a place where it can be loaded in big trucks and covered with sacks of rice. From there to rice barges that will take it down the Chao Phraya to Bangkok, at which point you may make your own arrangements."

"We will need coordination between us and the Khmer Rouge that we all attack the dog-eaters at the same moment and in the agreed sectors."

"What of the other Cambodian groups? The KPNLF, the Hmong, and Mith Yon's group?" Bhun Sa asked.

"We will handle these. When all is ready, we will signal you on the radio which we will give you. The signal to attack will be the one word 'Dragonfire,' which will be repeated until you signal back that the message has been received."

Bhun Sa looked curiously at Sawyer.

"Tell me, Soyah-khrap. You have confidence in this plan?"

Sawyer's stomach went queasy. For all that Bhun Sa was a primitive warlord, Sawyer had seen that he had an instinctive talent for military strategy. Or maybe it was that the question had aroused doubts within himself that he hadn't wanted to think about.

"Why does the Lord of the Shan ask?"

"Does the See-Ah-Ay truly believe that these mosquito stings will chase the dog-eaters from Kampuchea?"

Sawyer didn't say anything.

"Perhaps," Bhun Sa ventured, "you think only to keep the dog-eaters from crossing into Thailand and only make children's stories of a free Kampuchea for such as the woman who speaks for Mith Yon."

Sawyer hesitated. Darkness had come. He could not see Bhun Sa's face, only his silhouette against the light from the cave.

"More guns for Bhun Sa means more dead Birmans," he said softly.

Bhun Sa hawked and spat. In the silence of the shadows, it was as loud as a pistol shot.

"But suppose you make a success, Soyah-khrap? Have you thought what is your coalition? My war is in Burma and the Golden Triangle, not Kampuchea. As for the Khmer resistance groups, the Khmer Rouge and the others are like the tiger and a litter of kittens. If the dog-eaters withdraw, who will the tiger feed on next?"

"Not the Shan," Sawyer said stubbornly.

"Perhaps not today," Bhun Sa agreed. "But who can say what a hungry tiger may do? The kittens will be gone in one bite. "So!" he said, snapping his jaw shut so his teeth clicked loudly. "And then . . . it is said that once the tiger tastes of human meat he prefers it to any other."

"I have heard this," Sawyer admitted.

"The Yuessay people have given much to Asia peoples. But their gifts bring only sorrow, Soyah-khrap. You gave arms and gold to the Vietnamese, yet the Communists win. You gave arms and gold to the Lao and it brought them war and the Pathet Lao. You gave arms and gold to the Kampucheans and it brought them war and the Khmer Rouge. Truly, your gifts are most expensive, Soyah-khrap. And now you wish to give arms and gold to me?"

Sawyer spat. When those geniuses in Langley were brainstorming this beauty, they hadn't figured that a backwoods bandit could have seen through the whole thing. Bhun Sa had put his finger right on it. They were grabbing the tiger's tail, and once they did, they couldn't let go and there was no telling where it would lead. If the Khmer Rouge were to ever win again, they'd begin right where they left off. How many millions more do you want to see die? he asked himself. But if he didn't pull Dragonfire off, the war might engulf all of Southeast Asia.

Hobson's choice.

Time to vote.

Sawyer made as if to stand up.

"If you are not interested in beating the Birmans—or ten millions in gold . . ." He shrugged, bluffing like crazy.

"Neh, neh," Bhun Sa said hurriedly. "Mai pen rai. Rice is, how you say, rice. And a man must eat, neh?"

Sawyer grinned.

"As it is said, 'Rice gives strength, even to the king,' " he said.

Bhun Sa grunted and poured out the last of the Johnny Walker. They drank.

"I have one question, Soyah-khrap," Bhun Sa brought out

delicately. "A matter of some curiosity, but of a personal nature. May one speak?"

"There is no offense when so presented among peu-un, Bhun Sa-khrap."

Bhun Sa put the bottle down with a clink. He watched it roll a few inches before stopping against a twig.

"How did you come to lose your eye?"

"A mine. During the war in Vietnam."

Bhun Sa nodded.

"Then you were fortunate to have lost no more."

"Yes, though it was not I but a peu-un who stepped on the device. Had it been otherwise, your humble servant should not be here," Sawyer said, a shade too pompously. All at once the whiskey had hit him hard.

"But this covering over the eye. Is it not of a great handicap in your profession? Who can fail to spot a one-eyed man?"

Sawyer laughed.

"Sometimes it is of great value in my profession for one to be easily recognizable. Other times, no, in which case," he tore off his eye-patch.

Bhun Sa took Sawyer's chin in his hand and turned it toward the light from the cave.

"By the phi, there is no blemish!" Bhun Sa declared.

"The eye is glass. The skin took numerous surgeries," Sawyer said. "So you see, those told to look for a one-eyed man will not see me though I stand in front of them. Also, the fact that my right eye is still good means I can still use a gun."

"By the phi and all the nats, this is most rare. But if the eye of glass is such perfection, why wear the covering at all?"

Sawyer frowned. It was hard to explain, even to himself.

"Call it a romantic impulse." He shrugged. Then seeing the lack of comprehension on Bhun Sa's face, he grimaced and put the eye-patch back on.

"At first, after the war, I wore it as a thing to thrust in people's faces. To remind them of the war, because they treated us like lepers when we came home."

Bhun Sa's brow furrowed.

"Who would treat a warrior so?"

"Many did because we fought at all. Others because we lost. It seems strange, yet it was a common thing in those days."

"We say defeat is a child without parents."

"We say the same." Sawyer smiled.

"So this covering of the eye was not a thing of vanity, to say to men I was there. I was a warrior and you were not," Bhun Sa observed shrewdly. In the light from the cave his face looked like a profile on a frieze, a barbaric chieftain from an age when men became legends.

"It *was* vanity. I wore it to say to men, 'I am more of a man than you,' and to say to women, 'Here is a mystery,' for they love riddles better than food and drink," Sawyer admitted, his tongue growing thick from the whiskey.

"And did the farang women flock?"

"Some," Sawyer bragged. "There was a time when I wanted to fuck every pretty woman I saw. Sometimes I would follow one in the street, fantasizing how she would look, her ingyi opening to bare her breasts, and how I would raise her longyi and bend her over. I would contrive to meet her if I could. Yet no sooner did I have her than I wanted to be away and find another. After a time, I came to see the pointlessness of such a quest. I was no more than the animal that puts his injured paw in his jaws in order to bite the pain."

"Why? Does not the farang woman know how to give pleasure?"

"Yes, but they wanted something in return."

"Ah, money." Bhun Sa clucked his tongue in understanding.

"No, not money. Something else."

"What then?"

"I never knew," Sawyer confessed. "Perhaps they did not know themselves."

Bhun Sa made a face.

"Pah! I have heard that the farang women are big and pink and yet their female parts are tight and good to give pleasure. But now I see there is no difference. All women want the same."

"What is that?" Sawyer asked, feeling himself on that high drunken peak where the world is spread out to view and life is a thing that can be explained.

"I have had many wives of many tribes. And concubines without counting. Yet in this regard they were as one. What women want above all," Bhun Sa pronounced solemnly, "is to be envied by other women. Thus, they desire most what they think other women have. If it became the fashion for them to stick parrot feathers in their ears, not a bird in the forest would be safe!'' Bhun Sa hooted.

They laughed so hard the others looked up and smiled to see their "little flight," as a happy drunk is called among the hill people. As they staggered back toward the cave, Bhun Sa put his arm around Sawyer and pressed his lips to Sawyer's ear as though bestowing a kiss.

"Listen, farang. Your woman-who-is-not-your-woman, she is of another kind. A fire burns in her, but it is a dark fire that gives no light. Perhaps it is she and not that pig, Toonsang, who is most like the Hanuman snake. For the Hanuman is green like finest jade and most beautiful, but its kiss is death,'' Bhun Sa said.

Sawyer came awake all at once. The back of his shirt was damp with sweat. There had been no sound, but something had awoken him.

He sat up in the darkness, concentrating on his listening the way a blind man does. He listened to the sound of heavy breathing. The Shan who shared the cave slept deeply, and he wondered what it was like to be able to sleep that way. He listened to the others sleep and tried to think, and then he realized what had awakened him.

Suong's place was empty.

She had been curled around him, spoon fashion. She had felt good against him, the whiskey making him pleasantly tired, with that wonderful feeling that sleep was going to be as easy as closing his eyes. He touched the depression in the blanket where she had been. It was still warm. She couldn't have been gone long. She probably slipped out for a night call, he thought. She'll be back in a minute. Or maybe she's out there praying to that crazy shrine of hers, whatever the hell that was about. Before this thing was over, he'd have to get to the bottom of that, he told himself.

Forget it, his tired brain told him. He had a terrible taste in his mouth from the whiskey and just wanted to sleep it off. But there was something that had wakened him. Something bad. Stay awake, the Reptile insisted, the sweat prickling all over his body. Even his hands were sweating.

She had taken the Ingram.

His stomach lurched. He clawed blindly in the darkness, feeling for the M-16. Nothing. He felt all around, carefully so as not to awaken the Shan, his panic growing. Then his hands closed on the familiar metal shape. He started to heave a sigh of relief, then thought he'd better check it.

It was empty. All the clips were gone. He didn't bother to check the pack for more clips. Whoever had done it had been very deliberate. They wouldn't have left him a clip by mistake. Not "they," the Reptile whispered inside him. *She.* Even the tanto knife was gone.

Sawyer got up slowly. What was it his Recondo instructor at Nha Trang used to say? "The successful infiltrator moves as if he does not disturb even the air." He glided out of the cave on the balls of his feet like a shadow.

Outside, a wet mist had settled over the camp. Trees loomed like indistinct dark shapes only when they were close enough to touch, and he had to go warily so as not to trip. The ground was covered with wet pine needles, making it spongy underfoot and muffling the sound of his footsteps. It was like walking through a black cloud. It smelled of wet earth and smoke and yet was like nothing he had ever experienced except in dreams.

He moved smoothly, silently through the camp, remembering how they taught him. Remembering the Vietnamese sapper who taught him how to move like the butcher's knife in the story of Chuang Tzu. It was said the knife never needed sharpening because the skilled butcher always guided it through the spaces between the joints, so that it separated the bones without ever touching them.

The mist swallowed him up like a sponge. He saw no one, yet there were thousands of men all around. In a way it was good not having a weapon, for no one would question him even if he were spotted. He would just say he'd had to make a night call and had gotten lost in the mist. But he felt defenseless without a gun all the same. The very fact that someone—say "she," admit it, he told himself—had gone to the trouble of depriving him of it was a pretty good indication that he might have need of it.

Something made him stop. He reached out his fingers and touched a branch, its leaves glistening with moisture. Another step and he would have blundered into it. He was lost, not quite sure where he was going, except that he kept moving up the slight incline and to the left, where he believed Bhun Sa's command cave was.

He felt his way around the tree. He saw a gauzy glow shining in the mist like a marsh light from Bhun Sa's cave. A crack of light was peeking from the edge of the Shan blanket hung over the entrance. She was there, Sawyer thought, feeling anger and jealousy flare up inside him. He didn't know how he knew, but he was certain of it. Where else would she be?

Was she selling him out to Bhun Sa? Or was Bhun Sa trying to cut a separate deal with her? Hatred for both of them came easily. Fucking gooks! he thought. No—stop! Jai yen yen, heart cool cool, as the Thais say.

There was a sentry seated in the lotus position by the cave entrance, a rifle across his thighs. Sawyer froze. He listened intently. Was there some sound? He could hear nothing, but he could see the sentry turning his head to listen to something happening inside the cave. His stomach tightened like a fist. Suong and Bhun Sa! He had to get to her.

He might be able to circle around and take the sentry from the side away from the entrance, he decided. It could work if the sentry was still eavesdropping on whatever was happening inside the cave. He had to hurry, but with each step he would have to take care not to make a sound and to be sure that his silhouette always blended into a dark background. He began mentally to step his way and had almost worked it out when the swish of a twig sounded behind him. He started to turn. A dark figure with a long knife loomed out of the mist.

Toonsang.

For the briefest instant Sawyer saw the piggy eyes narrowed, the lips drawn back in a killing snarl, and then there was no time for seeing. Toonsang was very fast; he had already adjusted for Sawyer's sudden turning around. His blade thrust straight at Sawyer's throat.

Sawyer threw up his right forearm to block, the blade slicing through like fire. Sawyer held the block sideways for an instant, then still with the right hand clawed at Toonsang's throat. Sawyer grabbed Toonsang's shirt and yanked Toonsang forward in the same direction as the thrust, adding to his forward momentum. Bringing his right knee up in a high side kick, he slammed it solidly into Toonsang's chest. Toonsang grunted like a pig. As he stumbled over Sawyer's right leg, Sawyer, still adding to Toonsang's forward momentum, put everything he had into a left hook to Toonsang's kidney. Toonsang sprawled facedown on the wet ground. Yet he still had enough left to slash back at Sawyer's exposed right leg with the knife.

Sawyer just managed to dance out of the way with a quick half-jump to the right. The instant his right foot jarred on the ground, Sawyer raised his left knee high and kicked savagely down, his left heel smashing into Toonsang's face. He felt something crunch under his foot. Toonsang's jaw hung slack and twisted like a shoe with the sole ripped half off.

Sawyer reached down for Toonsang's knife. The action saved his life. The crack of a shot sounded in the air where his head had been. Out of the corner of his eye he saw the dark bulk of the sentry closing. Only one chance, Sawyer thought, his hand closing on the knife. He whipped the knife sideways at the blurred figure coming at him in the mist and dived beside Toonsang.

Two shots cracked the silence in quick succession, one of them drilling deep into the muddy ground only inches from Sawyer's hand, the other thudding into Toonsang, who groaned and stirred, even though unconscious.

The smell of earth and blood was thick in Sawyer's nostrils, and he cringed, waiting for the sentry to come and finish him off. His only luck had been that the sentry's rifle must have been on semiautomatic and in the excitement he must have forgotten to switch it over. Come on, Sawyer thought irritably. Get it over with!

There was a sound, but no shot. Sawyer cautiously raised his head, expecting the blinding explosion of a bullet in his head, but nothing happened. The sentry was seated on the ground, not fifteen feet away. His eyes were wide open, but not on Sawyer. He was staring stupidly down at the handle of the knife sticking out of his belly. He plucked it out and it was like turning on a faucet. The sentry watched the blood pour out of the wound, as if it were a curiosity of nature that had nothing to do with him. He put his fingers to the wound to stem the bleeding. He watched the blood flow over his hand and never saw Sawyer at all.

Sawyer heard sounds of stirring all around in the mist. There was nothing to be seen, but he could feel the darkness coming to life. The sentry's shots must have roused the whole camp. There wasn't much time.

He started for the sentry's rifle, lying on the ground, when he heard a woman's muffled cry coming from the cave. He raced for the entrance. That bastard! he thought, whipping aside the blanket.

The cave was lit by a single lamp on a table that cast the struggling shadows of Suong and Bhun Sa high on the cave wall, as though it were a battle of giants. They were fighting for the Ingram, twisted in someone's hand between them. Suong's face was terrified. Her shirt had been torn open. Sawyer could see her breasts, white and heaving, mottled red by angry finger marks.

Bhun Sa's face was scored by bleeding furrows from Suong's nails. His face was grim, a cruel light in his eyes. He had been forcing the muzzle toward her chest at the moment Sawyer entered. Yet his instincts were remarkable. Despite the intensity of the struggle, he had somehow heard Sawyer enter and had already started to turn.

There was no time. The only move Sawyer had was a chop to Bhun Sa's neck, but it was a killing blow. It would mean the end of the mission. Suong looked desperately at him. There were sounds outside.

The Ingram rang out loudly in the confined space. The shots pinged as they ricocheted off the cave walls. They had just missed Suong. Bhun Sa forced the muzzle against her chest, at the same time swinging Suong around to put her between him and Sawyer, when Sawyer let go a slicing right hand edge-on to the Adam's apple. Sawyer felt something give in Bhun Sa's throat. Bhun Sa collapsed like a thing made of rags, a ghastly strangled sound coming from his throat. His body began to twitch. His heels drummed against the ground for a few seconds and stopped.

Sawyer grabbed Suong with one hand and the Ingram with the other. She looked down with a kind of fascination at Bhun Sa, and Sawyer had to yank her toward the cave entrance. He didn't look back. He didn't have to.

Bhun Sa was dead.

17

The wind blows beneath heaven.
The prince shouts his orders
to the four winds.
A strong and willful woman;
do not embrace her.

SHE watched the young man enter the room. His hair was short and dark. He had knowing eyes and a handsome mouth. He was strongly built for a Thai, every muscle perfectly sculpted. His naked body was magnificent. It gleamed as though oiled in the low light, sending a shiver through her.

She stretched languorously, feeling the caress of the gold-colored satin sheets against her skin. She watched herself in the mirrors on the ceiling and walls, her sleek body white against the gold of the sheet. The mirrors made a hundred reflected images of her. She was woman, containing multitudes of selves, she thought. She liked watching herself, turning her firm white thighs this way and that, now concealing, now revealing the cleft hidden between them like a secret. She put her finger to her lips, wetting it, then touched the finger first to one nipple, then the other, stirring them erect. She shuddered, breathing deeply of the scent of jasmine. The soft, discordant, yet strangely stirring pi-nai music seemed to smooth out time like an iron smoothing cotton wrinkles.

He turned her over easily as if she were a child. He raised her gold curls away from the nape of her neck and nibbled softly at her neck and ears. Then he poured the warm oil smelling of sandalwood into his palms and began gently working on the sides of her neck down to her shoulders, his touch somewhere between a massage and a caress.

His hands glided strongly yet lightly over her body, the sensation warming and exquisite. He smoothed away the tension in her back, trailing his fingers around and under the shoulder blades and down the spine to her buttocks, pulling and kneading them till they were tingling; then down the back of her thighs and calves to the soles of her feet. He massaged her toes one at a time, and when they were done, he turned her on her back and began on her breasts, moving in circles spiraling inward toward the nipples, which grew hard as iron under his touch.

He dipped his handsome face to the soft mound of her belly, kissing and licking his way down through the dense triangle of hair to the inside of her thighs. Sighing, she parted her thighs and shivered as his tongue found the entrance, an exquisite warmth spreading from that thrilling point of contact throughout her body.

Now she wanted him inside her. Hard and strong and all male. As she started to reach down for him, she felt a weight around her head. She gazed up at a second man, strong and lean and sporting a magnificent erection. She reached up and took him hungrily in her mouth. A wave of sensation coursed like electricity between her upper and lower lips. She gasped as the first man entered her, and she clutched him to her, wanting him as deep as he could go, her nails digging red crescents into his buttocks.

She had them both inside her now and she wanted them everywhere. The feeling came stronger and stronger and just as she was about to go over the peak, they turned her over on her hands and knees; one of them in her mouth, the other in her from behind, building it in waves even stronger than before.

Her pulse pounded in her ears like the surf. Her breathing grew harder, faster. She began to go wild with the overpowering presence of the two men inside her, gnawing at the one as the other pounded against her squirming buttocks. And then she was spinning out of control and it was good, good, so very good. She felt them spurting into her, hard and hot, wet and salty to the taste, and she took it in greedily, only wanting more and for it never to end.

And the old man watching it all through the peephole felt the ancient stirrings as the lithe young girl at his feet, half a century younger than he, lapped like a dog at his semierection. He crooned softly with pleasure as she proudly held up for him the fruit of her labor, a tiny drop of sperm gleaming like a seed pearl at the tip of his penis.

The old man watched the woman through the peephole sprawl back on the gold satin sheets in utter, delicious exhaustion. He pressed a button, and the soft lights in the mirrored room slowly dimmed into darkness. After a moment he pressed it again, and they slowly brightened to a gentle glow.

The two young men were gone. In their place were two pretty young women, both naked, who began to gently wash the woman from head to foot with scented soap. As they sat her on a stool and began toweling her with big fluffy towels, the woman looked up at the hidden peephole and smiled sardonically.

"Well, Vasnasong-kha. Did you enjoy the show?" she called out in a husky voice that had a world of cigarettes and cocktails in it.

Vasnasong pressed a button and spoke into a microphone.

"More than ever, Lady Caroline. It is great regret for me that you leave Bangkok."

"And for me, old friend. London has its pleasures, of course, but I find them not sufficiently— Oh bother! What's the word I want? . . ." Lady Caroline said, lighting a cigarette.

"Raffiné," Vasnasong suggested.

"Yes, that's it!" she brightened, concentrating as though memorizing it for a quip at a future cocktail party. "Raffiné."

She got up and slipped on a sheer white silk peignoir held up by one of the women, and stepped into soft white slippers held by the other woman, kneeling at her feet. She walked with long purposeful strides through a mirrored door that swiveled open at her touch into Vasnasong's private room.

The young girl was gone and Vasnasong was already dressed and waiting. He was seated in a silk and blackwood chair in front of an exceptional black lacquer Chinese screen, inlaid with ivory. He gestured for her to sit in the facing chair, carefully positioned on a large red Tientsin rug, its intricate pattern and colors complementing the spare elegance of the matching Chinese blackwood table, and offered the iced gin and tonics and the sogo. She drank the gin and tonic greedily.

"Christ, I needed that," she said.

"After such exquisite performance, it is well earned," he said, smiling.

"Well, if you enjoyed watching half as much as I enjoyed doing it, then you bloody well had the time of your life, you old fart." She laughed.

Vasnasong laughed easily, his ample belly bouncing under his folded hands.

"Bangkok won't be the same without you, dear lady."

Her face turned thoughtful, moody.

"All because of that Yank bastard, Sawyer. A pity too. He was damn sexy. Even with that bloody eye-patch."

Vasnasong raised his eyebrows.

"You found his eye-patch exciting. How interesting."

Lady Caroline smiled.

"Don't go all bloody Asiatic on me, Vasnasong-kha. You're not a woman. He was damn sexy. That thing gave him an untamed look, like a wild hawk. Pity we couldn't turn him," she said, biting her lower lip as if she wanted to say more but wasn't going to.

"Mai pan rai. Who will not dip into the common bowl will have to go without." He shrugged.

"Unlike those of us who have learned to share. Haven't we, darling?" she murmured, her eyes sparkling.

"Parting gifts?"

"How wise you are, old friend. That's something else I shall miss about this place; having one's desires understood without even having to ask. The man who could do that all the time could have any woman on the planet," she said, laughing at herself. It was a good sexy laugh that pealed clear as a bell.

Vasnasong raised his glass to her.

"Wisdom bows to beauty, dear lady. Cha Yo," he toasted.

"Cha Yo yourself, you old fraud," she said warmly, and drank. Her face was flushed. It made her look not merely attractive, but pretty. For a moment he could see how lovely she must have been as a young woman.

Vasnasong put down his drink with slow deliberation.

"I take it London is not so much unhappy with Sir Geoffrey, despite his recall," he said carefully.

"Not at all, darling. There's even been some grumbling among the inner circle over the Americans being so heavy-handed about it. Lots of 'What can you expect?' handwringing. And now, especially with Geoffrey's last little coup, our final gift to 'the Cousins' "—using the MI6 term for their CIA counterparts—"it makes them look very foolish indeed."

"A coup, you say," Vasnasong said, not bothering to conceal his interest.

"Don't worry, darling"—she laughed, tossing her hair out of her eyes—"that's my parting gift to you. From Beijing via our Hong Kong network. The latest on the Vietnamese mobilization. Fifty-five thousand additional troops are being moved to the Thai border. The invasion is scheduled to coincide with the Loy Krathong Festival of the Floating Lights at the end of the monsoon season. Despite 'the Cousins' ' bloody-mindedness, Downing Street feels we've made a contribution."

"Ah, that is most interesting," Vasnasong said, in a tone that indicated the exact opposite.

"Really, darling. I thought you'd be a good deal more impressed." Caroline pouted.

"No, no. Independent confirmation will no doubt be much appreciated in Washington," Vasnasong hurriedly assured her. "It is only my parting gift to you which renders your news less of a surprise."

"Will it secure our position?" she pounced greedily, deliberately leaving vague whom she meant by "our."

"Oh, assuredly." Vasnasong smiled.

She curled up on her chair like a cat. She licked her lip as though there was cream on it.

"Come on, you sly puss. Don't be such a bloody fanny-teaser," she purred.

Vasnasong leaned forward. So did Lady Caroline. Their faces were within inches of each other.

"Most interesting refugee arrived in Bangkok yesterday. I only got all the details myself last night," he began.

"A solid source?"

"Ah yes. You see the refugee, his name is Pich, was the Khmer Rouge's top agent in Samrin government, the Vietnamese puppet regime in Cambodia. Apparently he was senior Khmer Rouge cadre who defected to Vietnamese with Samrin clique, but who actually go along under secret orders from Son Lot himself. When the Vietnamese conquered most of Cambodia in '79, he became the primary source for Khmer Rouge pipeline to Beijing. The Vietnamese began to suspect him, so Khmer Rouge brought him 'out of the cold,' as you Brits say, though I would have said it was really getting too hot! So you see, it all ties together."

"Is that the gift? A saved Cambodian mole?" she asked, her face falling.

Vasnasong shook his head.

"Fortunately, this Pich was foresighted enough not to come empty-handed. Otherwise," he shrugged, "his Khmer Rouge comrades maybe just leave him in Tuol Sleng."

"Did he confirm the Vietnamese mobilization?"

"Ah yes, but there is information of even more interesting nature," he said.

"Bhun Sa's morphine," she breathed.

"Ah yes, but it seems that Son Lot is now partner in the affair. Morphine for arms against Vietnamese. That was the Americans' game. Only they needed an intermediary, Bhun Sa, and—how one says?—'facade,' to be able to say, if it ever came out, that the arms were going to non-Communist resistance in Cambodia, the KPNLF, Sihanouk, and even Mith Yon's faction. Only Son Lot took first American, Parker, and now, according to this Pich, he also has the morphine."

"So Son Lot means to squeeze Bhun Sa out. Is that it?"

"Once your sexy one-eyed American, the Soyah, arrives on the scene, Bhun Sa's position becomes most precarious," Vasnasong agreed.

"But will the Americans actually do a deal directly with the Khmer Rouge, the perpetrators of the holocaust in Cambodia?"

Vasnasong picked up his drink and swirled it in his hand. The tinkle of the ice cubes made her think of temple bells. When he spoke, his voice was without emotion.

"In my experience, dear lady, nations do not have moralities, only interests," he said. "If Soyah does not wish to deal with Khmer Rouge, Son Lot will no doubt find a way to persuade him."

Even though she hated Sawyer for how he had treated her and Barnes, the thought of what persuasion by the Khmer Rouge might mean sent a chill through her. She shook her head to clear it. What happened to the Americans was no affair of hers, she reminded herself.

"Is that all?"

Vasnasong smiled like a hostess springing a surprise dessert.

"Not quite. According to this man Pich, Vietnamese also know about morphine," he said softly.

"My God!" she murmured.

"But they don't know where it is! They think they will find it on Thai side when they invade. Only by then it will be in our hands!" Vasnasong declared gleefully.

"How?" she asked, forcing a nervous smile. He smiled back, at that moment looking every inch a ruthless mandarin of some ancient Chinese court, despite his Western-style silk shirt and slacks.

"Among my various shipping interests is old freighter, name *Siam Star*. Vessel of Panamanian registry." He shrugged. "She is one of those ships that arouses no attention in any port and appears to be held together primarily by rust, but which is actually quite seaworthy. The crew, except for the captain, who is Swatowese, like my mother's people, are mostly Filipino scum.

"Because of my Thai connections and also the useful information I was able to supply from MI6, thanks to our connection" —inclining his head in her direction—"I was able to convince new CIA station chief, a certain Harris-khrap, that the *Siam Star* would be able to transport the morphine with the kind of discretion required for such a delicate affair."

"Just don't forget our share in this," she said.

"Ours?" Vasnasong smiled.

"Yes, ours, Geoffrey's and mine, as you bloody well know," she snapped.

Vasnasong laughed, holding his hand on his stomach as though it hurt.

"Ah, my dear lady. Bangkok is going to be so very boring without you."

"Well then," she said, slightly mollified.

"Well then," he teased. "Once morphine has been loaded, the *Siam Star* will leave Bangkok and head south into the Gulf of Thailand to swing well clear of Cambodian and Vietnamese waters. It is possible she may even go a bit too far south to the waters off Songkhla. Who knows what can happen there?"

"Pirates?"

"It is said the men of Songkhla are fishermen when their nets are in the water." He smiled.

"And the ship?"

"It is insured. The CIA will no doubt make sure insurance companies do not inquire too deeply into the nature of her cargo," he said, with a shrug.

"And I get ten percent, as we agreed, you sly puss," she said, reaching over and cupping his sex in her hand.

"As we agreed." He nodded complacently, taking a deep breath. "But you are already so wealthy, dear lady. What will you do with so much?"

Her gaze was level and absolutely sincere.

"Really, darling. Money is always useful," she said.

18

The wind blows above the earth.
The worshiper has washed his hands
but has not yet presented the
*   sacrifice.*
He examines his own life.

A temple bell sounded the end of meditation and just like that Utama was back with them. For hours he had sat in the lotus position without movement. All at once, his eyes were twinkling and they could see him breathe once more. He smiled at Sawyer, draped in the yellow robe of a naga aspirant, and Suong, dressed in peasant black. Around them were the sounds of bare feet on stone as the other monks in the uposatha wai'd to the golden Buddha on the altar and exited through the door that led to the hall of the achan.

"Why do you meditate?" Sawyer asked.

"Why do you Christians pray?" Utama replied.

"For God's help, I suppose." Sawyer shrugged, thinking that he was hardly qualified to speak for Christianity.

"Pah!" Utama said, waving the thought away with his hand. "That makes of God a celestial telephone operator. 'Yes, you may have that new phasin.' 'Saw at dee! So sorry! Tomorrow your father must die of cancer.' 'Hello. You want to kill your enemy. This morning he ask my help to kill you. So, so. You win today. But in two weeks your little girl will step on mine and lose her legs. Bye-bye.' You make of God a great stupidity. Once I studied in a Christian mission school in Chiang Mai, but they say so many so foolishnesses I wonder how the European manages to survive in this world."

"We manage." Sawyer smiled. "And you haven't answered my question."

Utama smiled back, the wrinkles making deep furrows around his eyes, buried deep in his face like almonds pressed into dough.

"One meditates to clear the mind, my brother. Always there is so much noise in one's head. Chitter-chatter. Chitter-chatter. Even at this instant there is a voice in your mind repeating every word I am saying, though there is no need, for it is I who am speaking, not you. One meditates to get rid of this chitter-chatter. Only when the lake is calm does the water reflect the sky. When the mind is quiet, one can see things as they really are. Then one's life can be purposeful and not of those that, as the Enlightened One said, 'are pushed and pulled this way and that like a twig in a drainage ditch.' "

The smell of incense tickled Sawyer's nose. He didn't know how to respond to Utama's oblique reference to the hash he had made of things. Suong sat beside him like an ikon. She had said little in the hours since their escape. There were moments when he thought he caught a look of fear or pleading in her eyes, but when he tried to say something, her eyes went blank. She had "gone inside," as the Asians say.

"You mean like me," Sawyer said.

Utama only smiled.

"Your karma brought you here. Perhaps so we could talk. Tell me, how did you escape from Bhun Sa's camp?"

Sawyer shrugged wearily. He was very tired.

"We walked out. The mist was heavy outside Bhun Sa's cave, and we were able to pull the sentry's body inside without being seen. Bhun Sa's men had heard the shots, of course, but by the time they found Toonsang and dared approach Bhun Sa's cave, knowing his standing orders not to be disturbed, we were able to get our packs and were well away. With the KMT out there somewhere and the night so dark and misty, they probably decided to wait till dawn before coming after us. The mist probably saved our lives."

"So you came here."

"So we came here," Sawyer agreed.

Utama got stiffly to his feet and beckoned them to follow. He led them to the vihara temple for lay people. The vihara dormitory hall was lit by flickering oil lamps. They were alone, though there was room on the floor to bed perhaps a hundred people. Along the walls were murals depicting parables from Buddha's teachings.

"I can give you sanctuary for one night, no more. This we do for anyone and also because I think your escape was most arhat-like, to simply walk out of the camp of your enemies. It is surely karma. But after dawn you must not be here, for we cannot take sides," Utama said.

"The Buddhists in Vietnam take sides."

"And look at Vietnam," Utama replied.

Touché, Sawyer thought as he wai'd, Suong waiing with a deep bow. Utama's face was working. He had something more to say. Finally he brought it out.

"There is a thing between the two of you that is festering in silence. It poisons not only your peace, but the space around you. There will be a half-moon tonight. Perhaps by its light . . ."

Sawyer frowned. He had prided himself on being a better actor than that. He peered deeply into the monk's eyes.

"We will talk again, afterward," Utama said, and was gone.

Suong and Sawyer looked at each other in the empty hall. The sound of a heavy tropical downpour drummed on the roof. A young naga came in with two bowls of rice. As he padded out on bare feet, they sat down and began to eat in silence.

After the rain, the brightness of the moon came as a surprise. It wore a halo of clouds, but was bright enough to cast a shadow. The hills were dark and featureless. Somewhere out there, Bhun Sa's men were hunting them, but here in a grove of betel palms outside the temple, Sawyer felt safe somehow. There was a whisper of wind in the palm fronds. It stirred the bamboo chimes hanging near the vihara gate to music.

"What do you accuse me of?" Suong asked. She had loosened her hair. It fell loose to her shoulders, framing her face, cameo white in the moonlight.

"Have I accused you of anything?"

"With words, no. But in your heart, yes."

"Do you feel guilty, is that it?"

Suong looked down at the ground. She didn't say anything.

"Why did you go to Bhun Sa?" Sawyer asked finally.

"He summoned me," she said, not looking at him.

"Why didn't you wake me?"

She took hold of a palm frond and tugged it.

"And the gun. Why did you take it?" he asked.

"Oh, So-yah," she said. The light of the moon glimmered in her eyes.

"What are you hiding?" he demanded, the softness of his voice only accentuating his anger.

"He wanted me alone," she said, looking down at the crumpled leaf in her hand. "The way he looked at me was the way you all look at me. Do you think I have not seen it before? I took your pistolet-mitrailleur so you would not do a foolish thing. For then he would surely kill you. I thought if I showed him the pistolet-mitrailleur, he would think you harmless and let you live. But he spat and said he could sell the morphine anywhere and that the Americans were fools to believe he would risk his men to fight the dog-eaters so far from the Shan mountains when his real war was with the Birmans."

Sawyer put his hand to her cheek. She pushed it angrily away. She looked up at him defiantly, silver sparks of the moon in her eyes.

"I thought the pistolet-mitrailleur would frighten him, but he only laughed," she went on. "He said if I was not his, he would give me to his men. He said they would chain me like a dog to a tree for the use of any who passed by; that the last female so used had spent six months that way, raving and talking to herself. Then he called for Toonsang and sent him to kill you as you slept. I tried to kill him with the pistolet-mitrailleur, but he was too fast for me." She shrugged. "The rest you know."

She looked at the leaf remnants in her hand and threw them away. Sawyer turned and walked to a rise near the edge of the palm grove. From here he could see the dark humps of the hills in the moonlight all the way to the valley of the Nong Lom, and in his imagination even beyond, to the Mekong. The wind came up and he listened to the sound of the chimes and the noise of the fronds—not idly, but with intent, as a sailor listens to the sound of canvas. He sensed her behind him. He turned and they were in each other's arms, kissing passionately. Her lips were warm and sweet and it was the best kiss he'd ever had.

"And now? What now?" she asked finally.

He made a face.

"It's over. Finished. Without Bhun Sa . . ." he began.

She shook her head. Her hair flared in the wind. A shadow passed across her face. He looked up. A cloud had covered the moon. It started to rain again, suddenly as someone turning on a shower. They stepped under a tall palm and listened to the rain on the leaves.

"Bhun Sa didn't have the morphine," she said. Her voice seemed to come out of the night itself. It had the sound of rain in it.

That was right, he thought. With so much else that had gone wrong, he knew that that part at least was right. If the morphine had been in Bhun Sa's camp, Bhun Sa would have shown it to him—and the camp's internal security would have been tighter. Bhun Sa might have been acting, but all his people couldn't have been acting too.

"Who does?"

"Son Lot. The Khmer Rouge. With your arms they could stop the Vietnamese," she whispered.

"How do you know?"

"Bhun Sa told me. He bragged about it. He was going to betray the Khmer Rouge to the Vietnamese and sell the morphine to them for Russian arms. Less trouble to him, and he needn't to risk his men inside Kampuchea. He was a snake, this Bhun Sa. For him you Americans were merely—how one says?—'d'astuces pour gagner,' to use as a stick in his bargaining with the Vietnamese."

"Plots within plots within plots. It's getting all mixed up," Sawyer murmured.

Suong wiped the rain out of her eyes with the back of her hand.

"This is Asia, my So-yah. Here nothing is as it appears."

"If only we knew where Son Lot has the morphine," he muttered.

"Why? Would the CIA deal directly with the Khmer Rouge? That is the question."

"I don't know," he admitted.

"You could ask."

"But without knowing where the morphine is . . ." He shrugged.

"But we do know," she said, smiling a secret smile.

"How?"

She showed him the crude map she had taken from Bhun Sa's body while Sawyer was dragging the sentry's body back in the cave. Rain splattered the map as she showed him the markings in Bhun Sa's own hand by the flare of a matchlight. The light revealed her clothes molded to her body by the rain.

"Inside Cambodia," he whispered, unable to take his eyes off her. She began to unbutton her blouse.

"In the ancient place of the gods," she murmured, the warm rain glistening on her skin as she pulled him down to the soft wet earth.

"How goes it with the woman?" Utama asked.

They were sitting in his tiny cell. A single candle burned on a low table. It created a close tent of light around them. Sawyer knew there were mosaics on the wall, though it was too dark to see them. The smell of incense permeated the air. Its sweetness was almost strangulating.

"Better," Sawyer said.

"But still . . ." Utama suggested.

Sawyer made a face. It was all falling apart in his hands like rotten cloth and he wasn't sure what was true anymore. "This is Asia. . . . Here nothing is as it appears," she had said.

"Women," he replied, the way men do among themselves to indicate the impossibility of the two sexes ever seeing eye to eye.

Utama laughed.

"Nonsense. You Europeans always see things in terms of success and failure, winning and losing," he said cheerily. "I win my lover. I lose my lover. I give you this much love, but you only give me that much. So maybe I give you less so that I am not losing. Everything is a contest. You even have to defeat death. So silly."

"Why silly?"

The darkness around the cocoon of candlelight created an odd intimacy. Sawyer felt as though he were talking to himself.

"Because it is not practical. Your thoughts make you what

you are. If they do not help in a most practical way, they are of no value. For instance, the mission priest told us that your Jesus of Christ raised a man from the dead. But of what value is that to you when your own wife or brother dies? Will Jesus come back and raise them too? Of what value, then, is such thinking? Or must you believe they have gone to live in a celestial Land of Bliss which you yourself have never seen and for which there is not the slightest shred of evidence? This the Enlightened One would never accept. Only what your reason can accept, only what you yourself experience, unclouded by emotion or wishful thinking, only this partakes of truth. This is what Buddha meant when men came to him and, recognizing that he was a different order of being from other men, asked him not 'Who are you?' but 'What are you?'

" 'Are you a god?' they asked. 'No.' 'An angel?' 'No.' 'A saint, perhaps?' 'No.' 'Then what are you?'

"Buddha answered, 'I am awake.' "

"What would Buddha have done?"

"A young woman named Kisagotami came to the Enlightened One hugging the dead body of her infant son to her breast," Utama related. "She begged him to raise the child from the dead. 'This I can do,' the Tathagata told her, 'but the special medicine I need requires mustard seed from a house where no relative, servant, or friend has died.' So Kisagotami went begging for the mustard seed from house to house, but nowhere could she find a place where death had not visited. Only then did she understand that all that lives dies; there is no permanence to things. Some lights in the village go out; others come on. It is not a contest. It is the way things are. She became, as we say, 'enlightened' and was able to bury her child in the forest. Which approach do you think more practical?"

"And I, how am I to be enlightened?" Sawyer asked hoarsely.

The darkness seemed to press close around them. Utama sat cross-legged, his pale skin almost translucent in the candlelight. Sawyer could see the veins crawling under the skin of his ancient skull like blue worms. Utama blinked like one waking up.

"Mai pen rai, my brother. You have the one eye and can see much more than those who are blind. It has taken you thus far. Yet without two good eyes, you cannot see things as they really ire. Then who does your action help, yourself or your enemy?"

"What is it that I should see, holy one?"

Utama reached up and pulled off Sawyer's eye-patch. He regarded Sawyer's glass eye with a kind of clinical appreciation, the way a surgeon might. The candle flame could be seen in it as in a mirror.

"You don't need this anymore, my brother. Besides, the men of Bhun Sa will not find you so easily without it. As for the path you should take, remember that your karma has brought you this far, it will take you to the place where you will see the whole truth. Though for you, I think it is a dark place, lit by a dark fire," he said uneasily.

"And then?"

"And then you must choose, like all men, even as your bowels turn to water with fear. And worlds will hang upon your choice," Utama said.

19

The marsh has risen over the earth.
The superior man puts his weapons
in order and prepares for
*   unforeseen emergencies.*
Confer with the great man.
Success
as long as you are willing to pay
*   the price.*

L IKE slow-motion dancers, the two elephants raised their right front feet in unison and with an almost feminine delicacy rolled the long heavy teak log forward a few feet. Their mounted mahouts lightly tapped the massive shoulders with short bamboo sticks, and the elephants repeated their dance, pushing the log along the ground until it rested against the pile being loaded onto the big flatbed truck. The loading of the logs created a temporary roadblock across Highway 107, and a line of gaudily painted trucks and carts had settled down to wait. One enterprising driver had even slung a hammock from the bumpers of two tractor-trailer rigs and had settled in for a nap. Other drivers were reading or eating beside the road, the hot scent of red Prek-kk-noo peppers shimmering in the steamy midday heat.

It was an ordinary enough sight in rural Thailand, but Sawyer was instantly watchful. Any roadblock was dangerous, but there was something about this one that didn't feel right.

It was too late to turn back. They'd already been seen by a small group of truck drivers sitting in the shade of an alocassia and gossiping over a shared bottle of Amarit beer. Not that there should be anything worth noting, Sawyer reassured himself, in a monk in a worn saffron robe, his hair cropped close, body shaved smooth and hairless as an Asian, skin stained with berry juice, and a young peasant boy of the Lisu, grimy from the road. Suong's breasts were wrapped down, her hair was pinned under a straw hat, and no one should have given them a second glance. But Sawyer's Reptile was wide awake as they approached the line of trucks, and he could feel the sweat prickling all over his body. His hand tightened on the Ingram, concealed inside the furled-up black umbrella he carried, like many monks, against both sun and rain.

There was something wrong, the Reptile was telling him. It was like one of those "Can You Tell What's Wrong" picture puzzles. At first you don't see anything, but finally your eye catches the cloud that actually turns out to be a fish in the sky. They walked past the driver on the hammock and the drivers sitting in the shade eating, and there was nothing. One of the drivers wai'd to Sawyer, but he remembered to ignore the wai the way a real monk would. He knew their disguises wouldn't stand up to much scrutiny, but they ought to get them through any casual situation. Bhun Sa's men were looking for a one-eyed white man and a beautiful female, not a two-eyed Asian monk and a Lisu boy. It was just an ordinary rural scene, the stalled trucks baking in the sun, except that his Reptile was getting very jumpy. There was a fish in the sky somewhere. But where?

Suong trudged beside him, head bent, as though weighed down by the packs on her back and the steamy afternoon heat. Then he had it.

The driver lounging in the hammock had positioned it so he was in the boiling sun, something no Thai would have ever done. His position was perfect for covering the road but not for resting. Of course the sun might have moved, but there were plenty of shady places where he could have strung the hammock. And there was something else. Sawyer let his memory reconstruct the image without forcing it, which always creates distortions. He didn't dare turn around and look back. That would have blown the monk cover there and then. Yes, he had seen it. The driver's shirt had been open at the neck and he had seen part of a Shan tattoo.

It was a trap.

Sawyer's eyes darted around, measuring the distance to the high grass and palms alongside the road. He could fire the Ingram through the umbrella, and once in the high grass, they could make a break for it. His heart pounded. Should they go for it? So far they hadn't been challenged. What were the chances on bluffing versus running? he wondered. Lousy either way. Go for it, he thought. Better to die moving. His legs tensed. The only question was how quickly Suong would react. Then he changed his mind.

Bhun Sa's men were lounging in the shade under the flatbed truck, covering the road with automatic weapons. They had no choice. They would have to bluff.

Sawyer's skin was shiny with sweat. He hoped to God it wasn't making the stain run. If only the men under the truck had never seen them before, they might have a chance. He felt Suong tense up beside him. She had made no sound or movement, but he felt it. The sun baked down on them. Sawyer felt exposed, as though the sun was an eye in a giant microscope peering down at them. He risked a glance out of the corner of his eye and was immediately sorry he had. He didn't recognize any of the others, but Timber Wolf and his M-1 was staring right at him.

The Ingram grip felt slippery in his hand. They were passing within ten meters of the flatbed. He didn't dare look, but he could feel Timber Wolf's eyes burning on the back of his neck. Just then there was a loud sound and Sawyer almost jumped out of his skin. The flatbed shuddered and Bhun Sa's men looked up. An elephant had dropped a big teak log from its trunk onto the pile on the flatbed. The animal smell was overwhelming. The elephant began to urinate. It splattered on the road with the force of a fire hose, and Bhun Sa's men laughed raucously as they scrambled out of the way. Sawyer forced an enigmatic Buddha smile, like Utama.

They plodded on in the burning heat. At every step he expected to hear them shout for him to stop, but it never came. Only after they had rounded the next bend and were out of sight did Sawyer and Suong both sink to the ground at the same instant, as though it had been planned. They managed a feeble smile between them. Their legs were trembling, too weak to carry them any further.

"Dragonfire" was the code intro, and Sawyer didn't have to go into a bunch of countersign bullshit because he'd have inserted the word "weather" into the first sentence or two if he were calling under duress. There was no need for security at this end since Suong was outside the noodle shop keeping watch and this was the only phone in Tha Ton, a tiny village on the banks of the Kok River. From inside the shop, Sawyer could see the hang-yao they had hired. It was tied to a wooden plank that served as a pier. The driver squatted in the stern, eating a bowl of noodles slowly, as though he wanted to make it last.

The shop owner, a hill Thai with flat features, stared goggle-eyed at the monk making the call, but there probably wasn't anyone within a hundred kilometers who could manage more than five words of English and a simple conversation code was more than adequate. The only real danger was bugging at Harris' end, but after the fiasco with Barnes, Sawyer figured he'd have that covered.

"What happened?"

Even through the god-awful Thai telephone connection, he could hear the tension in Harris' voice, waiting for the bad news. A field agent doesn't call his case officer from the red zone to wish him a happy birthday.

"It's our friend from the hills." He couldn't afford to use Bhun Sa's name.

"What about him?"

"He bought the farm."

Sawyer could hear the sudden intake of air through the earpiece. But Harris kept it under control. Maybe Harris was better than he had given him credit for, Sawyer thought. By rights he should be cursing Sawyer up one side and down the other.

"How?"

"A field decision."

"I see," Harris said quietly.

Sawyer waited, letting the implications sink in. He wanted Harris to see the whole mission dissolve before his eyes before he threw the son of a bitch a lifeline. Because he wanted them to understand, really understand, before they made the decision. Then it would be out of his hands. Then he would just be following orders, he lied to himself, knowing it was a lie.

"No, you don't see. It was necessary."

"Of course," Harris said, his tone clearly implying that of course it wasn't.

"It doesn't matter. He didn't have it."

"You mean 'the coconuts'?"

Jesus, Sawyer thought.

"Yeah, the goddamn coconuts," Sawyer said. He looked into the face of the shopkeeper, and the Thai had the kreng chai to look away. He looked outside at Suong, who never took her eyes off the Fang road. If there was any trouble, it would have followed them up that road.

"Where are they?"

Sawyer could hear the desperation in Harris' voice. He was grasping at straws.

"Our friends from the hills stashed them with another old friend of ours—from the Parrot's Beak," Sawyer said, hoping Harris would understand the oblique reference to Pranh, alias Son Lot, in the case file.

"Our *double*-jointed, rather famous friend," Harris said carefully.

He wasn't stupid, Sawyer thought. Whatever else you might think about the son of a bitch, at least he did his homework.

"That's a ten-four."

"Where?"

"Where do you think?"

"Inside Cambodia." Harris sighed. The implications were beginning to sink in. Sawyer could have taken him the next step. It was obvious what they had to do not to abort the mission. But he wanted it to come from them, dammit. He didn't want it to be his idea. Let it be karma.

He saw Suong straighten up outside. She was motionless, utterly concentrated.

"Could we," Harris began slowly, "implement Dragonfire using our Parrot's Beak friend?"

"In theory, I suppose."

"And in practice?"

"Who knows? They shoot on sight over there."

"But could you?" Harris pressed.

There it was.

"Is that what you want?"

Suong stood up. She had seen something.

Harris' voice was dry, matter of fact.

"If it can be arranged," he said.

"Jesus!" Sawyer exploded, talking openly and suddenly not

caring who heard him. "You know who these people are! You know what they'll do if they win. It's murder, for Chrissakes!"

Harris didn't say anything. They must think he had finally "gone Asian," to care about a bunch of gooks slaughtering a whole bunch of other gooks when there were important things like careers to worry about, Sawyer thought bitterly. He looked outside. He couldn't see Suong. The sky was ominous. Thunderheads were bundled over the gray river.

"It's murder if you don't. The Vietnamese have moved fifty-five thousand more troops into Cambodia. We've had more input," Harris said. He told Sawyer about Pich and the data from MI6. He wouldn't have done it if he hadn't needed to talk me into it. They must be going crazy in Washington, Sawyer thought. And then: God forgive us for the crimes we commit for our country.

"If I don't make it back . . ." Sawyer began.

Harris' response was immediate.

"Don't give me that crap! The good ones never talk that way."

"Good? That's a funny word to use on this one."

Harris didn't answer. He was smart enough not to pick it up. He was probably wondering just how spooked his agent really was at this point. Plenty, Sawyer thought. He shouldn't have brought it up. When it came to Asia, most round-eyes just couldn't understand. It was like trying to explain color to a blind man. The receiver crackled in his ear like a nest of insects. Sawyer waited. That was something Asia had taught him: how to wait.

"Anything else?" Harris asked. From his tone, Sawyer could tell he was anxious to get on the horn to Langley.

Sawyer hesitated. He had more, but his Reptile was working overtime. Where was Suong? He had to go. He eyed the bamboo curtain over the opening at the back of the shop. Whatever it was, it was coming. He should just hang up and go, except he had been damn lucky to find a phone and get through to Harris down in Bangkok somewhere.

And it wasn't clear. All he had were vague suspicions, nothing solid. If he'd presented them in a CTP case study, he'd have been laughed out of the room. But there was something there, all right. No smoking guns, but brick by brick, something was getting built.

"What is it?" Harris asked quietly. He was smart enough to know that not only do an agent's feelings and hunches matter, sometimes they are all that matters.

Sawyer told him.

"I'll check it out. Talk to that Cambodian resistance guy," Harris said wearily when Sawyer finished.

"No, I will." Sawyer didn't want to mention Mith Yon's name on an open line.

"I take it you'll be passing through the same place"—meaning Aranyaprathet, where they'd met the last time—"on your way into—"

Just then Suong came bursting into the noodle shop, carrying both packs. Her eyes were rolling like a crazed animal.

"Sawyer! Saw—" Harris' shout was like an insect chirp as Sawyer slammed down the receiver and, grabbing his pack, leaped through the bamboo curtain.

He landed in the muddy ground outside the shop and began sprinting for the riverbank and the waiting hang-yao. Suong pounded at his heels. Her breath came in sobs. She was trying to say something but couldn't get it out.

Shots rang out. Automatic fire. A lot of it. Coming from the direction of the Fang road. He could see small figures in a Land Rover bouncing over the rutted village street, racing to cut them off from the river. Bullets drilled into the mud around their feet. Suong started to dive to the ground. A natural instinct he had to fight in himself.

"No!" he shouted, yanking her arm with one hand as he fired the Ingram through the umbrella with the other. They were in open ground; hitting the dirt would be suicidal. He began to zigzag like a rabbit, firing back blindly and suddenly changing direction without pattern. After an instant's hesitation, Suong broke away and did the same. They were two separate erratically moving targets.

But the shots were getting closer as the Land Rover started to come within range. Sawyer could see it careening wildly through a flock of crazed chickens, the Shan barely hanging on as the Land Rover cut across the muddy track toward the wooden pier. One of them leaned far out and, balancing precariously, took dead aim at Sawyer's chest. Still running, Sawyer ripped away the umbrella handle and squeezed the trigger.

Nothing happened. He squeezed again and the sickening realization that the clip was empty hit the pit of his stomach. He ducked and the shots sounded very close. His breath came in great painful heaves, but he ran on even faster, Suong beginning to fall behind.

He yanked out the empty clip and reached into the pack for another. His hand closed instead on a grenade. For an instant, he debated throwing it for a diversion, anything to slow down the Land Rover, but with everything moving, it would take a miracle to even get near the Land Rover. He was almost to the riverbank, but the Land Rover was getting closer. It would be a near thing.

He blinked the sweat out of his eye. Christ! The hang-yao driver had dropped his bowl and was watching the chase wide-eyed. Sawyer could see the Shan in the Land Rover clearly now. They were grinning with betel-blackened teeth at the excitement of the hunt. They knew they had them dead to rights. Except the one next to the driver with the devil's eyebrows and bandages around his mouth and one arm.

Toonsang!

That must've been what Suong was trying to tell him. They had been recognized back at the roadblock all right. It was just that Toonsang wanted the pleasure of finishing them off himself.

His hand found another clip just as he reached the plank. He shoved it home and fired half a clip. There was a yelp of pain and the Land Rover swerved aside. Toonsang's men jumped out and started to run toward him. They were less than fifty meters away.

Suong ran out on the plank and jumped down into the hang-yao. Sawyer fired the Ingram again, and for a precious second, Toonsang's men hit the dirt. Sawyer jumped down into the bobbing prow of the hang-yao. He pointed the Ingram at the terrified driver.

"Go! Lee-oh! Now! Dee-o nee, you son of a bitch!" he ordered.

It seemed like an eternity for the driver to get the rusty little engine to turn over. Thunder sounded loudly, as though it were right overhead. Sawyer threw the Ingram to Suong. She fired blindly over the top of the bank. Sawyer's head was level with the plank. He pulled the pin on the grenade. He grabbed a big handful of mud from the bank and flung it on top of the grenade at the edge of the plank. Bullets smacked into the water around them. The second the engine caught, he released the spoon on the grenade and ducked.

"Dee-o nee!" he screamed, pushing Suong down as she fired the last of the clip.

Toonsang came up on the plank as the hang-yao started to pull into the fast-moving current. They were too close to shore for him to miss. His eyes were wide in anticipation. He winced slightly as he raised his AK-47, and just as the rain came pouring down, a deafening explosion hit the side of the boat like a battering ram. Hot metal fragments whizzed around them. One of them took away a piece of the driver's neck. He watched the blood pouring down his side, the rain washing it away as fast as it poured out. It soaked down to the bilge, turning the water in the bottom of the boat a dull pink. The driver leaned over sideways, as if he were going to lie down for a nap, and toppled out of the hang-yao.

Sawyer peeked over the gunwale. The plank was gone. There were things bobbing in the water, but the rain was like a curtain and it wasn't clear who or what they were. Someone was still firing from the bank, away from the plank, but the current was pulling them downstream very fast and the visibility was too poor for the shots to get that close. A good thing too, because the boat was going in spirals, across the current. Sawyer reached up and grabbed the long-tail tiller, fighting to bring her around and headed downstream.

Suong sat up. Her hair was plastered to her head like a black helmet. She reached into the pack and put a fresh clip into the Ingram. She looked up at him and smiled. It was a wonderful smile.

At that moment, in spite of everything, perhaps because of it, he was happier than he could ever remember being in his whole life. He smiled back. She placed the Ingram where he could reach it, and grabbing a bent tin can, began to bail.

The hang-yao raced down the river. Along this part of the Kok, the banks were high and rocky. The teak forest came to the edge of the river, the trees emblazoned with wildly colored orchids. The greens of the forest and the colors of the flowers were intensified, almost electric, by the warm rain. The beauty caught at his throat and stayed there.

The water was gray, gray as the sky and the rocks. It was

choppy and pocked with millions of tiny craters from the rain, except where the submerged rocks were. They made the water smooth as glass above them, and with the current running this fast, he kept a wary eye on them.

He watched Suong bail. The wet clothes clung to her body like a second skin. He watched the muscles in her back, delicate yet so strong. She was just keeping even with the rain. The pinkish bilge water sloshed around their ankles. There were supposed to be rapids coming up. Most were okay, but they might have to pull in and portage around the really bad ones near Keng Luang. If they could get past the white water, they ought to make Chiang Rai in about five or six hours, he thought. From there they could make connections to anywhere in Thailand. He could change the image, get back in Western clothes. They had to be careful of course, but the Thai army was far too strong in that area. None of Bhun Sa's men would normally dare venture into Chiang Rai.

So getting to Chiang Rai wasn't what worried him. Cambodia was what worried him. Ever since the Parrot's Beak it had scared him like nothing else. It scared everyone. Just thinking about it made his throat go dry, despite the water soaking him from head to foot. He tilted his head back, opened his mouth, and drank the rain. It was warm and clean. It tasted of wet earth. But no matter how much he drank, it didn't wash away the dryness.

Since the war, Cambodia had become the Land of Death.

No one ever came back from there.

PART THREE

*Dragons battle in
the wilderness.*

20

The lake in the volcano.
The superior man looks inward
and cultivates his virtue.
Remain on friendly ground
and avoid hostile territory.

THE market was already bustling when they got to Sisophon, just an hour or so after dawn. The main street was lined with stalls selling black market goods smuggled across the border from nearby Thailand. Although the sun was still low, it was starting to get hot and most of the stallkeepers had their umbrellas and cloth awnings up. Dogs prowled the dirt street for scraps. A goat settled in a patch of shade provided by an old motorcycle piled high with baskets of oranges. Suong had gone off to try and find a kong dup to take them the fifty or so kilometers to Siem Reap.

Sawyer stopped at a money changer's stall to change some Thai baht into the new Kampuchean riels. Then he went across the street to a café consisting of a few crude tables under a coconut palm. It smelled of buffalo manure and dust and the sweet fermented smell of home-brewed daom thnot, sugar palm beer. The proprietor, who seemed very young, stood behind a wooden table lined with bottles that looked like they'd been buried in the earth for a hundred years. For decoration, he had hung a cracked mirror with a peeling Byrrh advertisement on it on the palm tree.

Two young soldiers in green uniforms with RPK emblems

on their caps were sitting at a table. They looked up guiltily when they saw Sawyer and saluted. It surprised him because he was in civilian slacks and short-sleeved shirt. He hesitated for a second, then returned their salute. They both got up and slinging their AKMs over their shoulders, walked quickly away, leaving their bottles of daom thnot half finished.

Sawyer watched them go. They were very young. In fact, now that he thought about it, everyone that he had seen on this side of the border was young. Maybe it was only the young who had managed to survive the Khmer Rouge, he thought.

"What was that all about?" he asked the proprietor in French.

"You Russki?"

Sawyer shook his head.

"International Red Cross representative."

"Nye Russki?" the proprietor asked doubtfully.

Sawyer shook his head again.

"Canadian."

It was always good cover for an American. The Canadians didn't have so many people in the world angry at them and the accent was virtually indistinguishable from American, except for the double-dipthong on words like "out." But the proprietor still didn't look convinced.

"Not French, not American?"

"Canadian."

"The Party says the Americans are imperialist enemies of the people. Americans, French, very bad."

"We Canadians have had some problems with them ourselves," Sawyer remarked.

"Where is Canadian?"

"Far away near the top of the world where there is much snow and cold."

"Like Russki. You want vodka maybe?" the proprietor asked suspiciously.

"Beer. Thai, if you have it."

"Only Amarit," the proprietor said mournfully.

"Amarit is fine," Sawyer said.

The proprietor rummaged in a wooden box and brought out a dusty bottle. He opened it and poured it into a glass fogged with fingerprints. It was warm and flat as bath water. Sawyer drank it anyway as the proprietor watched him with interest, as though drinking Thai beer was an exotic skill. It tasted stale. Sawyer wondered how long it had been in the bottle.

"Why'd they run off like that?" he asked.

The proprietor sniffed contemptuously.

"They think you are Russki officier. They are not supposed to be drinking during the hours of service. They have fear you will report them."

Sawyer wondered what there was about him that made them take him for a Russian. He looked at himself in the Byrrh mirror. Maybe it was because he'd cropped his hair so short for the monk disguise. It made him look younger, thinner, but it also made his nose stick out more, like a bird's beak. He didn't like the way it made him look. His glass eye stared fixedly back at him. He looked away. Maybe they just assumed he was Russian because Soviet advisers to the Heng Samrin government were virtually the only foreigners allowed in Cambodia.

"You want woman?"

"It's too early in the morning," Sawyer smiled.

"Never too early. You make baisage in morning, you feel good all day," the proprietor said with great seriousness.

Sawyer just smiled.

"Young girl. No clap. You no like, I get you other one." The proprietor leaned confidentially across the table.

"Some other time," Sawyer said.

"No. No other time. You not want woman. I see you come with pretty woman. Maybe you need papers, cross border."

Sawyer put the glass down.

"What kind of papers?"

The proprietor poured the rest of the bottle into the glass.

"All kinds. RPK. KR. Even Thai. Also, if you need to cross border you will need guide. Many mines. Many objets piégés. Very dangerous."

That was true enough, Sawyer thought. The night crossing from Aranyaprathet through the jungle to the road near Poipet had been harrowing. The border was heavily mined and there were vine and pungi traps on all the trails. It had brought back Nam with a vengeance. He remembered the call of "Lock and load" and the terrible reluctance at every step to put your weight down on your foot because of the mines, until the green stink and heat finally wore you down and that's when it happened. This time he had done it in darkness, following one of Mith Yon's teenage guides as he moved cautiously through the underbrush, while Suong and Sawyer had tried to follow exactly in his footsteps. Sawyer brought up the rear, one hand touching Suong's pack like a blind man, sweat pouring into his eyes, and feeling graceless as an elephant.

Suong had thought that Mith Yon and his men would be crossing with them, but after Sawyer had spoken privately with Mith Yon, he had reluctantly agreed to wait ın Aranyaprathet for the time being.

"What makes you think I'm heading for the border?" Sawyer asked, taking another sip of the beer.

"Your Omega," the proprietor said, indicating Sawyer's watch. "Only high officers and contrebandiers wear Omega. You are not Russki, so you have problem on every side. From RPK, Vietnamese youn, KR. Business never easy without friends."

Damn! He'd have to get rid of the watch, Sawyer thought.

"I don't need papers or a guide. We're going to Phnom Penh," Sawyer said loudly, in case anyone else might be listening. He finished the beer.

"By train or road?"

"Train," Sawyer lied.

"Train better," the proprietor agreed. "The road near Siem Reap is very dangerous."

"Khmer Rouge?"

The proprietor looked around. He wet his lips.

"Many dangers. No person goes there. And in the villages are the Old People."

Sawyer had heard the term before. The "Old People" were the peasants favored by the Khmer Rouge. The "New People" were those tainted by Western ideas. The Khmer Rouge had slaughtered the New People by the millions.

"Do the Old People still support the Khmer Rouge?"

The proprietor began wiping the table with a rag.

"The Party denies this, so it cannot be so."

"No," Sawyer agreed, wiping his lips with the back of his hand. An oxcart rumbled by, its big wooden wheels squealing loudly. The peasants purposely never greased them so the noise would frighten away the evil spirits.

Sawyer watched the dusty street. A young woman with a

baby at her breast haggled over a brightly colored length of cloth. A small band of barefoot children noisily chased a partially deflated soccer ball in between the stalls. The sour taste of warm beer too early in the morning was already backing up in his throat.

It was worse than he had thought and not just because he stuck out like a sore thumb, Sawyer decided. If half of what the proprietor said was true, it meant that Angkor and the area around Siem Reap and even the villages were crawling with troops from every faction. It sounded like a no-man's-land, where every peasant in a rice paddy might be an informer and where they were all running scared and trigger-happy. And no matter who they ran into, even if they survived the first encounter, they would be treated as enemies.

And then there was Suong. Just thinking about her started that tingle at the base of his groin. He had never wanted a woman so much, and yet, ever since they had gotten together, he had been on the defensive, always reacting, never initiating. Somehow, whether with Toonsang or the Akha or Bhun Sa, it was always her forcing the issue.

All right. Maybe it was always for the good of the mission, and she had been proved right time and again. And whenever he ordered her to do something, she obeyed instantly. Maybe it was just masculine pride, he admitted to himself. Maybe that was it. But he was still uneasy. All he knew was that they had run out of options. There was no time left and he had somehow been maneuvered into dealing with the one person he wanted to least in the world. Pranh, who called himself Son Lot.

The memories started to come and he pushed them away. He had learned how to do that a long time ago. That was then, this is now, he told himself. He was thinking so hard that at first he didn't notice Suong standing under a sugar palm down the street, waiting for him.

He handed the proprietor one of the new riel bills.

"Remember. If you need a friend . . ." the proprietor began. He really couldn't have been more than fifteen, Sawyer thought.

"Friends are always good to have," Sawyer agreed, getting up.

The proprietor cleared away Sawyer's bottle and glass and wiped off the table.

"The dog-eater soldiers come to the market at ten every morning to check papers," he whispered, not looking up.

Sawyer put another bill on the table.

"My papers are in order, but I thank you for your concern."

"A thousand pardons, oun. I thought only for your convenience," the proprietor said, slipping the money into his pocket.

"For the convenience, then," Sawyer said.

He walked down the street to where Suong was waiting. He could feel eyes on him as he passed the stalls and shoppers. The sun heated the air into shimmering waves. Though it was still early morning, it had to be at least 110 degrees already, he thought. He could see the tiny beads of perspiration on Suong's face as he approached. He heard a rooster crow and it was like a warning. He took a deep breath. The air was hot and rank with the scent of mud and vegetation and spices. Asia, he thought. It gets us all in the end. But before it got him, he'd get the truth out of her if he had to tear it out.

Suong fell into step beside him.

"I found a kong dup. But the driver is very frightened. He wants three times the normal rate and even then, he will only take us part of the way to the Siem Reap," she said.

Sawyer nodded. He was going to get control of this mission if it killed him. And the first damn thing he was going to do was to get inside that goddamn black box of hers. His blood boiled. Love wasn't enough. He wanted her very soul.

Suong looked at him, concerned.

"So-yah. Are you okay?"

"I'm fine," he said. "Everything is fine."

21

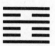

*The teeth of the lightning illuminate the majesty of the
  thunder.
The man bites through dry meat;
he encounters something rotten.*

THEY shot the young boy in the rain. From where he
was hiding, Sawyer could see the whole thing. They had
emerged from the pointed arch of the Lokeshvara, the
high stone tower surmounted by the giant faces of the
Boddhisattva. There were four faces, each staring out in one of
the four cardinal directions, all identical. In the Bayon temple
alone, there must have been more than fifty such Lokeshvara towers, all of them with the same face repeated over and over, wearing
the same unending smile for all eternity. The heavy stone slabs of
the columns and arches were carpeted by green mold, and vegetation sprouted in the crevices. A silk-cotton tree grew out of the
Boddhisattva's head, sending its white roots deep into the stone
structure. Sawyer had watched the small black-clad figures come
out of the shadow of the arch one by one, like ants emerging from
a crack in a wall. They crept out cautiously, turning their heads
from side to side, looking more like a patrol in enemy territory
than a firing squad.

They stood the boy against a carved wall. All along the wall
bare-breasted devata goddesses stood in graceful poses, their feet
pointed sideways in a style characteristic of a civilization that had

not yet perfected frontal drawing. Rain slid down the carvings in tiny rivulets. There were fallen palm fronds and puddles all around the ancient courtyard, and they had to walk some way along the wall to find a place where they wouldn't have to stand in a puddle to shoot him.

The boy wore black pajamas like the others, but his hands were tied behind him. Sawyer squinted to see him better. He was very young. He looked like he was ten years old. They were all young, but the boy looked extremely young. Sawyer didn't want to watch it, but he didn't know how not to watch it. The boy's eyes bulged from their sockets as if he couldn't believe it was happening to him.

At one point, he tried to run away. Two of them clubbed him to the ground with their rifle butts and then tied his feet together before they marched him back to the wall. He had to hop to keep up with them and some of the others laughed. They left him swaying in the rain in front of the devatas, and he started to shout something in Khmer in a high childish voice till the volley of shots blew him off his feet.

Some of the bullets knocked chips of stone off the carvings. For a lark, one of them fired again at the wall, the shots mutilating the stone breasts of one of the devatas. Then one of them shouted an order and the one who had fired just shrugged. Sawyer watched them go back the way they came. They left the body behind them, lying in the rain. After they had gone, Sawyer discovered that he had clenched his fists so tightly that his nails had left deep crescents in his palms.

Sawyer crept over the tumbled rocks back to Suong. When he had left her to reconnoiter, she had been sleeping. The shots must have awakened her, he thought, moving silently and with great care. The rocks were slippery with the rain and the slightest noise could be fatal. Khmer Rouge troops were all around the area. And the crevices between the rocks were favorite hiding places for snakes.

Why'd they do it? Sawyer wondered as he scrambled over a fallen column. What possible crime could a ten-year-old have committed that warranted death? Why shoot a fucking wall, for that matter? Why do anything?

He remembered an argument between Brother Rap and Major

Lu the time they had found the mutilated bodies of an entire family killed by the Viet Cong.

"What kind of a motherfucker would do something like this?" Rap had demanded truculently, as if he were looking for an argument.

"Oddly enough, they are men just like you and I. They laugh; they cry; they love their families," Major Lu had replied.

"No way, man! Don't you lay that gook jive on me, motherfucker! They ain't no way the fuckers who done this are like me, man," Rap had raged, his eyes rolling white in their sockets.

But Major Lu had simply looked calmly up at him.

"You have not been in Vietnam long enough," Major Lu had observed mildly. "You do not yet know what you yourself are capable of, what you yourself may do."

When Sawyer crawled back to the dark niche inside one of the myriad temple corridors, he was surprised to find Suong still asleep. He had thought she would have heard the shots. He listened intently. The air inside the niche was dank and dead, as though it had been there for centuries. He couldn't hear the rain. Maybe the sound couldn't penetrate the thick stone walls, he thought. Maybe.

He looked around at the walls in the dim gray light filtering from chinks in the outside corridor roof and wall. They were covered with intricately carved bas-reliefs of an army of dvarapala, the immortal guardians of the temples. He hoped they were keeping watch, because Christ knew he didn't want to get caught unawares by the Khmer Rouge. Still, they should be all right here, he thought. The Angkor Thom complex was a vast maze overgrown by heavy vegetation. An army could comb the place for months and not find them, as long as they were careful.

He watched Suong sleep. She slept like a child, curled on her side. But it wasn't an easy sleep. He could see her fingers and toes twitch every once in a while. She must be exhausted, he thought. He wasn't feeling so great himself. He couldn't get the execution out of his mind. And now he had to find a way to get to Pranh before they got to him, and convince him to do the deal. And if he made it, if he actually pulled it off, he would have succeeded in putting some of the best weapons in the world into the hands of those animals who just killed a ten-year-old for no goddamn reason.

You better not think about that, Sawyer told himself. That's not your job. Leave that to Washington. Sure, he answered himself. Only how do you not think about it?

He watched Suong's deep regular breathing, the rise and fall of her breasts. What are you going to do about her? the Reptile whispered. Remember what Bhun Sa said. She was like a Hanuman snake, beautiful and deadly. And now Bhun Sa was dead because of her. And you're alone in KR territory. Shut up, he told the Reptile. Just shut up. But what are you going to do?

"Find out the fucking truth once and for all," he said out loud, digging the black box out of her pack.

He set it on a rock that had once been part of a column plinth. It was a rectangular box about six inches square made of laquered black wood and locked with a simple key lock. He took out the tanto knife, slid it into the crack near the lock and hit the knife handle with his hand. The lid came open with a loud snap. He heard Suong stir behind him, but he didn't care.

Shoes. Just a pair of toddler-size shoes, for God's sake. And a stump of candle. There was nothing else in the box. His eye hadn't deceived him back at the clearing. He started to examine the box more closely when he heard her suddenly sit up. He whirled and grabbed her, the knife at her throat.

"Don't say it. Don't say anything! I'm tired of this shit! Ever since we met, everything's gone wrong and I can't afford any more mistakes," he hissed.

"Oh, So-yah," she said. "Couldn't you wait?"

"No. No more waiting. They kill kids here. What do you think they'll do to us?"

"I know what they do," she said softly.

"I want it all. Now," he said, pressing on the knife. The point made a dimple in the skin of her throat.

"Put away the knife, So-yah. There's no need for it anymore," she said, a terrible weariness in her voice.

"I was married before," Suong began. "My husband's name was Khieu Phat. He was a colonel in the Cambodian army. We had a little boy, my chouchou. I named him Jean-Pierre after my father, but that was before the Khmer Rouge came and made the having of a farang name a crime. How could I know when I named him for my cher papa that this would someday be a bad thing, So-yah? How?" She paused.

Sawyer didn't say anything. What was there to say?

"When the a khmau, the soldiers of the Khmer Rouge, came, we said his name is Little Khieu. At night we would coach him and tell him we make a game to call him Little Khieu and that he must never tell anyone his real name. But he insisted on being called Jean-Pierre, and we had to spank him very hard. I will never forget him crying, 'I sorry, Maman. No more Jean-Pierre. Little Khieu be good boy. Jean-Pierre bad.' But sometimes he would forget and not turn around when someone say 'Little Khieu,' and it would make a blue fear for me that he would say his true name.

"But all that comes much later, when it was already too late."

"Where was this?"

"In Phnom Penh. We had a villa there. It was very pretty. The garden was shaded with banana palms, and there was jasmine and bougainvillea that made the evenings sweet as in the Land of Bliss, where the thewada are said to dwell.

"We did not always live in the villa. It was the war that made us rich, and even then, only late in the war before we could afford to move. Before then we lived in a flat near the Pochentong market in a building owned by my mother.

"I believe my husband loved me, for he did not maintain a putain in a separate apartment later when he could afford one. Although I believe he also married me because my father had left me a little money and also through my mother I was related to Sirik Tamak, who later helped Lon Nol oust Prince Sihanouk. You see, although my husband came of good family, he was the eighth son and he had not the money to buy himself a high rank. But my mother told me, 'Khieu is a good man, also very shrewd, which is better sometimes than money. And he will put your interests and those of your sons, if the Lord Buddha smile, before his own.' And so we wed.

"It was good for us, as my mother foretold, though Khieu advanced so slowly in the army that it made a pain inside him. He rarely spoke of it. Then Lon Nol and Sirik came to power. And with them came the Americans. And the war.

"And with the war came Khieu's opportunity at last. Through our connection to Sirik, he was given command of a brigade. And this made us rich, for with the Americans came a river of money. It would have taken Boddhisattva to resist, for the wealth of the Americans overflowed like the Tônlé Sap in the time of the monsoon, so that even fools could not help becoming rich. And Khieu was no fool.

"Like nearly all of Lon Nol's officers, he came to command battalions that did not exist and put the pay for thousands of men into his pocket. He made his ball of string, as the French say. But even here he showed integrity, for he did not, though some brother colonels called him 'fool' for it, keep also the pay of the soldiers he did command, so they must steal food from the peasants. Nor did he sell the guns and tanks the Americans gave him to the Khmer Rouge, as many others did, so that often an empty-handed battalion was wiped out by its own guns in KR hands.

"Yet, the higher he rose, the sadder he became. The lines in his face became deep and bitter. He would sit for hours staring at nothing, ignoring the baby, and at night in bed, I could give him no comfort.

" 'We came too soon or too late to the war, for we have not the knack of it,' he would complain to me sometimes. 'Our soldiers bicycle to the front straight down the highway into ambushes. They march with flags in front as though it were the nineteenth century and many do not even know how to switch off the safety. The artillery stops for lunch and dinner precisely on the hour, even in the middle of a battle, and among the sergeants it is whispered that the enemy can set their watches by the timing of our attacks.'

" 'The Americans will save us,' I told him. That was the common belief in Phnom Penh in those days. He made a face.

" 'That is what Lon Nol and Sirik Tamak say. That is what the Americans tell them. But they are all fools if they believe the American is willing to die forever to save Asians from each other. The President Nixon promises much, but every day there are fewer American soldiers in South Vietnam. And someday here also, the Americans will get tired and go home and there will be no one left but these incompetent weaklings and the Khmer Rouge. Then who will stand between us and what is to come?'

"I told you he was no fool. The American B-52's came and dropped many bombs till the land was cratered like the face of the moon, and yet each day it was not Lon Nol's army, but the Khmer Rouge forces who advanced.

"We spoke of fleeing the country, but at that time we were not so rich yet. Also, Khieu did not like this idea.

" 'Where would we go? L'Amérique? La France? Where is there a place in the world where the stranger of a different race is not despised in the heart, no matter what governments may say? And for this we forsake our ancestors? Is this my heritage to my son, to make of him a refugee? We are Khmer. Where is a Khmer to live if not in the land of the Khmer? Who is to save Kampuchea if we do not?'

"Also my mother was ill then and I did not want to leave her. So we stayed on in Phnom Penh. So perhaps Khieu was a fool after all, because afterward, when we might have thought of getting out, it was too late.

"All that week he did not say much, except to complain bitterly over the stupidity and corruption of Lon Nol's men. A new American 'adviser' had joined his unit and had told him in the casual way of a conversation banale that most American peoples did not even know they were fighting a war in Cambodia! To Khieu this came like a thunderclap!

" 'I was right,' he told me that night in bed. 'If a government keeps such a matter secret from its own people, it means they fear what the people will say if the truth comes out. Such a government will not save us if the wind should shift—whereas the Khmer Rouge will fight on if it takes a thousand years.' He paused. 'Perhaps it is they who have the will of heaven, after all.'

"And then he said a strange thing.

" 'When I was a boy in French-Catholic school, I was like a brother to Ieng Pranh, who now calls himself Son Lot and sits at the right hand of Pol Pot.'

"I believe it was at that moment that he decided to become a spy for the Khmer Rouge.

"But of this he told me nothing for a time. Now he no longer complained of corruption and failure. He moved through the days with purpose. He believed, I think, that he had found a way to save his family. He began to teach me of the revolution and the angkar in secret. It was a new language he taught me. The ideas were most strange. Buddha was only a man long dead, who spoke in useless riddles. Forget Buddha. Forget the neak ta. Do not speak the français. Enemies were 'CIA spies' and 'imperialist lackeys.' The peasants were the 'tools of the revolution.'

" 'Does my husband believe these thoughts?' I asked him.

" 'When the time comes, we must make others believe we believe it,' he whispered, his eyes big in the night.

"Perhaps he believed a little. He wanted to, I think. Also it was easier for us as Buddhists of the Little Raft. For the object of angkar and Buddhism was in some way the same: the annihilation of one's own selfish desires. Yet there was a difference. At the core of Buddhism is the eternal; at the core of the revolution was hate. But we did not see into the core.

"When he thought me ready, I became a courier. I would leave messages, hidden inside a fish wrapped in newspaper, with a sullen peasant who had a shack on the mud flats along the Bassac River. The peasant never said a word to me, but his eyes watched me as though I had come to steal something. Although I trembled inside on these trips, no one ever questioned me. Who would suspect a senior officer's wife with a small child? Meanwhile, we buried more gold every week in a secret place under the house.

"By the spring the fighting had come close enough so that sometimes people would stop what they were doing and children would stop in the middle of the playground to listen to the distant rumble of the guns, like dry season thunder. Then they would go back to what they were doing, but with a strange hesitancy, as if what they were doing no longer mattered.

"Sometimes a rocket would hit a house. But there was little panic in the city, for it happened too quickly. It came out of the empty sky without warning, and afterward passers-by would look away because the craters and smoldering ruins left behind had not an air of war, but of misfortune. Bad karma. Such a thing may happen to anyone and it is best not to arouse the interest of the phi. At night you could see white flashes in the sky, like an electrical storm. It was strangely interesting and sometimes I would sit and watch for hours.

"Then one night, not long before dawn, Khieu came home directly from the front, an M-16 in his hand. We spoke in the darkened kitchen, for he had warned me not to turn on the lights. His face was dirty and gray with exhaustion and his uniform was stained and smelled of sweat.

"I stared at him. He was my husband, yet like a stranger almost. I was not used to seeing him like that because he had always been so fastidious about his clothes. We spoke in whispers. His eyes were shining as with fever, and I did not know if it was from excitement or fear or both peut-être. Or maybe it was something else. In Paris as a girl I read a poem by a Greek, I think. Catafy or Cavafy, or some such name. There was something about waiting for the barbarians to take a city and people being disappointed when they did not come because the barbarians were some sort of a solution. So perhaps what Khieu felt was a kind of relief that the storm he had built a dike for was no longer threatening but had broken at last.

" 'The hour has come,' he told me. 'At dawn the forces of the revolution will attack Neak Luong. From there, Phnom Penh will be under constant artillery bombardment. The city cannot hold out. You must leave.'

" 'When?'

" 'Tonight. Now.'

" 'I'll get Jean-Pie—Little Khieu.'

"He grabbed me by the hair and twisted till it hurt. His face was contorted and ugly. I had never seen it so and fear stabbed at my heart like a knife.

" 'Never say that name again,' he hissed. 'Never! French is dead. Phnom Penh is dead. Anything that ever happened before tonight is dead.'

" 'What of my mother? She has only the old woman to take care of her.'

" 'Mother is dead,' he whispered. 'You must choose between the old one and our son. I have a jeep downstairs waiting. I will drop you off on this side of the Tônlé Sap. A comrade will row you across. Go on foot, you and the little one, on Highway Four toward Kompong Speu. The a khmau will stop you within two or three kilometers. Say at once, "Cheyo yotheyas! Long live the liberation!" Say, "Greetings to Comrade Son Lot from Comrade Khieu and tell him I will bring him a present at Neak Luong." Tell them to guard well the family of Khieu or Comrade Son Lot will put them with the sambor bep, the fat cats, when we take the city.'

" 'What should I take?'

" 'Dress yourself and the Little Mouse in black peasant garb, krama, and sandals. Take a small sack of salt and rice. Nothing else. If you are seen, say nothing to anyone.'

" 'Should I take identification papers? Money?'

"He shook his head.

" 'What of the gold?'

"He gave an odd laugh. It sounded almost like a cough.

" 'Take nothing!' he hissed again. 'Leave the gold in the ground from where it came. It will be a long time, if ever, before it sees the light.'

"His words made a blue fear in my heart and I trembled. What kind of a world is it where money and gold have no value? I touched his grimy cheek as a small child touches a mirror to see if the image before him is real.

" 'Where do you go?' I whispered.

" 'Back to the front. I am bringing a gift that should secure our future, if anything will,' he said grimly, his eyes shining like a beacon. And suddenly I had an inkling of how terrible it was for him and also how dangerous.

"At that moment I had never loved anyone so much as I loved him. He was our savior, which is the most thing a man can be, and I threw my arms around him and clung desperately to him. I trembled like a leaf in the dry monsoon and I thought how wise my mother had been in advising me to marry him.

"He caressed my hair and for the first time in our marriage I felt I am utterly his.

" 'Why do you tremble. To show fear now is very danger-ous,' he said at last.

" 'Yesterday our neighbor Sath Chung was cleaning and a bat came flying out of the closet screeching and attacking. Sath Chung hit it with a broom and killed it. And when she picked it up, she saw that a baby bat had been suckling at its breast and it was also dead. That is a terrible omen.'

" 'It means nothing anymore. Superstition is illegal under the new regime,' Khieu said, an odd expression on his face. He kissed me one last time.

"Later that night, because Khieu was as good at being for the Khmer Rouge as he had been against it, he succeeded in surren-dering his entire brigade intact to Son Lot. This left Neak Luong's flank open on the river side. The Khmer Rouge took Neak Luong, and the nonstop bombardment of the city, swollen with refugees to more than two millions, began.

"When the city was taken at last, there were white flags fluttering at every window and then a big celebration with people shouting 'Vive la paix!' and 'Vive la révolution!' or so we were told, because by then Khieu and I were manning a barricade on Highway Five leading north from Phnom Penh. The poor fools! How could they understand, when even with Khieu's teaching I myself did not understand, because at first I tried to keep my Little Mouse with me. A cadre, a young man with lips thick like they were pumped full of air, snatched him from me and sent him marching into a field with the other children. Jean-Pierre started to cry and it tore at my heart.

" 'But he is my son,' I started to say.

"The cadre screamed at me in a voice as shrill as anything I have ever heard.

" 'You must cease such revisionist thought. He belongs to angkar, not to you!'

"I looked to my husband and saw a look in his eyes I will never forget.

" 'Forgive this woman, Comrade. The closeness of these filthy sambor bep'—pointing at the endless line of people on the road, stopped by the barricade—'has confused her,' Khieu said smoothly. 'But she knows her duty. Comrade Pol Pot has said that only unflagging energy will root out counter-revolutionary tendencies.'

" 'I know what Comrade Pol Pot says as well as you,' the cadre said sullenly, then looked across the barrier for someone to take out his frustration on.

"He spied a young man in a nice shirt and slacks, who looked like a bank clerk, and a pretty girl. They were holding hands and the cadre screamed for them to make room at the barrier. The young man looked confused. There were too many people for him to move even a centimeter. 'Make room, sambor bep!' the cadre screamed, and clubbed the young man with the butt of his rifle. The young man fell to his knees, his eyes stunned, and then the cadre was all over him, pounding his head with the rifle even after he lay dead on the ground.

" 'Sok!' the girl called the boy's name. She started to cry and the people pressed away to make room for the cadre.

" 'Shut up, city whore!' the cadre screeched. 'You find new boy to'—here he say something very vulgar—'in country.'

"I did not want to see this. I looked over at the field where the children were drilling, the little ones running to keep up with the bigger ones, looking for my little one. A terrible feeling caught at my heart when I saw him marching with the others, all of them like tiny, clumsy soldiers. This feeling was not to leave me, waking or sleeping, ever again."

"What was happening at the barricade?" Sawyer asked.

"The barricade was a kind of tribunal. We were judges, Khieu and I. There were others, perhaps ten of us at a table to check identity papers and around us and all along the road, many a khmau, all heavily armed, with hand grenades hanging all over them like green mangoes on a tree. Every now and then, one of the a khmau would shoot his gun, sometimes in the air, sometimes at the crowd, for no reason, and a few more bodies would fall. People would step around the bodies, not daring to look, for there were many bodies scattered all along the road. In one place, many soldiers still in the uniform of the Cambodian army had been shot with their hands tied behind them.

"It was a thing not to be imagined, my So-yah. For as far as the eye could see were people and carts jammed along Highway Five. Some had water buffalo or oxen to pull the carts through the heat and dust, for the heat was terrible and the dust was in your nostrils at every breath. Some people pulled carts like beasts. The carts were piled high with belongings, and sometimes old people or children hanging precariously to the top. Others pushed rickshaws or velo-cabs, and once I even saw a whole family pushing a Toyota crammed with furniture and even a television, for it was forbidden to drive. Others just walked, often carrying babies or sick relatives.

"There were all kinds of people. City people in smart clothes now wrinkled and caked with dust, ragged refugees, Buddhist bhikku in their orange robes, army deserters in city clothes, children still in school uniform. There was no end to it. The procession went on forever. I did not know there were so many people in the whole world and still they came.

"And yet, there was an eerie silence, despite the presence of so many. You could hear the babies crying and crying and sometimes a dog barked, but that was how it was, heat and dust and crying babies.

" 'Where do they think they are going?' I asked the cadre sitting next to me. He was short, smaller than I, and plump, with a smooth face like a young girl, and he spoke with a pursing of the lips, comme un pédé, tu comprends? But he had three ballpoint pens in his shirt pocket, which was a sign of high rank among the cadre. Khieu also had three, I one.

" 'They have been told that the Americans are coming to bomb Phnom Penh,' he said. 'After, they will be permitted to return to their homes. Look! Who would have believed it? The city has been emptied.'

"It was true. The entire city had been turned inside out like a shirt for the laundry.

" 'But will any be allowed to return?' I asked.

"He pursed his lips disapprovingly, touching his tongue to his lips like a woman checking her lipstick. His eyes showed plainly that he thought my question a stupid one.

" 'Why for? The sambor bep of the city produce no rice; they devour it. Without cities, angkar gains twofold,' he went on, as though reading something from a poster. 'No city people means there is none to exploit the peasants and steal their rice. Thus less consumption. Also, by turning the city people into opakar, field-workers, there is more production,' he said, motioning the next applicant to come forward.

"With horror, I saw that it was Monsieur Van Sophan, my old lycée teacher of the mathematics. He recognized me at once and started to say something, then seemed to think better of it. He stood straight like a soldier, as he always had at the blackboard, but his eyes had dark circles under them and his shoes that had always been so brightly polished were scuffed and covered with dust. Mathematics was my most bad subject and I failed my examination. All my friends were going on to the next grade and I pleaded not to be left behind. So he gave me the chance to take the examination again. For a week he came every night to tutor me. I could not understand the fractions, so every night he would bring me cakes and cut them up into the fractions, and when I would finally solve one, he would applaud and we would both cram the pieces of cake in our mouths, giggling like small children, and my mother would come in and say, 'Fine lessons!' but she would be smiling and then have a piece of cake too. He was a bachelor and lonely, I think, and after my lesson, he and my mother would talk over tea. But he was always most correct, no roublardise, and I think he made the second examination easy for me and I passed, though I never became very good at the mathematics.

"Now he stood there looking like he had not slept in days. The cadre next to me asked him his name and Monsieur Sophan told him.

" 'Identity card?'

"Monsieur Sophan looked at me and I managed to shake my head the most small bit to indicate no. The cadre must have noticed something, because he darted a glance at me. But I ignored him and motioned a woman with a child and a crying baby to come forward. She had her identity card ready and I pretended to busy myself with it. I overheard Monsieur Sophan tell the cadre that it had been lost in the shelling. There was a trembling in his voice.

" 'No matter. Angkar will give you a new one,' the cadre said smoothly, reaching for a blank card.

" 'What is your profession?'

"Monsieur Sophan looked again at me and I smiled, because our orders were to be firm but reassuring—but my eyes were not smiling. I put fear in them, hoping he would see and understand, but the other cadre was watching and all it did was make Monsieur Sophan hesitate.

" 'Do not be afraid,' the cadre said, now smiling reassuringly himself and looking at me with approval. 'Angkar is in desperate need of the skilled and the educated. We are fighters, yes, but have no experience as administrators. There are many opportunities for those with the right skills and the willingness to work.'

" 'I have always worked,' Monsieur Sophan said, with a touch of pride.

" 'Excellent.' The cadre beamed. 'At what please?' His pen poised over the new card. I could not look any longer and motioned the woman with the children to go through the gap in the barrier and past the a khmau in jeeps with machine guns mounted on them.

" 'I am—was—a teacher of the mathematics,' I heard Monsieur Sophan say, and my heart plummeted.

" 'Tant mieux, Monsieur le Professeur!' the cadre declared heartily, and pointed Monsieur Sophan toward a nearby field already filled with thousands of people squatting in the heat like cattle among their bags and possessions. Some had already been waiting for many hours, but when one of them had gone up to a guard to ask for water, the guard had shot him on the spot and screamed at them to be quiet. After that, there was little talking there.

"Monsieur Sophan looked back hesitantly, clutching his new identity card in his hand as if it were a winning lottery ticket.

" 'Go on! Those will be the first to be allowed to return to the city,' the cadre said, waving the next one forward. It was a hatchet-faced man who claimed to be a construction worker, but his hands were soft and the blisters on them too new. The cadre called over the guards. They shoved him into a jeep and drove him away.

"As for those sent into the fields to wait, they were marched away in small groups and no one saw them after that. Yet new ones were continually added, so that the field never emptied, but was like a rice paddy filled and drained by water ditches of the same size. Some remained there for days, living without shelter and staring mindlessly into space, like the animals in the Phnom zoo, where I used to take my Little Mouse, until they too were taken away. When I asked Khieu at night what happened to them, he told me, 'Do not ask. You do not want to know.'

"But two nights later I was eating and I saw one of the guards come to the communal pot to take rice, but his face was sick and he went away without taking any. I sat beside him. He was very young. They were all young, but this one looked too small to carry his gun. His uniform was far too big on him, and he wore his cap with the brim tilted up, the way children sometimes do. He looked like he wanted to run away.

" 'To e na bong? Where do you go, little brother?' I asked him. He would not look at me.

" 'Do you want rice?' I asked. A spasm passed across his face.

" 'I cannot eat,' he whispered. I could see sweat trickling down his face. A cadre with one pen sat down on his other side.

" 'Are you sick?' I asked.

"He shook his head.

" 'I have never killed anyone before,' he said in a guilty voice. 'It makes a sickness in my stomach, Comrade.'

" 'You will get used to it,' the cadre said.

"The boy swallowed and nodded, but he did not look convinced. Two more guards, older boys, came over. I knew one of them. His name was Mam and he wore two watches, an Omega that had stopped on one wrist and a woman's diamond-studded Piaget on the other, though he told time by the sun like everyone else. These boys were not like any Khmers I had ever known before. They liked to wave their guns about and would grab for each other's privates when they roughhoused.

" 'It would be easier with guns. I am too little for the hoes,' the boy offered hopefully.

"The cadre's face was smooth. His eyes were like black stones.

" 'Bullets are precious. Angkar will not waste arms needed against imperialist foreigners and their dog-eating Vietnamese lackeys on such as these sambor bep.'

" 'I like the hoes, though it is tiring. There is a sound when one hits the head just right that is most satisfying,' Mam volunteered. 'Like a coconut, though the inside of the head is gray, not white.'

" 'Try the iron bars,' the other guard suggested. 'With these one only needs a single blow on the back of the neck, while with the hoes, sometimes two or three are required to make them stop jiggling and sometimes these are thrown in the pit still moving.'

" 'What difference if they are still moving?' Mam shrugged.

" 'The iron bar is better,' the other insisted. 'Did you see me hit that sambor bep with it today? The one who wet his pants with fear and Chhung laughed and say he must be spanked for such naughtiness? We pulled his pants down and used bamboo sticks till his buttocks bled, and all the time the sambor bep's face is more and more red and tears are coming from his eyes, though he is not saying anything. Then Chhung says, "You learn your lesson good, sambor bep?" He shake his head, the tears still coming, and then I hit him with my iron bar and he is finished. Only the one time,' he sneered to Mam.

" 'It was a most excellent hit,' Mam agreed. 'Though Chhung was funny about the lesson,' he said, turning to us. 'You see, the sambor bep was a professor of the mathematics,' he explained.

" 'Try iron bars tomorrow. Once you get the way of it, it is as easy as breaking eggs,' the other guard advised the boy.

"The boy's face had gone white with the telling. I could see he had witnessed it all. I was glad they were looking at his face and not at mine.

" 'If only the enemy looked more like an enemy. They look like us. They might be anybody,' the boy whispered.

" 'Do not be fooled,' the cadre warned him harshly. 'These are what Comrade Pol Pot calls "Khmer bodies with imperialist minds." These were whoring with the American murderers while we were suffering in the jungle for the revolution. Now eat the rice. Tomorrow you must do better.'

"The boy smiled weakly and managed to swallow a few mouthfuls of rice as though it were dog meat, while over his head the cadre and Mam exchanged a glance.

"The boy did not come back from the fields the next evening.

"Meanwhile, the endless parade went on in the broiling sun, day after day. I was seeing my life passing by, for I saw almost everyone I had ever known. Some looked at me with sudden hope when they recognized me, for by then everyone had seen enough to be always in fear. Others could not keep the contempt out of their eyes.

"Such a one was Keo, an old army friend of my husband's. Khieu always said that if Lon Nol had had only twenty like Keo, the Khmer Rouge would have been of no greater matter than the evening mosquitoes in our garden. But when Keo saw my husband, his face fell momentarily. When he looked up, the certainty of his own death was in his eyes. He straightened like soldier, and when he spoke, it was as one who has decided to die.

" 'I would have believed this of any before you,' Keo said.

"Seeing that Keo had condemned himself with his own words, my husband leaped to denounce him.

" 'It is you who speak with the jaw of traitor!' Khieu cried, pointing an accusing finger at Keo.

"Late that night, Khieu told me, 'It was impossible to save him. Better to use his death to secure our position.' But his eyes held a shame in them and he would not look at me. But at the time he accused Keo, his eyes were blazing with revolutionary fervor.

" 'Comrades! Here is one of the worst of the sambor bep cowardly trying to escape the justice of the revolution!'

" 'If you are going to shoot me, do it. But kindly do not insult my intelligence with such merde,' Keo said, looking disgustedly at Khieu.

" 'We will not shoot you,' the plump cadre next to me said. There was a silky quality in his voice, like the touch of a spider thread, that made me shiver.

"The a khmau grabbed Keo and staked him out on the highway, where their trucks would go. The trucks drove over him for hours, till Keo was nothing but a red smear perhaps forty meters long.

"And still they came. All except my mother. Most of the sick ones never made it that far. Each time I saw one I knew, I trembled inside at the contempt I thought must be in their minds. But none reproached me, and I even managed to save some of my old neighbors and family by giving them new identity cards that said they had been lowly workers and passing them through. Only once did someone challenge me. Sath Buth, a girl I had known at school.

"She stood there, her makeup caked with dust, a large Louis Vuitton handbag slung over her shoulder as though she were on her way to tea at the Hotel Phnom. Her identity card identified her husband's profession as fonctionnaire publique, but when I tried to give her a new card saying she was a seamstress, she lashed out at me.

" 'Don't you dare write such a thing! It is you and your husband who are the true parvenus. Ever since we were in school, you have been jealous of me,' she sniffed.

"I could see the plump cadre looking curiously at me. If I did not close her mouth, her imbecile vanity would condemn me too.

" 'It is you who lie and claim to be an honest worker. Go there with the others of your kind!' I screamed, tearing her card to bits and flinging the pieces at her.

" 'You will never be anything but a petite bourgeoise,' she snapped triumphantly, as she gathered her skirt and stepped to the side of the road, her Louis Vuitton clutched in her hand like a weapon.

"It took weeks before the endless procession became a trickle, and then it stopped, comme ça. The cadres and guards broke up the camp. Nothing remained but some bodies scattered here and there along the road, slowly turning black in the sun. As a reward for his good work and because of his friendship with Son Lot, Khieu was allowed to return to Phnom Penh as the new commandant of Tuol Sleng prison. What went on there, Khieu would not say. But in this time we call the peal chur chat, Kampuchea was the worst place on earth, and it was said that Tuol Sleng was the worst place in Kampuchea. Nor could Khieu do anything to improve conditions. For Pich Sam, his second in command, was a spy, planted there by Pol Pot for no other reason than to report on Khieu himself.

"Save for a few fonctionnaires and senior cadre of the angkar, Phnom Penh was utterly empty. There was a strangeness to it that cannot be told. Abandoned cars and overturned kong dup littered the streets, so you would have to pick your way around them. Bodies had been left to rot, and there were streets you could not go because the smell was so bad. Weeds began to sprout in the cracks in the sidewalks, and sometimes you would come upon piles of now-worthless paper riels, swirled like leaves by the wind. You could walk the main boulevards for hours and hear nothing but the sound of your own footsteps. You would pass the places you knew, the park by the Phnom where I used to take my Little Mouse to play, the Tuol Tumpoung market, the shops on Monivong, the Monorom, near the station, where Khieu had sometimes taken me for drinks, many places, and there would be only silence.

"But the silence was not blank space. It had a presence like the silence of an empty theater, and you found yourself talking very loudly as a way to fill it. We were like ghosts in a graveyard, unable to touch the world. The city had become so unreal, it was we who felt unreal.

"We lived in an apartment house with other fonctionnaires. There was no electricity or running water, but we were well off compared to most. In the first days after the barricade and at Tuol Sleng, Khieu said little. But he no longer reached for me in the night.

" 'I cannot now. The things I have seen are before my eyes. They take the desire away,' he confessed.

" 'Mai pen rai,' I told him. 'You are a man of strength and it will be with us as before.'

"But it never was. Each day there was less and less between

us. His eyes grew hard, and when he spoke, it was in the slogans of angkar, as into a loudspeaker. Perhaps he slaked his desire at the prison, for there were female prisoners whom the guards would use for pleasure or torture as they pleased. I know not. Only this I do know, So-yah: if you give one human too much power over another, it will end with neither of them being human. This happened to Khieu.

"But at night sometimes I would see something in his eyes. It reminds me of the eyes of one who wears the monkey mask in the Khon dance. The face is the face of a monkey, but the eyes trapped in the mask, the eyes are human. So with Khieu. The face was the face of angkar, but his eyes in those moments were full of fear.

" 'Tell me your heart,' I begged him.

" 'Soon it will be our turn,' he said. 'At first at Tuol Sleng, there were those of the Lon Nol regime. Then any of the intelligentsia or those singled out for special punishment. But these are long gone, though they all signed confessions and, at the very sight of the electric wire, would invent even more hideous crimes to confess. But now, almost all of our prisoners are traitors from within angkar itself. The Revolution has become like the snake that swallows its own tail. Bite by bite we consume ourselves.'

"And then later, as I lay there listening to him be awake, I heard him say, 'If I do not get Pich Sam, he will get me.'

"One day he came home in great excitement.

" 'We have captured four Americans in a sailing boat off the coast. They claim they are yachtsmen, but Pol Pot wants them to confess their CIA plotting.'

" 'Are they CIA men?'

"The look on his face was the look of the new Khieu. It frightened me. His voice was the voice of angkar.

" 'Without a signed confession, we will not let them die so easily.'

"Weeks later, Khieu reported that Pol Pot himself had been pleased with the Americans' confessions, but Khieu himself seemed disappointed.

" 'What is the matter?' I asked him.

"He made a face.

" 'The Americans died badly. They screamed at the electrics like neang instead of men. I used to think them so powerful. They came among us like gods, telling us do this and that, but without their machines and their dollars, they are as crying babies. I expected more of them.'

" 'What did you expect? When they use the wire, everyone screams.'

" 'A Khmer dies better. He knows there is more to the world than his own khwan. But now I see the Americans are only poseurs.'

" 'What matters that to us?'

" 'Because poseurs could never have saved us and now nothing can save us. The tiger begins to devour his own cubs,' he declared, and would say no more.

"In the days that followed, there was the feeling that time was running out for us. One morning I passed a shoe store and on an impulse walked inside. The shop had been smashed, of course, they all were, but still sitting on the counter was the most beautiful pair of blue children's shoes. They were the perfect size for my Little Khieu. I looked around to make sure no one saw me, though that was silly, because there was no one to see, and slipped the shoes into my sack. There was no reason for it. All the children had to wear rubber sandals. But the shoes tugged at my heart, like a memory of all that had been.

"Meanwhile we were having trouble with Little Khieu. He was running away from his indoctrination classes. In my heart I was proud of him. He is only a little boy, I longed to tell them. He is too bright and full of life to sit for hours listening to your endless deadening lectures. But I pretended to be angry and scolded him. When that didn't work, Khieu slapped his face many times. Our Little Mouse no longer laughed. He grew sullen and began to silently watch us from corners like a wary animal.

"The food situation, even for cadre, was becoming very bad. The rice harvest was disastrous, and Pol Pot secretly shipped almost all the rice that was harvested to China, to trade for arms for our war against the Vietnamese. Once more you could see fresh bodies in the main boulevards, as a khmau suspected of being spies for the youn, as the Vietnamese were contemptuously called, were shot down like dogs. Our next door neighbors got so desperate, they took to making fires in deserted villas to smoke out the bats, who would tumble dizzily to the ground. Then we would all have bat soup.

"One by one, families began to disappear. No one would speak of it, but Tuol Sleng grew more and more overcrowded and each night the lines in Khieu's face grew deeper.

"He had, he told me, enjoyed the great pleasure of seeing Pich Sam being tortured by his own subordinates. But Khieu's triumph was short-lived. A week later, we were arrested and taken to the school. Our son had denounced us for sometimes speaking French at home. Also for hoarding food, which we did, of course. Everyone did.

"At the school, Khieu acted outraged. He accused the boy of running away from indoctrination class and making these pretexts to cover his own guilt. The senior cadre hesitated.

"I watched horrified, not knowing which was worse. If they were to believe my husband or my son. I felt like I was being torn apart.

" 'That is true. Little Khieu is always running away. We will fix him so he does not run away again,' the senior cadre said. He motioned for them to take Little Khieu away. They grabbed him. One of the guards was carrying an ax.

"The other children stood and watched. They had no expression. They were angkar's children. One or two even smiled.

"I looked desperately at my husband. The ghastly monkey look was in his eyes. But he said nothing. The look of angkar was painted on his face.

" 'No!' I wailed. Someone grabbed me.

" 'Maman!' came Little Khieu's cry.

" 'Little Khieu!' I cried and I felt a blow. I fell to my knees, the world spinning around me. But I saw Little Khieu break away and stand alone in the schoolyard for a moment.

" 'No! I am not Little Khieu!' he announced in a loud clear voice. 'I am called Jean-Pierre!'

"A sickly smile came to my husband's face. Then they grabbed him and my Little Jean-Pierre too and marched them away. I never saw either of them again.

"Two days later I was sent north to a work camp near Siem Reap. I managed to take the little blue shoes with me. When the Vietnamese youn attacked, I escaped from the camp. Mith Yon saved me and we made our way to the mountains called the 'Oder Mean Chey,' the Way Beyond, and into Thailand.

"Now every night I pray to my Lord Buddha for a kindness.

That the shoes my little one never got to wear on earth, he can wear in the Land of Bliss."

Sawyer tried to swallow and couldn't. He reached out his hand to touch her, but his hand fell into his lap as though the gravity of Jupiter was pulling on it. He leaned his head back against the stone wall and closed his eyes. They burned, and he saw veins of white in the blackness and kept them closed. He heard the swish of her moving and felt her pulling his head to her breast. His ear was against her chest and he listened to the beating of her heart.

"Rest now, my So-yah. You need rest. I will keep watch. Later, we will find Son Lot and finish it," she soothed. He thought it was odd that she was comforting him. It should be the other way around, he thought. And yet it was right, somehow. It was what they both needed, he thought, drifting off.

He heard shooting, automatic fire, faint and far away. He wasn't sure if he were dreaming, or if he really heard it. He opened his eyes. The niche and the temple corridor were empty. He heard nothing. It must have been a dream, he thought. His eyes were burning from lack of sleep. He couldn't have been out for more than a few minutes. He felt for the Ingram. It was gone.

Then he remembered. Suong had taken it when she went on watch. He started to relax when he heard footsteps scraping over the stone paving of the corridor. More than one person, coming fast toward the niche. Christ! he thought, grabbing the knife. It hadn't been a dream!

Suddenly there were three shadowy figures in front of the niche. He raised the knife to the throwing position. A flashlight clicked on, almost blinding him.

"Drop it, Jack!" a voice snapped in English. It was familiar somehow. He had heard it before. He could see that two of them had SKS carbines aimed right at him. The knife clattered on the stones.

"Put your hands on your head," the same voice ordered.

"Get that fucking light out of my eyes," Sawyer said.

"Of course," Pranh said, coming nearer and pointing the flashlight down at the floor. Flanking him were two young Khmer Rouge. They kept the SKS's pointed at his head. Their eyes showed nothing, like the eyes of the dead.

22

The earth contains and sustains;
the qualities of a mare.
The dew has frozen.
Winter approaches.
The sack is tied up.

THEY walked atop the stone wall of the great baray. The ancient reservoir had long since dried and been overgrown with jungle. Sawyer had to step over thick vines reaching out over the wall from the dense greenery below, like octopus arms from a B horror movie. He had to be careful not to trip and couldn't use his hands to steady himself. They were tied behind his back. The sun was brilliant and the heat was becoming unbearable.

"Water," Pranh said, indicating the overgrown baray. "That was the secret of Angkor. By building the baray with dikes and canals above the level of the surrounding plain, our Khmer ancestors could use the force of gravity to irrigate the land during the dry season. This enabled them to grow two or three rice crops a year instead of one, and with the surplus of rice came trade and the ability to support armies and a great civilization. Once this," he said, with a sweeping gesture that took in the ruins and the vast sea of vegetation, "was the capital city of a great empire. The population of the city alone was well over a million. All this when London was a mud village and Paris a squalid fortress town confined to the Île de la Cité."

"Pranh, I'm hot and tired and history bores me, so if you want to play tour guide, I'd just as soon wait in the bus," Sawyer said, running his tongue over his dry lips. He was very thirsty, but knew better than to ask for a drink. A request from a captive is a lever for the jailer; it always puts the captive at a greater disadvantage.

Pranh stopped.

"I am called Son Lot now," he said.

"You're called a lot of things now."

Pranh looked at Sawyer. His face was still handsome and unlined. He had an air of power, despite being dressed like the others in black shorts and shirt. His hair was neatly combed and parted. He hadn't aged a day in all these years, Sawyer thought. His eyes were yellow, like a lion's eyes, and he still moved with the grace of a big cat.

"You haven't changed, Jack."

"You have."

"No," Pranh shook his head. "You just never really knew me. You foreigners never knew us at all."

Sawyer didn't say anything. It was true. They stood in the blazing sun so high overhead they barely cast a shadow, staring out at the crumbling ruins snared in tendrils of advancing vegetation like long-dead flies in a vast green spider web. One guard stood near Pranh, his eyes never still. The other stood behind Sawyer, his finger on an SKS's trigger. A leather thong had been tied from Sawyer's hands to the muzzle, so that if he tried to run or jerk the weapon, it would automatically fire into his back.

"You should care," Pranh said.

"Why?"

"Because this is where it all began."

Pranh nodded to Sawyer's guard, and they began to walk again along the wall and down huge stone steps to a road unevenly paved with big sandstone slabs. Sawyer could feel the heat of the stone even through the soles of his sandals.

"Comrade Pol Pot came here when he was young. It fired his imagination. In Paris, where he went to study radio mechanics, they treated him as an inferior, comme tous les asiatiques. For Kampuchea to regain la gloire perdue, we had to return to the ways of Angkor. One leader: like the Buddharaja; one religion: the party; one goal: rice."

"But you failed."

"We have had a setback," Pranh conceded.

"You were too ruthless."

Pranh's reply sent a shiver down Sawyer's spine.

"No. We were not ruthless enough."

He looked into Pranh's yellow eyes and saw what he had never seen before and it terrified him. Pranh was utterly insane.

"What about Suong? What have you done with her?"

Pranh whirled suddenly, his hand raised as if to slap Sawyer. The front guard pushed his SKS at Sawyer's face till the muzzle touched his forehead. Sawyer tensed. He could see the desire to pull the trigger in the guard's eyes.

"That is none of your affair! You are not to mention her!" Pranh shrieked.

Sweat trickled into Sawyer's eyes, but he didn't dare blink or look away. His eyes were locked with Pranh's. Sawyer licked his lips. They were already beginning to dry and crack.

"What about Parker?" Sawyer croaked.

Pranh looked at him sharply. A faint smile hovered on his lips.

"You will see him soon enough. We will have a—how you say?—the big reunion."

"Where are we going?"

"That too you will see, very soon."

They passed through a Lokeshvara gate, the shade under the arch a brief relief from the blazing heat. There were soldiers in black shorts and shirts lounging around the gate, until they saw Pranh and snapped rigidly to attention. Even their eyes were rigid. The open area beyond the gate was swarming with Khmer Rouge. They had set up hootches and cooking fires among the fallen lingams and broken statuary. It was a combat lager. They went through the camp and through another Lokeshvara gate.

Beyond the gate was another ruined temple. It had a long, high, central staircase surmounted by the remains of what must have been a tower. The temple was very old; the design of it more primitive, less ornate, than the Bayon. It was surrounded by Khmer Rouge dug into positions facing the temple.

Pranh motioned to one of the guards, who handed him a canteen. He sat down on a giant stone head of Buddha staring straight up at the sky. It might have tumbled from the clouds, for there was no headless statue nearby that it could have come from. Pranh took a long swallow. He looked at Sawyer for a moment, then pulled out a knife and, motioning Sawyer to turn around, cut his hands free. He handed Sawyer the canteen.

"You see how it is. We have to do business, you and I. That is why we treat you so well," Pranh said seriously, not conscious of any irony.

Sawyer drank the tepid water greedily, never taking his eyes from Pranh. This was a man who shot ten-year-old kids for nothing, he reminded himself.

"Where is the morphine?"

"In there," Pranh said, tilting his head to indicate the temple.

"We trade arms for the morphine. You coordinate an attack on the Vietnamese with the other Cambodian resistance forces. The Viets have moved their troops to the Thai border. We both know you couldn't hold this area if they hadn't. You can hit them from behind. They'll be caught between you and the Thais. It's a classic hammer and anvil operation, but the timing is everything. It must occur as soon as you have the bulk of the arms, before the end of the monsoon. That's the deal," Sawyer said, rubbing the ache out of his wrists where they had been tied.

"The monsoon is better for us. It makes it more difficult for them to use their tanks."

"We'll give you all the antitank weapons you need."

"Good. That is our understanding too. And one thing more—"

"What?" Sawyer asked nervously. The fact that he had been expecting something didn't make it any easier.

"We naturally expect the U.S. government to officially recognize us as the only legitimate government of Kampuchea."

This was the part Sawyer really hated. Fuck Harris, he thought. Fuck all of them.

"Those are my instructions," he said.

Pranh smiled. It was the same eerie smile that the Boddhisattva wore. You couldn't get away from it in this place.

"Then there is no problem. Your morphine is there," gesturing at the temple with the canteen. "Take it."

Sawyer could hear the water slosh in the canteen. He shook his head. He wasn't ready yet.

"Why did you take Parker?"

Pranh's smile broadened to show perfect teeth. He really was very handsome, Sawyer thought.

"Ah, Jack. You want more than morphine for your guns. You want wisdom too," Pranh said.

Sawyer stuck his hands in his pockets and just stood there, head cocked to one side. At that moment, he looked very American.

"Why? That's all I want to know."

Pranh's eyebrows went up.

"So little. Only that. That is only a little wisdom," Pranh mocked.

"You didn't do it for fun. You had to come into Bangkok to do it. That was a big risk for you. Why was it so important?" Sawyer insisted.

"So we could deal directly with the Americans, of course," Pranh said, as though it were perfectly obvious. "We had to find out first how serious you were. When Bhun Sa said the U.S. government now wished to buy morphine, naturally we were skeptical. Also, to eliminate Bhun Sa."

"Why?"

"Bhun Sa was hors de propos, you understand. He was no longer needed, so why should he have a share? We do the fighting. We have the morphine. You should deal directly with us. By taking Parker, we bring you to us. By questioning him, we find out your true intentions."

"He didn't know our true intentions, dammit. They don't tell field agents everything," Sawyer said, trying to suppress the anger in his voice.

"Unfortunately, it took a great deal of questioning before we were able to ascertain that," Pranh said, a bland expression on his face.

You bastard! Sawyer thought. You miserable bastard!

"When I leave, he goes with me," Sawyer said, keeping his voice under tight control.

"As you like, Jack. C'est du pareil au même. Only neither of you is going anywhere until the arms have been delivered. We have the radio from your pack. The one disguised as an electric razor. Once you have explained all your codes to us, we will allow you to call your people to arrange the delivery."

Sawyer leaned against the Buddha head and looked at Pranh. He had to squint in the strong sunlight.

"I guess I did you a favor by taking Bhun Sa out, didn't I?" he observed.

"Most people in this world are necessary only to themselves. We were not sorry to hear of his death, but it has left us with one little problem."

"Ah," Sawyer said, like an Asian. Pranh's brows beetled and Sawyer smiled inside. He had gained a little face on the bastard.

"Inside the temple are a squad of Bhun Sa's men. The morphine is wired to explosives. If you cannot convince them to surrender, they will . . . pouf!" Pranh said, throwing his hands into the air.

"Me!"

"Who else?" Pranh shrugged. "For some reason they will not believe us."

"I can't imagine why not," Sawyer said.

Pranh climbed down off the Buddha head. His men tightened in expectation of orders.

"Do not fail to persuade them, Jack. For if there is no morphine, then there are no arms, no attack on the dog-eaters, and no reason to keep you and Parker alive," he said.

Sawyer just looked at him.

"Tou!" Pranh ordered. Go ahead.

Sawyer turned and started to walk toward the temple. Pranh called him and he turned back.

"Eh bien, Jack. Why don't you just say it?"

"Say what?"

"Whatever it is that is going on behind your forehead."

Sawyer stood there, sweating. He wondered if he should tell the truth. Then it struck him that it didn't matter. Pranh was an utter pragmatist. He could say anything he liked.

"I'm sorry we're on the same side. I'd prefer you as an enemy," Sawyer said.

"Because of the Parrot's Beak."

"Because of a lot of things."

"Poor Jack," Pranh said, lighting a cigarette. "You always were a sentimentalist."

★ ★ ★

The air inside the temple was hot and stale. It was air with the oxygen taken out of it. They had taken him to a storeroom somewhere in the center of a maze of narrow passageways. Stacked against the walls were thousands of wooden boxes covered with red Thai and Chinese lettering. They had made no attempt to hide the plastique and wires placed around the boxes. Sawyer almost gagged on the smell of chemicals and unwashed bodies confined for too long in a narrow space. There were candles burning on boxes all around the room, giving it an almost churchlike feel. The room was bright with their light and hot as a sauna. Stalactites of wax dripped from the base of the candles down to the stone floor. It made Sawyer nervous, so many candles so close to the plastique, even though in theory he knew it should be safe enough.

The leader was a fat bare-chested Shan, his tattoos stretched over a bulging belly and pointed womanish breasts. He motioned Sawyer to sit, gesturing with a rusty .45 automatic that looked like it hadn't been cleaned since the Second World War.

"The khrap will take cha," the fat Shan said in Isan Thai, pouring Sawyer a tiny cup of jasmine tea. It was not a question.

"A thousand of thanks, Khob khun khrap," Sawyer replied, taking a sip. It was very sweet and good, despite the heat.

The fat Shan took a sip and smacked his lips loudly to show appreciation. He put his cup down.

"So now they send a farang to try to persuade us," he said, speaking not to Sawyer but to the others in the room. They did not respond, only stared blankly into space.

"You mean you do not burn with the desire to put yourselves into the hands of the Khmer Rouge?" Sawyer asked facetiously.

The room exploded with laughter. The fat Shan slapped his thigh loudly as a pistol shot.

"By the nats and phi, this one is a jokester!" the fat Shan wheezed when he could catch his breath. He put the .45 down on a wooden case as if to signal that he was ready to talk, nevertheless being careful to place it out of Sawyer's reach.

"No, Jokester-khrap. Though we have had no orders from Bhun Sa, yet we have no great trust of the Khmer Rouge," the fat Shan said.

"What have they told you?"

"That Bhun Sa is dead, but we do not believe."

"Bhun Sa is dead," Sawyer said.

The fat Shan looked away. No one met his glance. When he looked back at Sawyer, his eyes showed that he believed Sawyer but that he didn't want to believe it.

"How do you know this? Have you seen the body?"

"Yes," Sawyer said, wondering what it was that made them believe him. Then he realized what it was. "You haven't been able to raise Bhun Sa's camp with your radio, have you?" he asked.

The fat Shan didn't answer. All at once a cunning light came into his eyes. Somehow he had guessed!

"Did you kill him?"

The room was deathly still. Sawyer wondered if they would kill him if he told the truth. He remembered Utama. It was karma, whatever happened.

"Yes," he said.

A breath of air entered the room as though the temple itself had sighed. The fat Shan tapped his thick fingers on the butt of the .45 as though trying to decide whether or not to use it on Sawyer.

"We are dead men," the fat Shan said.

No one spoke. There was no answer to that.

"We have orders . . ." one of them said, coming forward. He was tall for a Shan.

"Of what value loyalty to a dead man!" a thin-faced Shan broke out.

"How do we know this? On the word of a farang?" the tall Shan objected.

"And this of the radio? Does this one presume that is no proof? Or that we hear nothing from Bhun Sa? That too is nothing?" the thin-faced one demanded.

"Radios can malfunction. This is known. This one's mother's sister's son bought a radio at the market in Kengtung, and within a ten of days it made only noises like the crackling of burning wood."

"That was a different kind of radio, imbecile!"

"A radio is a radio," the tall Shan insisted.

"And a fool is a fool."

The tall Shan started to say something, then thought better of it. He paused at the doorway, drawing himself up.

"My brother is a good man, but he knows nothing of the modern mechanics," he declared impressively and walked out.

The fat Shan looked at Sawyer as he sipped his tea. His hand was as big as a ham. The cup disappeared in it.

"Son Lot says he will let us keep our arms and all the morphine we can carry. He says he will guarantee our safe passage out of Angkor. That is what he says," the fat Shan said.

Sawyer sipped his tea. Behind him he could hear the thin-faced Shan snort in disgust.

"Can we believe him?" the fat Shan asked.

Christ, what do you do with that? Sawyer thought. How the hell should he know? And why should they believe him? It was their lives balanced against the mission. The goddamn mission. And who made him judge and jury? And maybe it didn't even matter what he said. They would make their own judgments. There was no answer. There was only karma.

"I don't know," Sawyer said.

The fat Shan nodded as though Sawyer had told him exactly what he needed to know.

"I think he will kill us. The Khmer Rouge kill everyone, even their own. I think they will kill us too. That is what I think," the fat Shan said.

"What shall I say to Son Lot?"

The fat Shan looked up.

"Tell him we stay. If we go outside, we die. If we stay here, we die. So we might as well stay here."

"Inside, outside. What difference? We are dead all the same," the thin-faced Shan snapped.

"Mai pen rai. There is no difference," the fat Shan shrugged. "I prefer to die fighting. It is a man's way to die, that is all. But there is no difference."

The sunlight was very strong and it made him blink as he came out of the temple. The walk down the ancient stairway seemed to take a long time. Pranh was waiting for him, crouched behind a battered army deuce-and-a-half truck that he kept as a shield between him and the temple, though no shots had been fired on either side. Pranh looked expectantly at Sawyer as he came around the truck.

"They're not coming out," Sawyer said.

Pranh's handsome face twisted with sudden violent hate.

"It is you who failed!" he screamed, struggling to pull his

pistol out of the holster on his hip. Something exploded inside Sawyer too.

"No, it's you they don't trust!" he shouted back, jabbing his index finger toward Pranh as though it were a gun.

"Now you die!" Pranh shouted, freeing the pistol. He pointed it straight at Sawyer's head and cocked the hammer. A voice cracked out of the truck cab like a shot.

"Wait!"

Pranh froze like a machine when the plug has been pulled.

"I am sure So-yah-oun can be persuaded to try again," Suong said, leaning her head out of the truck cab, her long hair falling to one side like a black cape.

Sawyer looked, unbelieving, from Suong to Pranh, then back to Suong.

All at once, everything was clear.

23

The sun sets behind the earth.
He enters the belly of the dark
  regions.
The dark times of Prince Chi.
He ascends above the roof of
  heaven;
he will descend below the crust
  of the earth.

HE couldn't stop shaking. His mind bounced off the inside of his skull like a Ping-Pong ball, finding no place to rest. The thing he had feared most in the world had finally happened. He was blind. They had sewn the lid of his good eye shut.

She was smiling as she ordered them to do it. She, not Pranh! She was the stronger. She who guessed his most secret fear. What could be hidden from her? They had all felt it and obeyed her instantly. The sight of her bronzed face glowing in the sunlight, its beauty still tugging at him, had been the last thing he had seen before they wrestled him to the ground and blotted out the sky.

That and the image of her next to Pranh, the two of them like mirror images of each other. A blind man could see they were brother and sister.

No, he told himself bitterly. A blind man sees nothing. How fitting that he should see nothing, he thought. Because he had seen nothing all along, even before. Utama had been right. If you can't see, who do your actions help, your enemy or yourself?

A groan escaped him. He put his fist in his mouth and bit the knuckle to stop it. Oh, Christ! He had loved her! He felt polluted, as though she had infected him with a venereal disease. But it was worse than that. There would be war now. No way to stop it. And those two would feed off the carnage like hyenas. No wonder Pranh had outsmarted them all. No, Pranh, the great Son Lot, was a front. *She* had outsmarted them all! First she eliminated Parker. Then she got him to eliminate all the other players one by one, Barnes, Vasnasong and the Brits, and finally Bhun Sa and Toonsang, till there was no one left to pick up the pieces but her and Pranh. And Pol Pot.

She must have been in constant touch. The shoes! Those baby shoes—and the nightly prayers, always alone! He should have torn that black box apart long ago, but every time he got close, she had suckered him. How it must have galled her to have to feed him that story about the shoes when she was so goddamn close to home. Christ, what an actress! They were all actors. That's what agents were. But she was in another league. She could win an Oscar with her hands tied behind her back. That story about the kid and the Khmer Rouge—she couldn't have made all that up. No one could. A chill passed through him.

She hadn't invented that stuff about the killing fields and her son. It had all happened. It was like an optical illusion puzzle where all you see is a rabbit and then you somehow look at it another way and see that it's a nude. She had told the truth, the way the best liars do.

Except for one thing. She wasn't an unwilling participant in angkar's reign of terror.

She was one of the perpetrators.

And if he completed his mission, she would do it again.

And if he didn't, there would be another Vietnam war.

The old monk had foreseen it. What was it he had said? That he would have to choose. And that worlds would hang upon his choice. And that he would be afraid. That was true too, because—oh, Christ—he was scared. He couldn't stop shaking. And they had sewn his eye shut just for openers! He lay on the hard floor of the pit, or whatever place they had thrown him in. It smelled of wet earth and something rotten. Something had died in here. His hands were tied behind him. He tried to get himself under control, but he couldn't. A whimper escaped him. He couldn't help it.

"Jack? Is that you?"

A voice groped in the dark for him like a blind man's hand. At first it startled him. And then he realized that he had heard it before, a long time ago.

"Mike? Mike?"

"Yeah, it's me. Can't you tell?" Parker croaked. His voice was weak and Sawyer could hear the pain in it.

"They blinded me. I can't see."

"Is it really you, Jack? Or am I talking to myself again?" Parker's voice faded away.

"It's me, Mike. Harris brought me in after they snatched you."

Sawyer waited. Parker didn't say anything. He wondered if Parker had passed out. He sounded bad. Talking when you are blind is like tapping out a telegraph message, he suddenly realized. Until someone responds, you're never sure if the message has been received.

"Mike, you still there?"

"So she got you too, huh?" Parker croaked.

She. Not Pranh. Not they. *She.* What was it Bhun Sa had said? The Hanuman snake is beautiful and its bite is fatal.

"Take it easy," Sawyer said.

He heard a curious sound. It sounded like Parker was choking or gagging.

"Mike? Mike?"

The sound got louder, wilder, and then he recognized it. Parker was laughing, but it was like no laughter Sawyer had ever heard before. It sounded insane. It tapered off with little hiccups of sound like an arpeggio.

"Of all the fucking agents in the whole fucking Company they had to send you, you one-eyed son of a bitch," Parker said, the laughter starting up again. Only now it degenerated into something else, a kind of deep-throated gasping, and all at once Sawyer understood. Parker was crying.

"You got to help me, Jack. You got to," Parker blubbered, unable to keep an awful whine out of his voice.

"All right, Mike. All right," Sawyer said, the lie sticking in his throat like a bone. He couldn't even help himself. Talk about the blind leading the blind! He almost laughed aloud himself, before he caught it. Jesus, what was happening to him? Was insanity contagious? He didn't know. He didn't know anything, except that unless he held tightly to something, he was as lost as Parker. Then it hit him. That was what she was counting on. That was why she had put them together. She had to break Sawyer without physically incapacitating him in order to use him to get the morphine. Clever little Suong!

He wouldn't let her do it. That was what he could hold on to.

"Don't bullshit me! I know what you're thinking. You're thinking Parker can't hack it. Parker fucked up!" Parker lashed out, his voice breaking.

He was going off the deep end, Sawyer thought. He had to do something, but he didn't know what. And then he understood what the monk had been trying to tell him. When you're up against the wall, the only thing that works is the truth.

"Maybe you can't hack it," he said quietly into Parker's tirade.

"Oh, Christ! I can't take it anymore! It's my feet, Jack. Look what they did to me," Parker's voice degenerating back into that awful whine.

"I can't see, goddammit. What did they do?"

"My feet are killing me," Parker whined.

"I'll help you, Mike. I swear," Sawyer said. He knew what he had to do. He just had to get Parker to cooperate.

"Help me, Jack," Parker pleaded, a crafty note creeping into his voice. "You know how."

"No," Sawyer muttered in a strangled voice. They had sworn never to speak of it again.

"You promised," Parker's voice sulked like a child.

"I didn't promise that, goddammit. Don't you understand? The mission is over. Everything is over. We lost. There's nothing left except for us to try and save our own asses. We're getting out, man. We're gonna get out of here. Okay?"

At first he thought Parker was coughing. Then he realized he was laughing again, laughing hysterically.

"You blind son of a bitch! You don't understand a goddamn thing! Christ! You think Langley will ever understand this? Do you?" Parker said.

Parker was right about that, Sawyer thought, summoning up Langley in his mind. The big square buildings, white as sugar cubes in the sun, white inside and out, sterile as a hospital, with their endless cubicles and computer terminals and everyone with their little badges clipped to white shirt pockets. Langley was an enclosed, rigorously ordered world, and the view out of the windows was of other white buildings, identical amid the greenways and the parking lots. Langley could no more understand the reality of a pit in the Cambodian jungle than they could admit to a belief in witches and dragons.

"Fuck Langley," Sawyer said.

"I'm not leaving here. I can't," Parker whispered.

Parker was pushing all the buttons, Sawyer thought. He was bringing it all back now. The Parrot's Beak and the Twelfth Evac and Zama. Out of habit, he slammed the door shut in his mind, the way he had learned how to do it. Tell him anything. Just get it going, Sawyer thought.

"All right, Mike. But I'll need your help."

"You know how," Parker insisted sullenly.

You always were a gutless bastard! Sawyer thought.

"I'll need my hands free," he said.

"Try to get over here and turn around. I'll use my teeth," Parker said. He had obviously been thinking about it.

"Where are we? Describe it," Sawyer said, struggling to his feet. He used Parker's voice to find Parker.

"We're in a pit about ten feet deep. Dirt floor and walls all around. They got bamboo bars over the top like the tiger cages back in Nam."

"Are we open to the sky?"

"Yes."

"What time is it?"

"Almost dark. If it wasn't so cloudy, you could see the first stars."

"What about guards?"

"There's always one. They look in during the day, but it's pretty dark down here at night, so they don't bother much. Be glad you don't have the midday guard."

"Why?"

"He likes to piss down on my head," Parker admitted, starting to cry, and then it changed to a laugh and then they were both laughing.

"Hey, remember Brother Rap always said Asia was a fucking toilet," Sawyer managed to wheeze. They laughed harder, and for an instant they were on the same side again.

"Yeah, Brother Rap," Parker said finally, and they both stopped laughing.

"When do they change the guards?"

"They already did. We're okay for now. There's only one up there and half the time I think he's sneaking in a nap."

"Won't they hear us talking?"

"Sure, but it doesn't matter. They don't know English, and anyway they're used to me screaming and talking to— Aaaah!" Parker screamed.

Sawyer had bumped into something.

"Don't hit me anymore. Please, I'll tell you anything. Please, please," Parker whimpered.

"Hang on, man," Sawyer urged.

"I can't."

"You're better than you think. Now just shut the fuck up and use your teeth for something useful," Sawyer said brutally.

He waited, listening to Parker's whimpers. Listening to him try to fight it. The smell was very bad by Parker. It was almost overpowering.

"It'll take a while. It's pretty tight," Parker managed to get out.

"That's okay. We've got all night."

Sawyer felt a tug and then a series of tiny jerks as Parker began to gnaw at the rope binding his wrists. It felt like a fish mouthing a baited hook. He could hear wet chewing sounds behind him. He tried to stand utterly still and get himself under control. "Yeah, Brother Rap," Parker had said. There was nothing to do except stand there and try not to think, only shutting the door wasn't working this time. This time there was no way not to remember. No way at all.

They were coming out of the jungle—thousands of them, crawling into the rice paddy like black worms. Sawyer had been expecting it, but still, it was spooky to see it in the ghostly light of a flare. Sawyer glanced around the lager, sensing the ARVNs stirring along the night defensive perimeter. They wouldn't hold this time, he thought. Ever since the firefight earlier, he had known it was only a matter of time.

Pranh had led them all the way into the jungle, insisting that the real VC headquarters, COSVN, wasn't "the City," uncovered by American troops in the Fish Hook, but was in the Parrot's Beak. Since he was supposed to be S-2 for Cambodian intelligence and since the enemy kept melting into the jungle ahead of them, Major Lu had gone along. They kept marching deeper and deeper into the Parrot's Beak, seeking a COSVN becoming increasingly mythical, like Spanish conquistadors seeking El Dorado. Then— was it only yesterday morning that it all happened?—Brother Rap had laid it on him.

"Pranh's di-di'd, man."

"What are you talking about?"

"I mean the motherfucker di-di'd. He's gone, man."

A queer feeling came over Sawyer.

"Maybe he bought it. Maybe . . ."

"Forget it, bro'. The LP saw him go out through the NDP wire. They asked him what he was up to, and he gave them some slope jive about 'LRRPing' it. That fucker never even touched a gun before. It's a fucking trap, man," Rap said, squatting next to Sawyer. He bent his head forward as if he were praying, and his love beads swung free.

"We've got to get out of here," Sawyer said.

"Hey, tell me about it," Rap agreed.

"What about Major Lu?"

"He called it in and HQ told him to stay put. They say they ain't no Charlie worth worrying about in the Parrot's Beak, any-ways. Lu's called in a slick. He's gonna debate it with 'em face to face." Rap grinned, spitting in little squirts through the spaces between his teeth.

They both looked out at the terrain. The lager was on a rise that overlooked the rice paddies down to a stream bordered on the far side by the jungle. The sky glowed with the milky light that comes before the dawn, and the trees beyond the stream had begun the change from shadow to green. A veil of mist lay over the fields. Soon the sun would come to burn off the mist and reveal the emerald green forest that stretched to the rim of the world, and it would be light enough to light a cigarette. Sawyer shook his head.

"That won't work," Sawyer said. "MACV's already called the Parrot's Beak a big goddamn victory without hardly a shot being fired. How in hell are they going to allow us to retreat?"

"Yeah," Rap agreed, shaking his head dubiously, as though getting screwed was what life was all about.

They waited all morning for orders, the air shimmering in the rising heat. It wasn't until they finally heard the slick coming in that the VC opened up with rockets and mortars. Brother Rap started shouting at the ARVNs, trying to organize return fire. Parker was with the RTO, a small ARVN named Phuoc, whom everyone called Fuck, trying to call in air support. Someone screamed "Incoming," the cry that got to you like nothing else, and Sawyer hit the dirt. The ground seemed to slam him in the face as an 82 mortar exploded nearby, and in the sudden glare he saw a head soaring in a high arc through the air like a punted football. Parker! Sawyer thought and started running.

Parker's arm was bleeding. The upper part of Phuoc's body was gone, and the radio was a twisted piece of smoking metal, though as a shield it had probably saved Parker's life.

"It's okay, Mike. It's a beauty, man. No real damage and free drinks in the bars when you get back to the World," Sawyer said. For a moment, Parker clutched at Sawyer's arm with his good hand.

"Tell me the truth, Jack. I can take it."

"I wish it was me," Sawyer said, hauling Parker to his feet, half dragging him to the slick, as the chopper dropped to the ground, blue green tracers from an RPD machine gun disappearing into the dust storm churned up by the rotor.

They saw Major Lu scramble on board. The slick started to pull up. RPD machine gun bullets were hitting the ground all around them, and Sawyer thought he was going to go crazy. He heaved Parker into the hatch.

"This ain't no dust-off! We got no—" a crewman screamed, his eyes wild with fear.

"Take him or I'll shoot you myself," Sawyer screamed back, aiming his M-16 at the crewman as the slick pulled heavily into the sky with an incredible clatter.

Sawyer was already on the ground. He watched the chopper go, resisting a sudden panicky impulse to call it back and jump aboard, as though it was his last chance. He watched it fly above the stream of tracers into the sun, the door gunner still working his M-60 on the tree line. A rocket exploded nearby, bringing him back to his senses. He headed for the NDP in a jerky but rapid four-legged lizard crawl.

After about an hour the firefight began to die down, but it wasn't until weeks later that he learned that although the slick had made it safely back to Division, Major Lu had disappeared without ever having made a report. They settled down for the night, still waiting for orders that never came, knowing that the VC would hit them seriously after dark and that without the radio they couldn't even call for help. They were utterly cut off.

They could feel it coming. Everyone had his weapon switched to automatic. The grenadiers loaded their M-79s with canisters. Sawyer went along the line, warning them to be sure the claymores hadn't been turned around before using them. The ARVNs just looked at him with despairing eyes, but the safeties clicked off their weapons as he passed.

"Now I know how Custer felt—and I always used to root for the Indians," Rap tried to joke, but his grin was unreal, like the smile painted on a doll's face.

They hunkered down to wait. Knowing it was coming made the night pass very slowly. Still, when it actually came, it was a surprise. An RPG rocket exploded somewhere off to the left. RPDs and AK-47s opened up. A flare went off and the paddy was swarming like an ant hill in the harsh white light. A few M-16s started to return ragged fire, though Sawyer shouted at them to wait. A nervous ARVN set off a claymore prematurely and blew himself into bits of wet confetti. VC sappers had turned it around in the night. Suddenly, Brother Rap was beside him.

"They ain't gonna hold, man," he whispered, his hand jiggling the sling on his M-16, too nervous to keep still. Sawyer shouted, "Fire!" and the intensity of firing got very heavy. It was like a wind with all long bursts and no breaks in the firing.

Sawyer had never been so afraid. The VC were coming through the wire. He screamed at the ARVN for them to use grenades, not the claymores, but it was too late. The claymores went off tearing holes in the NDP where two-man ARVN teams had been. The claymores had all been turned around! That was what set it off. The ARVNs broke. Screaming in panic, they began to run. The LZ was a mass of confusion, dark figures running everywhere.

Sawyer and Rap were running too. Shadows rose up from the ground near the far paddy dike. Sawyer didn't know if they were ARVN or VC. He heard shouts over the roaring in his ears. He fired, cutting down three of them. The shouts became screams. Rap was firing too and then they were running again. Somehow they made it over the dike and into the jungle and the endless night.

They gathered up the remnants of the ARVN Ranger battalion in the morning. They barely made up two squads. Lieutenant Qui was the only ARVN officer left, and they agreed the only chance they had was to try and walk out through the bush, avoiding the trails as much as possible. The afternoon sun was a blinding glare that filled the sky with a blue white haze. Rap took the point and Qui the slack as they made their way through a band of razor-edged elephant grass. Sawyer brought up the rear, spending half his time walking backward, because that was where the VC would most likely hit. The exhausted ARVNs crashed noisily through the elephant grass like a band of apes. The noise made Sawyer cringe, but shouting at them would only make more noise—and worse, if they didn't obey him because they were that far gone, it would mean that nobody would follow orders anymore.

Drops of sweat stung Sawyer's eyes and he blinked to clear them. Up ahead he could see Rap emerge from the elephant grass uphill into a clearing. He was carrying his M-16 across the back of his neck, both arms wearily draped over the carbine, his head lolling with fatigue and the heat. He looked like a Black Christ with his arms like that, and Sawyer was stabbed with a sudden pang of fear. He better take the point himself, he thought, getting ready to call a halt. The line of ARVNs shuffled wearily as pilgrims on an endless journey as they made their way across the clearing back toward the jungle.

"Oh God, I'm on it!"

Sawyer heard the sudden anguished cry and was torn with the realization that it was Rap's voice even before he hit the ground.

"Freeze, dammit! Freeze!" Sawyer screamed as the ARVNs hit the dirt, the sudden silence deafening as an artillery salvo.

"Jack! Where's the EOD! Where is the motherfucker!" Rap screamed in a high thin voice, and Sawyer knew Rap must have panicked, because the Explosive Ordnance Disposal, an easygoing sergeant named Minh, had been wounded by a booby trap two weeks earlier and hadn't been replaced yet. Sawyer raised his head, but couldn't make his legs support him. He was terrified. He finally managed to shout.

"Rap, is it pressure or a Bouncing Betty?"

Because if it was a Bouncing Betty there was no way to get off it without setting it off and all you could do was pray that the explosive charge got bounced up high enough to finish the job.

"Jesus! I can't tell! Jack, help me. Please help me!" Rap wailed.

And then, without knowing how—or why, because it wouldn't do any good—Sawyer was running toward Rap. And all he could think of was that he couldn't let Rap die thinking that no one even tried to help.

"Coming," Sawyer shouted, his voice quavering as he pounded toward the clearing. He could see Rap balanced like the ball on a seal's nose, the sweat pouring down his brown face in rivulets. Only a few more yards now, Sawyer thought.

"Oh shit, it's a Betty," he heard Rap whisper.

And then it went off.

You know how, Parker had said. And Sawyer was back in the hospital ward in Japan. He remembered the hospital smell of disinfectant that somehow couldn't disguise the stink of the factories and the polluted river nearby. But Sawyer couldn't see them. His eyes were bandaged. Only one was gone, but they had bandaged both. Something about sympathetic nerves or something.

Zama Army Hospital. And the night on the ward when Parker, his arm still in a sling, found him and took him to see Brother Rap.

Parker led him down endless corridors. It seemed to take a long time. Sawyer wasn't sure if it seemed so far because he was blindfolded or because the hospital was so spread out. "All army hospitals are spread out, in case of attack," the ward master, a lifer, had told him. "Why? I thought we were in Japan. Or are the Japs after us too?" Sawyer had said.

If he had known how bad it was, he would have let Rap die out there. That's what he always told himself, although even now he didn't know if he would have gone through with it. The medic had given Rap some morphine and albumin, and maybe Rap would have just died there in the clearing if the dust-off hadn't spotted them and the desperate ARVNs hadn't waved it in. At the time, Sawyer remembered thinking that it was good luck.

Brother Rap was awake, Parker said. That was the worst part. He was looking at them, although Parker wasn't sure he saw them. Rap's eyes were squinted to slits with the pain. His face was untouched. A white sheet covered him up to the waist. His upper body appeared to have escaped injury, Parker whispered in his ear.

"How is he?" Sawyer asked.

"He's bad," Parker said.

"How bad?"

"He's bad, Jack. Real bad."

"Take the bandage off my right eye. I can still see with that one."

"You're not supposed to. The doctor said—"

"Fuck the doctor!"

"It's the regs, man. If they catch us—"

"Take the fucking thing off!"

"All right, Jesus! Just keep it down, will you? You'll get the night nurse in here," Parker hissed.

"Jack. Is that you, man?" Rap called out.

"I'm coming," Sawyer said, pulling the bandage off his eyes. Although it was night and the only light came from a single dim night-light, he was almost blinded by it. He squinted his good eye desperately trying to see.

They were in a small surgery recovery room. Rap was hooked up to so many tubes he looked like something from a science fiction movie. His upper body seemed unmarked, but the white cotton sheet covering the lower part of his body was flat below the hips. Sawyer winced at that. Although the left leg was gone below the knee back in the clearing, the right leg, though covered with blood, had still been attached and he had hoped they could save it.

He glanced down at the chart at the foot of the bed. It was as thick as a small-town phone book. It was all unreadable medical gobbledygook, though words like *nephrectomy, ureterostomy,* and *traumatic amputation* leaped out at him. Then he noticed that Rap's arms were strapped to the bed. They looked very black against the white of the sheets and the bandages.

He could see Rap's lips moving. He motioned Parker over to the door to watch out for the night nurse. As he approached, he could feel the heat from Rap's body. It was like standing next to a hot stove. Rap's eyes were glassy with fever and pain. Sawyer felt sick to his stomach. He bent over till their faces were almost close enough to kiss.

"I tried to kill myself. Pulled out the tubes. The fuckers stopped me," Rap croaked.

"Can't they give you something for the pain?"

Rap grimaced.

"They give me so much fucking morphine and Demerol now, in Bedford Sty the junkies be sucking my blood like Dracula if they could."

"And the pain's still that bad?"

"Oh man," Rap whimpered.

"Oh shit, man. Oh shit," Sawyer murmured, not knowing what to say. He watched the blood drip one drop at a time from a hanging bottle into a catheter inserted into the back of Rap's hand.

Rap closed his eyes tight and Sawyer watched him struggle with the pain, Rap's hands clenched into fists. He was supposed to say something, but he didn't know what.

"It'll get better, man. They got all kinds of shit now. Artificial limbs you wouldn't believe, all kinds of stuff," Sawyer said.

"They ain't got anything."

"Yeah, they do. And you'll be getting plenty of money from the army. Maybe get a new Mustang with one of those special hand controls they got. Drive the chicks crazy, man. So you won't be a hotshot at the discos. So what? Men dancers are all kind of faggoty, anyway," Sawyer babbled, conscious of how inane he sounded.

"I ain't a man no more," Rap said.

Sawyer stopped. He felt like throwing up. He could hear someone groaning down the ward, but just by the sound he couldn't make out if it was pain or a nightmare. Vietnam was portable, he realized for the first time. You could take it with you wherever you went—whether you wanted to or not.

"I didn't know," he said.

Rap managed to raise his head an inch from the pillow. His neck tendons were like ropes; the liquid in his eyes looked like it was about to boil.

"You gotta help me, man. I can't go back. Not like this," Rap whispered.

Sawyer shook his head.

"Come on, Rap. Come on, man."

"Look at me, motherfucker! Look at me!" Rap raged, his voice barely a whisper. "I got no insides anymore. I be hooked to machines forever, man. No way to take care of myself. And what for? I ain't anything anymore, 'cept somethin' in pain that even morphine can't help. Can you picture me like this in a fucking Brooklyn tenement, man? Don't do this to me, Jack. For Chrissake, man."

Sawyer looked helplessly at him.

"I . . ." he began, and then he saw it come into Rap's eyes. Don't say it, he thought. For God's sake, don't say it.

"You owe me, motherfucker. You the one who talked me into going back," Rap said, not looking at Sawyer.

That's when it hit him: the picture of Brother Rap sitting in a wheelchair by a window in his mother's apartment in Brooklyn. Only he wasn't Brother Rap anymore. He was back to being Harold Johnson. He was hooked up to some kidney machine and staring out at the gray street, at the battered cars and the dudes jiving to a ghetto blaster and the girls in their short skirts, cheap and tight and hot with color. And Harold just staring, his eyes glazed with boredom and drugs. He was only nineteen. The doctors were good. They were very good. They might be able to keep him alive like that for a long time, Sawyer thought.

He put his hand on Rap's shoulder, then he went over to Parker, near the door. Parker's face was terrified.

"You're not going to listen to that, Jack. He's crazy. The fever's put him out of his mind."

"He's right."

Parker started to back away, shaking his head. Sawyer grabbed his hospital robe near the throat.

"It's wrong, man. Don't do it. And besides," Parker said, his eyes darting around suspiciously, "if they caught us, it's murder. They'd crucify us."

"Look at him. Just look at him, for Chrissakes!" Sawyer hissed, hauling Parker to the side of the bed. "Can you see him back in the World? Can you? What are they keeping him alive for? To suffer? Because they're scared shitless to kill him. They weren't scared to send him out to get his legs and balls and cock blown off! They weren't scared to do that!"

Parker squirmed in Sawyer's grasp. He tried to look away.

Sawyer grabbed a handful of hair and forced Parker to look into his good eye.

"I can't, Jack," Parker whispered.

"What if we were still in Nam? Still in Indian Country. What then?"

"We're not in Nam. This is Japan, man. It's all nice and clean here. They don't understand anything here."

"Uh-uh." Sawyer shook his head. "The hospital may be in Japan, but we're still in Nam. You don't believe me, just look inside the head of every poor fucking grunt in this whole fucking place. We're in Nam right now."

Rap stirred behind them.

"Sweet Christ, hurry! I need another shot," Rap said.

Parker blinked. He looked straight into Sawyer's eye and Sawyer could see him remembering. Maybe he was seeing Sawyer picking him up, heaving him into the slick. Sawyer and Rap staying behind, diminishing to the size of ants as the slick rose into the burning sky.

"If they catch us, we've had it," Parker managed, his mouth dry.

"Nobody'll catch us if you watch by the door and keep your fucking mouth shut," Sawyer said, shoving Parker toward the door.

Parker crouched by the door. They heard footsteps approach, and he signaled with his good hand. Sawyer knelt by the bed, listening. He recognized the ward master's tread by the slight shuffle of one of the feet. Blind people learn how to listen, he thought. If someone comes in, he wouldn't have to do it, he thought, not sure if he wanted to be stopped or not.

The footsteps receded down the corridor. Parker looked across the dim room and nodded. His face was white as a sheet. Sawyer knelt over Brother Rap. Rap's breathing sounded loud and harsh. Sawyer could hear the congestion rattling in his lungs.

"You gonna do it, honky?" Rap whispered, his eyes wet with pain.

Sawyer nodded.

Rap took a deep rasping breath, then another.

"Okay," he said, closing his eyes. "Okay."

"I'll take the watch. You go to sleep," Sawyer said, leaning over Rap, a pillow in his hand.

★ ★ ★

He felt the rope start to loosen even before Parker said any-thing. Parker spat out a mouthful of something, and then it was only a minute or two before it was loose enough for Sawyer to pull free.

He felt Parker slump against him and turned to hold him up. Then he felt the ropes holding Parker up and the bad feeling he'd had when Bhun Sa had dragged the KMT officer behind the Land Rover came back.

"You okay?" he whispered.

"No. I'm not okay," Parker whimpered.

Sawyer felt his way down Parker's body. Parker had been tied in a sitting position that held him upright even if he slept. They had seated him on a block of stone that couldn't be knocked over. As soon as Sawyer touched Parker's thighs, Parker screamed.

"Shut up!" Sawyer hissed.

He quickly slid his fingers down Parker's legs till he encoun-tered something metal. Parker gasped with a sudden intake of air as he tried to stifle his scream. Sawyer touched the metal. It was round and smooth and felt like brass, with a round opening and a wide lip. The shape was like an old-fashioned spittoon, maybe that's what it was, and then he felt the crudely sawed piece of wood. Parker screamed again, and Sawyer had to wait till it be-came a groan before he could talk. The bastards! he kept repeating to himself. The bastards!

"How'd they break your feet, Mike?"

"What?" Parker's voice was small and far away.

"Your feet. What'd they use?"

"An iron bar. On a rock. They smashed them again and again. I begged them. They were like bloody rags and they kept hitting them"—Parker's voice broke.

"Take it easy. Just take it easy," Sawyer said, feeling the twinges in his own feet. He could see it now in his mind. They had broken Parker's feet and jammed them into a brass pot, forcing him to sit there as his feet swelled against the sides, the pressure creating an incredible agony. But that still wasn't enough for Pranh. He'd wedged in a two-by-four for them to pound anytime they wanted to raise the pain a few degrees.

There was still something he had to find out. He would have to hurt Parker to do it. He prodded Parker's legs with his fingers.

Parker groaned. The flesh was hot and soft and held the impression. He could smell the rot. It was like sticking his fingers into thick oatmeal mush. The mushiness extended all the way to above Parker's knees. At every touch, Parker screamed.

Sawyer slapped him hard across the face.

"Shut up, for God's sake! Just shut up!"

"You fuck! You lousy fuck!" Parker said suddenly, quite distinctly.

"I'm sorry. I had to see what it was," Sawyer said. He gave a short sharp laugh, harsh as a cough. He could see nothing. He moved around Parker and began plucking at the knots that tied Parker's hands behind him.

"Jack? Jack?" Parker whispered into the darkness. His voice was very weak.

"Yeah, Mike."

"I can't move. I'm a liability. You can't get me out."

"I know."

Parker hesitated.

"If you leave me here, you know what they'll do to me." Sawyer could hear the fear in his voice.

"I know that too."

"I can't take it anymore, Jack. Please. You promised. Like Brother Rap, okay? Okay?"

"Don't beg, Mike. Just don't beg," Sawyer muttered.

If only he could see! And then he felt it, working on Parker's hands. Parker's fingernails hadn't been cut for a month, maybe more. They were long and sharp as claws. He could use one of them to cut the stitches that sewed his eyelid shut. It would probably infect, but that didn't matter. He needed to see now, not later.

He knew what he was going to do. It was a war all right, but it had nothing to do with America or Cambodia or Vietnam anymore. It was down to just him and Pranh.

And the bitch.

24

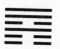

A tree on the mountain.
The wild geese reach the desert.
The husband leaves on an expedition
but will not return.

THE wind came up and blew out the moon as though it were a candle. Sawyer could hear it moving in the trees with a continuous murmuring sound like a fast stream over rocks. When the first drops of rain came, he had looked up in terror and fury, thinking that the night guard was pissing on him; but it was just the rain. It wasn't a heavy monsoon rain, but a light rain that just goes on and on until you think it will never end.

It was a good omen, he thought. Not even the Khmer Rouge liked sitting out all night in the rain, and it would help give him cover. He wasn't sorry about losing the moonlight either. He needed the dark, and at least he wouldn't have to look at Parker anymore. He didn't have to. The image of Parker, made black and white by a single ray of moonlight, retied to keep him erect, his head slumped down on his chest, his swollen legs primly tied together with the feet inside the brass pot, was seared in his brain as though put there by a branding iron.

You know how to do it.

Don't beg, Mike. Just don't beg.

And then the agony of Parker plucking out the stitches, and

he could see. His eye stung like crazy, but he could see. Parker was worse than he had imagined. If Sawyer had passed him on the street he might not have recognized him. Parker looked like an old man. There were black streaks running up his legs and his calves were swollen to the size of thighs.

"Spend my share, Jack. Have the biggest goddamn blowout the bastards ever saw," Parker croaked.

"What share?"

Parker went dead still.

"What share, Mike? Barnes and the morphine?"

Parker sighed. It might have been relief.

"Yeah. And Vasnasong and Harris. You didn't really think they were gonna just destroy all that lovely valuable skag, did you?"

"Harris too?"

Parker bit his lip. The pain was getting to him. He wouldn't be able to hold it much longer, Sawyer thought.

"Ask Barnes."

"Barnes is dead."

Parker turned away. In profile in the moonlight his face looked like the head on a silver coin. He looked almost the way Sawyer remembered him. They'd been friends once, and he changed his mind about pushing Parker on Harris. It didn't matter anymore. He had quit the team. They just didn't know it.

"Asia," Parker mumbled. "Fucking Asia."

Sawyer got up and started to retie Parker's hands. He didn't want to hear any more.

"She gets us all, Jack. She lifts her skirt and you think it's gonna be a quickie, but once you're in, it's like a tar baby and you can't ever get unstuck. You're the last one, Jack," Parker gasped over his shoulder, the pain harsh in his voice. "You better di–di or it'll get you too, man."

"Go to sleep, Mike," Sawyer said, the echo of Zama loud in his ears.

"Hurry, man," Parker whispered.

Sawyer put his left forearm at the back of Parker's neck and locked it on his right bicep, the right arm coiled around the throat.

"Jack! Jack!" Parker whispered.

"Yeah, Mike."

He could hear Parker swallow in the dark.

"Don't tell them how it really was with me, Jack."

Sawyer felt as though he had just stepped into something left by a dog on a pavement. Why'd he have to do that? he thought. He remembered Parker in his Class A's on hospital leave in Japan, wearing every ribbon he had, even the little bullshit ones that even the REMFs got, like the Vietnam Service Ribbon and the National Defense Ribbon. You pathetic bastard, Sawyer thought, feeling sorry for Parker and hating him for making him feel that way.

"They wouldn't understand," Parker mumbled, only making it worse.

It was a lousy way to go out, Sawyer thought, and felt ashamed for both of them. He wished he didn't have to be such a self-righteous son of a bitch. All he wants is his version of extreme unction, he told himself. You're in the wrong business. You're too good for this world. You should have been Saint Francis in a cave. And then he realized the joke of it all.

"Don't worry, Mike. You're a fucking hero. They'll put your name on a corridor in Langley. There'll be a whole new generation of CTP shitheads who'll bust their balls to try and live up to the standards you set."

"Thanks, Jack." Parker sighed, completely missing the irony.

Let it go, Sawyer thought. For Chrissakes, let him keep something. Maybe their believing he was a hero will make him one. Maybe that's what heroes are.

"Don't mention it," Sawyer said, tightening his grip relentlessly like a vice.

The rain was heavier now. He stood on Parker's still warm lap and, slipping the wooden pin, cautiously raised the bamboo lattice. He could see the black silhouettes of the palms and a crumbling temple wall against the dark clouds. It was still dark, but the sky had begun to acquire the faint glow that signals the pre-dawn.

The sentry was dozing against a sugar palm just a few feet away. He kept jerking his head up to try and stay awake. Sawyer waited, debating whether to let the sentry fall asleep or get him closer. A look at the sky decided him. Once it became light enough to see, he wouldn't stand a chance. He needed to bring the sentry closer, but how? He had ignored their voices all night. Then he thought of a sound that would wake any Asian in a second.

Sawyer hissed softly like a spitting cobra. The sentry jerked upright like a marionette. He got up cautiously, his eyes glued to the ground as he walked step by step to the edge of the pit.

Sawyer moved. In a single motion he threw open the bamboo lattice and yanked the rifle muzzle down, toppling the sentry head-first into the pit. Sawyer jumped down after him, right hand raised shoulder high for a killing blow, but there was no need. The sentry lay in the kind of uncomfortable sprawl unique to death, his head twisted sideways at an impossible angle against the dirt wall.

Sawyer checked the rifle in the dark. It was an SKS, and going over it brought back Nha Trang and the times they had to do it blindfolded, Sergeant Willis screaming in his ear, "Come on, turkey. It's not a tit. Don't diddle with it!" Now it was starting to come back. Simonov SKS. Chinese-made 7.62mm semiautomatic carbine. He checked the clip and magazine. Safety off. All right.

He stood back up on Parker's lap and slid the SKS butt-first up onto the ground. He eased the bamboo lattice open, grabbed a handful of wet grass, and swung himself up and over the edge.

He stopped, listening, the SKS ready. He was in a small clearing between a carved temple wall and dense jungle. He could see the outlines of things, but it was still too dark to distinguish details. The rain cut the visibility further, plastering his clothes to him. The rain felt good on his eye. It still stung, but he could live with it. After all, it wasn't anything compared to what Parker had gone through.

He heard something. It wasn't coming from the temple area where the KR defense perimeter had been set up, but from the jungle. A sound of branches scraping and the Reptile was wide awake. Christ, what was happening?

He waited till the sound faded, then scuttled on all fours into the dense foliage. He found the track only a few meters in. It had all come back now. He didn't have to think about how to do it anymore. He found a muddy heel mark. It was deep, water already pooling in it. So whoever they were, they were heavily laden. There were no scraps, cigarette butts, or garbage of any kind. So they were probably far from their base and were porting everything they needed. They were good, leaving nothing behind, and that also meant they would be setting up MA's and ambushes. Further on, he found more footprints. A lot of them. They were fresh, superimposed upon each other. It was a patrol in force.

He fingered a broken twig speculatively. It was chest high,

so they were holding their weapons at port arms, ready for combat. Further down the trail he found a few ripped thorny tendrils, about midsection high. It suggested that they were carrying AKMs or AK-47s because the AKs are long and the banana clip has a tendency to catch on vines. Just underneath he found a faint circular imprint in the mud where someone had set down what was probably the base of an RPG-7, to rest for a moment. All Soviet arms, Sawyer thought. He'd done this before. He knew who they were.

North Vietnamese regulars. Charley.

He moved carefully now, one step at a time. About twenty meters down the trail he found the first one. A vine stretched across the trail, about twenty centimeters above the ground. He followed it into the undergrowth to a claymore aimed at anyone coming up the trail from the direction of the temple complex.

He'd found his war. The one the Company wanted him to start. Only the Khmer Rouge wasn't going to attack the Vietnamese. It was the other way around. The Vietnamese had surrounded the Cambodians. They were in a trap.

Based on the size of the lager and the perimeter Pranh had showed him, Sawyer figured Pranh had to have at least three thousand men with him. The NVA had to have a full division, maybe more, to pull it off. There was no way Sawyer was going to be able to walk out through a whole damn army. He was trapped right along with the KR.

Parker had been right, he thought. Asia always gets you in the end. There was only one thing left for him to do. Karma. He wondered if he'd ever really had a choice. He got ready. There was damn little time left. The NVA couldn't stay undetected by Pranh's patrols forever. They would probably attack at dawn. He would have to hurry.

He made his way back toward the temple complex. It would be faster going there, with little likelihood of mines and booby traps within the defense perimeter.

He came to the edge of the tree line and froze, scarcely breathing. He had heard something. He waited, watching the temple wall and the eternally smiling face on a Lokeshvara gate. Then he heard it again. Conversation. It was somewhere off to the left. A Khmer Rouge two-man listening post.

He moved away from them, careful not to make a sound. "Combat is a misnomer," Sergeant Willis used to say. "The idea is not to confront the enemy, but to evade him. The whole thing is to get around the bastards. You don't want to fight 'em, just kill 'em. Preferably by surprise from behind. If you have to fight the fuckers, that means they have a chance to get you too, and nobody ever won a war by getting killed."

The rain was easing by the time he made it to the outside temple wall. There wasn't much time left. He crouched low beside a long line of spear-carrying warriors carved on the wall. I've done this before, he thought. Everything twice, like the fool who had to climb Mount Fuji. Cambodia twice. Charlie in the jungle twice. Having to terminate my own twice. "All this meditating and incarnations, how long do you have to do it?" he had asked Utama. "Until you get it right," the monk had replied. He heard something and whirled, but it was just a hawk rising over the trees.

He crept closer. There was sure to be a sentry covering the Lokeshvara gate, but he couldn't spot him. Take your time, he cautioned himself. The guys who bought it in Nam were the ones who lost patience, who didn't make sure. He tried again, quartering the area and using the side of his eye, because peripheral vision is better in bad light than straight on. He worked his way up, starting at ground level and still couldn't spot him.

"Come on, turkey," Sergeant Willis used to snap on the "boom-boom" course. "You'd find it fast enough if it had a triangle of hair above it."

There was just the tip of a muzzle sticking out of the foliage on top of the wall to one side of the arch. The first time he had mistaken it for a twig. Avoid confrontation, he reminded himself. He looked along the length of the temple wall away from the hidden sentry till he found what he was looking for. He slipped through the foliage alongside the wall till he came to the silk-cotton tree whose roots had already begun to push the stones apart and breach the wall. He slung the SKS over his shoulder and was about to climb the tree when he stopped and looked around. Something had changed in the landscape.

The rain had stopped.

He climbed the tree, then using the uneven handholds and footholds, climbed down on the other side of the wall. The Khmer Rouge camp was just beginning to stir. He would have to go quickly now.

Langley doctrine. Worst-case situation. When you are where

you don't belong and don't have adequate cover, act as if you own the joint. He unslung the SKS and began to walk openly across the bivouac area, past the hootches and the smoldering cooking fires, the massive pyramid of the temple ruin now clearly visible against the reddening sky.

A soldier in black pajamas came out of a hootch, yawning and stretching. He stopped when he saw Sawyer. He stood there, watching Sawyer cross right in front of him. Sawyer acted as if the soldier didn't exist. He felt the soldier's eyes burning holes in his back, but he kept moving till he saw what had to be Pranh's command post tent, still shielded from the entrance to the temple ruin by the deuce-and-a-half truck.

By now, there were others beginning to watch him. He kept going. A Khmer Rouge officer and a squad of men approached diagonally from his left. The officer shouted something at him. Sawyer ignored him and kept his eyes straight ahead. It was all happening very fast. He saw the uneven paving stones of the ancient courtyard, the weeds sprouting in the cracks, the fallen stone carvings and the giant head of Buddha still staring up at the empty sky, and at the edge of his field of vision, the KR officer and the squad cutting him off from Pranh's tent. He wasn't going to make it.

The officer shouted again. The carbines were pointing at him now, and like a man in a dream, he turned slowly toward them, the SKS coming into firing position as though it were a part of his hand, and Pranh's still-closed tent just out of reach, as though it were on the other side of a border.

The whistling sound was the same sound that could still snap him bolt upright, sweating in the night, even after all these years. He flung himself to the ground even before he consciously identified it as the sound of an incoming artillery shell.

The KR never got the chance to fire. The blast, hot and smelling of cordite, rolled over Sawyer, and then the rockets and mortars began to explode all around. Big ones, he thought. One-twenty-two's and 82-mortars, and then everything went crazy. Small arms fire and black pajamas running everywhere, and as Sawyer started to get up, he saw the KR officer struggling to point a heavy RPD at him. Sawyer dropped him with a single shot from the SKS.

He ran to the tent, expecting to get hit by a fragment at any second. He threw the flap open and had just an instant to take it all in. Suong was sitting up on a cot, her breasts exposed, her eyes dominating her face like the eyes of a starving child. Pranh, brow furrowed, was jumping naked from the cot for his pistol. And Sawyer thinking—her own brother! She even did it with her own goddamn brother! He was so stunned he actually waited till Pranh started to turn. Pranh's eyes, black as a snake's, were fixed on his as Sawyer fired. The first shot hit Pranh in the shoulder, spinning him around. The second opened a hole in his back, the blood immediately starting to trickle out of it. Sawyer's third shot smashed into the back of Pranh's head even before he toppled to the ground.

"So-yah, no!" Suong screamed as he pointed the SKS at her. "I did it for you, So-yah. I had to. It was the only way to save you. The only way!" she cried.

Sawyer pointed the muzzle at the valley between her heaving breasts. He could hear the explosions and fighting outside, but none of that mattered. His war was here.

"You lied!" he said through clenched teeth. "You always lied. You lied about Parker. You delivered him to Pranh on a silver platter. You lied about how you found me at the warehouse. That was you and Vasnasong. You got to him because you didn't want the buyer killed off. And me, the big jerk, I was so glad to be alive, I didn't look too closely at how you found out about the warehouse. Then you killed the Akha to force the issue with Toonsang, because you knew he was a thief and you couldn't afford to let anyone see what was in your pack, could you?"

She shook her head wildly, but Sawyer wasn't listening.

"Then you got us captured by Bhun Sa's men because you didn't want me cutting any separate deals with Bhun Sa, and when that didn't work, you went to see him that night. Then you lied about Bhun Sa. He wasn't trying to kill you. You were trying to kill him! So you could have it all. Cobras don't share, do they? And you lied about Bhun Sa's map. You had it in your pack all the time, didn't you. Then the shoes. There was a radio hidden in them, wasn't there?"

Her head hung down, sleek black hair shrouding her face.

"Wasn't there?" he shouted.

"No, I told you! They were my little Khieu's," she cried, tears starting down her cheeks.

"Little Khieu's, my ass. That's how you were able to stay in touch with Pranh all the time. That's what made him so fucking smart, and that's what you couldn't let Toonsang find. Or me."

"No, So-yah, you—"

"No wonder everything went wrong on this mission. With Little Miss Fixit sabotaging it every step of the way," he shouted, spittle flying.

Outside, the crump of rockets began to die down. The rattle of small arms fire grew closer. The Vietnamese were moving in. The tent canvas trembled like a sail in a rising wind.

"By then I began to suspect, so I connected with Mith Yon in Aranyaprathet. But I wasn't sure, so I took you along figuring that, worst-case, you might be a link to Pranh once we got here. But you fooled me again with that fairy tale about your kid and husband."

"I was married! I did have a baby!"

The shooting was getting closer. He didn't have much time left.

"And who betrayed them to angkar? Who? Who?"

She looked at him in utter horror. Her mouth dropped open. There was no mistaking the truth written on her face. Her naked breasts rose and fell rapidly, as if she couldn't get enough air.

"I had to," she whispered. "Pol Pot himself ordered me. He made me marry Khieu in the first place."

"You're a mole. Just a lousy mole. You've been one all along," he accused. "Only I was getting too close, so you signaled Pranh to come and get me. I thought I'd heard shots. Pranh! Your own brother! Look at you! You even fuck your own brother!" he screamed.

"Pranh and I are"—she faltered—"were one. From birth we were one. The world is very old, my So-yah, and these are things you know nothing of," she said, her perfect chin jutting out like the prow of a boat.

"Tell me one thing. Just one," Sawyer said, coming closer, the muzzle of the SKS almost grazing her nipple, strangely erect.

"The killing fields. Why the killing fields?"

Her face twisted, almost in contempt.

"Ah, So-yah. Don't you kill for your country? I too. What difference?"

"There's a difference."

"No difference, So-yah. My Lai. Kampuchea. No differ-ence."

"There's a difference," he insisted.

"So what now? You kill me now? Pourquoi? Who will fight the Vietnamese for you?"

"Fuck the Vietnamese!"

"Look at me, So-yah! Look at me!" she cried, throwing off the sheet. She lay naked on the cot, tracing the exquisite curves of her body with her long expressive fingers. She trailed her fin-gernails across her breasts and down the rib cage to the swell of her belly and down to the silky black hair where her middle finger disappeared.

"All this is yours, So-yah. Yours! Why destroy?" she breathed, parting her legs to give him a better view.

Sawyer's finger tightened on the trigger.

The shock wave and debris from the explosion hit the tent like a hurricane.

25

The man stands alone amid conflict.
Something approaches;
a pig covered with mud;
a carriage full of ghosts.
He draws his bow then relaxes it;
it is not an assailant,
but a close relative.

YOU will want this back," the Vietnamese officer repeated, raising his voice. He handed the electric razor with the transmitter concealed inside to Sawyer.

"Yes," Sawyer said, looking at it as though he had never seen it before. His ears still rang from the explosion.

They walked around one of the numerous square pillars that had once supported a corridor roof. The temple roofs had been made of wood and had decayed into dust centuries ago, but the stone pillars remained. The Vietnamese paused to study a bare-breasted relief of Lakshmi, the royal consort of Vishnu, carved on one of them.

"Exquisite," the Vietnamese murmured, as though talking about a living woman.

"Too fat." Sawyer shrugged.

"Like me," the Vietnamese said, looking down and ruefully patting his bulging stomach.

"That's what happens to conquerors. They get fat, Major."

"General, s'il vous plaît," General Lu reproved Sawyer. "I'm a general now."

They began climbing the steps to the vast stone terrace, carved with images of elephants on the walls and railings. Even the banister supports were carved to look like elephant trunks. The sun was high and very hot, throwing sharp-edged shadows across the crumpled courtyard below.

"You've come up in the world."

"We all have."

"No. Not all of us," Sawyer replied, pausing on one of the steps.

General Lu nodded. They continued up the stairway to an elevated platform that allowed them to overlook most of the temple complex. In the distance smoke was rising from the burning thatch roofs of a village to the north, almost hidden in the green carpet of jungle.

"Your men?" Sawyer asked, indicating the smoke.

General Lu shook his head.

"Some of the escaping Khmer Rouge. They probably grabbed everything they could carry and then set the fires as a warning to the other villages, comme d'habitude."

"Some got away then?"

"Ah yes. No operation ever goes perfectly."

A rattle of machine-gun fire echoed from a jungle clearing. Sawyer felt the old tightening in the pit of his stomach. Christ, how he hated Asia. It was difficult to swallow and he had to force down some saliva in order to be able to speak.

"You're taking no Khmer Rouge prisoners?"

General Lu looked at him as though he didn't understand the question.

"Whatever for?"

Sawyer looked away. For a time he stared at a wall carved with ancient battle scenes, myriad limbs wielding spears and swords, without seeing it. Then he realized what it was. The old monk had been right, he thought.

"Plus ça change . . ." he murmured.

"What?"

"Nothing," Sawyer said. *How long do you have to do it? Until you get it right.* "So you'd call it a success?"

General Lu's brown eyes twinkled and his smile had nothing of the mystery of the Buddha in it.

"Ah yes. Two thousand and five hundred enemy dead. Son

Lot, the Khmer Rouge's ablest commander, killed. A good ten percent of Pol Pot's effective force destroyed in a single morning. A success is certainly what I shall be reporting to the Politburo."

"You couldn't have done it without me. I handed it to you on a silver platter, didn't I?" Sawyer said bitterly.

"You were, one might say, invaluable," General Lu agreed.

"Who tumbled me? The café owner in Sisophon?"

General Lu nodded.

"After you were spotted in Sisophon, we stopped every train heading south to Battambang and set up roadblocks on Highway Five. But I had a hunch about Highway Six, because we'd had reports of increased Khmer Rouge activity near Siem Reap. So we left it open, and when you didn't show up elsewhere, we moved in on Angkor during the night."

"I should have waited. Taken the café owner out."

General Lu shook his head.

"It would have made nothing, Jack. You were seen by others. Also, you would have had to surface for the rendezvous with Son Lot. You cannot keep an entire army and four thousand kilos of morphine hidden forever. It was the reports that Son Lot had been spotted in the area that first alerted us, in any case. Also we made the time very short. If you force the timing, the enemy must expose himself."

"So you won again. Just like the Parrot's Beak. Is that why they made you a general?"

"C'est la guerre, Jack. In the end, we were all of us involved in the espionage: you, I, Parker, Pranh. Ho Chi Minh once said that a spy in the right place at the right time is worth ten times ten divisions. That is why we all do what we do."

"But in the Parrot's Beak, you and Pranh actually worked together to sucker us in, didn't you?" Sawyer said, squinting into the sun to look at General Lu. He rubbed his eyelid where it had been sewn. They had put antibiotic ointment on it, but it still hurt.

General Lu looked out at the stony temple spires poking out of the endless foliage like Aegean islands in a bright green sea.

"There was a brief moment when the NVA and the Khmer Rouge actually worked together," he admitted.

"And so you and Pranh became generals and Brother Rap got his balls blown off," Sawyer said. He hawked and spat over the railing. "Tell me, as a matter of historical curiosity, where was the Viet Cong COSVN anyway?"

"Ah, you Americans," General Lu said, shaking his head. "What arrogance! You always see the world in your own image. Because you had a Pentagon, you assumed we must have one too. We were never that sophisticated. COSVN never existed. It was a myth, like all these gods and goddesses," he said, vaguely gesturing at the ruins all around. "Like the myth of this very temple, about some Khmer king who mated with a she-dragon. What nonsense! C'est une bêtise!"

Sawyer thought about Suong and didn't say anything. He stared at the blackened ruin, amazed that so much of the temple had survived. There were new fissures running down the pyramidal sides, and a big jagged gap, like the opening to a cave, had been blown in the main stairway leading up to what was left of a tower that had vanished in some other invasion, centuries ago. It had been the blast from that gap that had blown away the tent.

He watched a long line of Vietnamese soldiers going in and out of the gap, trying to salvage what was left of the morphine base. So far it looked like they had found barely a dozen of the wooden boxes intact.

"Why'd they blow it?" Sawyer asked.

General Lu took off his officer's cap and wiped his sweating brow on his uniform sleeve. He watched the soldiers working on the ruin with his lips pursed, as though they were performing an act of great stupidity.

"When the shooting started, they probably thought the Khmer Rouge were attacking them. They had no hope of escape . . . et voilà. Now no person gets Bhun Sa's treasure. If you can take the satisfaction, that part of our operation was not a success," General Lu said, turning to Sawyer.

"Would you have really sold us the morphine?"

"Of course," General Lu snapped, peering shrewdly at Sawyer. "I thought surely you would have guessed by now what our operation was all about?"

"Most of it. There's not a damn thing wrong with my hindsight. God knows, it's better than my foresight," Sawyer said, shaking his head to refuse a cigarette. General Lu lit one for himself. The smoke drifted out over the ruins as the machine gun opened up again. Neither said anything. They waited for the sound to stop so they could resume their conversation, the way people do when a jet plane passes overhead.

"American," Sawyer commented.

"Quoi? The cigarette? Ah yes. You addicted us to them. You addicted us to more things American than you ever knew. After the war, we found whole warehouses of American cigarettes at Tan Son Nhut and Bien Hoa. For a time, the Cholonaise used them for currency until we could get them to accept the dong."

"Money," Sawyer said, with a little snort of laughter. "The mother's milk of politics. That's what it was all about."

"We are a poor country, mon cher Jack. And while our Soviet allies, toward whom we feel great gratitude and the strongest of fraternal Socialist ties, have been most generous," General Lu recited, glancing around as though he feared he might be overheard, "just between you and me, the Russians are what the bargirls used to call 'Cheap Charlies.' "

"That's tough," Sawyer said, without conviction. He leaned on an undulating stone balustrade carved to represent a giant serpent. The old Khmers had mixed it all together, he thought. Ancient tales of dragon goddesses and Buddhism and Hindu myths about a giant snake who churned up the Sea of Milk to create the world. The stone was hot under his forearms. He watched the soldiers piling up white chunks of morphine, crumbling like cheese, on the stone paving below. At least the machine-gunning had stopped for a while.

"Yes, it is—how you say?—tough," General Lu agreed carefully, watching Sawyer intently out of the corner of his eye.

Sawyer turned and looked sharply at the Vietnamese.

"Are you saying what I think you're saying, Lu?"

General Lu smiled happily.

"I told them you were good. If you were not good, it would have been a disaster. It was like the jiu-jitsu, you see. It is the enemy's own strength which defeats him."

Sawyer's face twisted.

"We made the one crucial error. We just didn't know there was another player on the field. You," Sawyer said.

General Lu smiled, and it reminded Sawyer of a snapshot Pranh had taken of them all in a jungle clearing a long time ago.

"Tell me. This Cambodian, what was his name?"

"Pich, I believe. A certain Pich Sam," General Lu said.

Sawyer sighed. It was Khieu's second-in-command. The one Suong could not afford to let Khieu terminate, so she turned in her own husband. It all fit.

"This Pich. Was he a 'double' or just a 'mole' that you were feeding disinformation to?"

"A 'mole,' as you Americans so colorfully put it," General Lu said, smiling. "He thought he was passing the good information. He was a true believer. It was much better than to try and 'turn' him. We made great efforts to supply corroborating evidence. It was essential that he be believed about our invading Thailand."

"Who'd he pass it to?"

"A true 'double,' as one says. One of the so-called 'Old People.' A peasant living in a shack on the river who was really one of ours. That was how we first got on to Pich. We knew it was the kind of thing the Khmer Rouge would surely pass on to their allies in Beijing. From there, one way or another, it was inevitable that it would eventually reach the Americans." General Lu shrugged.

"All right." Sawyer nodded. "Here's the scenario: there never was going to be a full-scale invasion of Thailand. Maybe just a few raids on Cambodian resistance camps. But the satellite confirmed mobilization and lots of troop movements. Where'd you really send them?"

"Against our real enemies," General Lu said, his lips tightening.

Sawyer whistled silently to himself.

"North, then. To the Chinese border," Sawyer said.

General Lu nodded again.

"Okay. Our operation was to forestall an invasion that was really never meant to happen. But your operation had at least two objectives: to bring Pranh, alias Son Lot, out into the open, so you could nail him, and to grab Bhun Sa's morphine for yourselves to acquire good old Western hard currency."

"Exactement," General Lu agreed. "You see, we found ourselves in a somewhat similar position in Cambodia to the situation you Americans had in Vietnam: fighting a guerrilla war in a country where the masses, although we ended the 'holocaust' for them, would be happier to see us go home. It is a racial problem. We consider the Cambodians slow-witted and backward, the way some of your white Southern officers used to talk about les noirs, while they secretly call us 'youn' and 'dog-eater.'

"However, we were determined not to repeat your errors. Pranh was a tiger on his own home ground. If you want to kill a tiger, you don't go beating around in the bush, for that is his game. No. You tether a goat in a clearing and wait for him to come," General Lu said.

"And Bhun Sa's morphine and the chance to sell it to the Americans for arms was the goat to tempt Pranh into the open."

"Just so. It was the rumor about Bhun Sa's opium and a possible connection between Bhun Sa and Son Lot that first gave us the idea."

"So you fed Pich the story about invading Thailand, figuring it would get back to us."

"How did it?"

Sawyer shrugged. It didn't matter now what he told Lu.

"The Khmer Rouge, Pranh, sent the information to their friends in Beijing. They deliberately let it slip, possibly to a 'double' of their own, who got it to Hong Kong, where the British MI6, which is strong there, picked it up and passed it to their 'American cousins.' Because it was Sir Geoffrey's network, he got the credit for passing it to London," Sawyer said.

"Fascinating."

"That set us into motion. You were counting on us somehow getting through and leading you to Pranh and the morphine. You didn't hunt the tiger, you trapped him. So your operation was at least half a success. Ours was a total failure," Sawyer said, making a face.

"Pas du tout, Jack. Your job was to stop our invasion of Thailand and you performed it brilliantly. You may even get a medal, mon vieux. There will be no invasion."

"Only because you never intended to invade in the first place. What a joke! What a stupid joke!" Sawyer said.

He watched the soldiers coming empty-handed out of the gap in the temple stairway. They were standing around, waiting for orders. There was obviously nothing more to salvage. A pile of about thirty kilos' worth of morphine lay on the hot paving stones. Some of the boxes were covered with rust-colored splotches. Blood, Sawyer thought. The Shan had stayed Shan to the end.

"You know, Lu, there's enough there to keep us both in comfort for the rest of our lives," Sawyer said, gesturing at the pile.

"And go where?" General Lu smiled.

Sawyer shrugged, his hands in his pockets.

"Switzerland. Hong Kong, maybe."

"Neh, Switzerland. What would one do? Watch them make the cuckoo clocks?"

"And yet half the putains in Asia have a poster of the Alps over their beds."

"A fantasy," General Lu observed. "Haven't you yet learned that the worst thing you can do with a fantasy is try to make it come true? Besides, they get the posters free from the airline offices," he added, putting out the cigarette and carefully field-stripping it.

"And Hong Kong?"

General Lu looked seriously at Sawyer.

"No Vietnamese ever feels comfortable surrounded by Chinese."

The two men began to walk down toward the Lokeshvara gate Sawyer had bypassed only that very morning. Far down the long stone pathway a dark puddle shimmered like black silk. A heat mirage, Sawyer thought. It's just a heat mirage.

"I'm leaving the woman, Suong, with you. Call it a gesture of goodwill," General Lu said.

"Don't bullshit me, Lu," Sawyer said, stopping. "North Vietnamese goodwill is like a present of mangoes with a hand grenade hidden in the basket."

General Lu's smile broadened.

"Eh bien, mon vieux. Let us just say that I prefer not to execute her and risk making her a martyr of the Kampuchean cause." His smile faded. He lightly touched Sawyer's arm. "She was the Madame LaFarge of their revolution, vous comprenez. She has the blood of millions on her hands."

Sawyer didn't say anything. After a moment, they resumed walking, their shadows stretching ahead of them.

"But I say this in all seriousness, Jack. You will deliver our very unofficial offer to the American government, eh? That is why I let you live," General Lu said, poking Sawyer with his pudgy fingers, knowing Sawyer didn't like it, to emphasize his point.

"Now we're getting down to it. The real reason for your operation, eh, General. Pranh was just a sideshow, icing on the cake, n'est-ce pas?"

General Lu nodded.

"This invasion was a threat. To let you know what we could do. Next time it might not be a feint, Jack. Next time we might really do it."

"Oh for Chrissakes, Lu! Just say what the fuck you're after," Sawyer spat out.

"We want help, Jack. Aid. Also trade. We're broke. We need money. This occupation of Cambodia is very dear for us."

"Then go home, Lu. We did."

"Mais oui. And what did you leave behind? Killing fields and concentration camps. Tell me. How can you still support these people? How?"

Sawyer looked away.

"You do business with plenty of Communists, Jack. The Russians, the Chinese, even the Khmer Rouge. Why not Vietnam?" General Lu insisted. He stopped walking.

Sawyer walked on.

"You owe us, Jack! Our whole country was devastated. Children still die from mines you left behind. You have an obligation!" General Lu shouted, his voice rising at the end.

Sawyer stopped and turned back. He looked at General Lu and thought of the Parrot's Beak. Of Brother Rap and Parker and a black wall in Washington.

"We already paid," he said.

They passed a Lokeshvara gate and down a long lane bordered on either side by giant stone heads, one after another. Each of the faces was identical.

"These faces. Always the same. Pah!" General Lu grimaced in disgust.

"It's supposed to be the face of God."

"Yes, well, the Khmer god repeats himself. It is boring."

"The Khmers aren't the only ones who keep repeating themselves," Sawyer said.

They walked down the aisle of great stone heads that cast

shadows across the road, so that they kept alternating between shadow and sunlight as they went. The hot sun had bleached much of the blue from the sky, and in the distance an island of gray monsoon cloud floated over the jungle.

For a time they walked side by side without talking. They passed Vietnamese soldiers clearing the area, preparing to evacuate. They came to the place where the giant head of Buddha had fallen facing the sky. Suong was seated on the giant forehead, guarded by two Vietnamese soldiers. With her long black hair and her hands tied behind her, she resembled a hawk, its wings folded, on a perch. Her eyes were hooded. She didn't look at either of them, yet they sensed her watching.

"How does this rasoir-machine march?" General Lu asked, gesturing at Sawyer's electric razor.

"If I release this button, open the head, raise the antenna, and turn this screw, it sends out a 'squirt,' a compressed transmission which will be picked up by an SR-71 Blackbird somewhere up there, too high to see or hear," Sawyer said, pointing at the sky. "Once it's received, they'll home in on the location and there'll be a chopper here in two to three hours to pick me up."

"So you don't need to talk."

Sawyer shook his head.

"Suppose someone else were to take it from you and use it?"

Sawyer grinned in a way that reminded General Lu of long ago.

"If anything else is pressed or opened, it sends another 'squirt.' Within a couple of hours the location will be hit with an air attack, followed by the Delta Force. That's a little something for *you* to watch out for next time."

General Lu looked warily at Sawyer, the smile frozen on his face.

"You had this—how you say?—in the pocket all the time! If the Shan had not destroyed the morphine, either Pranh or I would have unwittingly called in a strike and you would have gotten the morphine anyway!"

"Why bother?" Sawyer shrugged. "There never was a real invasion. That was a very dangerous lie, General."

General Lu once more took off his cap and wiped the sweat from his face with his sleeve. His hair was beginning to thin, Sawyer noticed. When Lu looked back at Sawyer, his smile was

Buddha-like, indifferent. No, Sawyer corrected himself. To Asians, the smile of the Buddha is compassionate; it's only to us Westerners that it seems indifferent. General Lu put his cap back on and straightened his uniform.

"That makes nothing, Jack." He shrugged. "You lied to us. We lied to you. Your failure was that you also lied to yourselves. This we did not do. That is why we won." He hesitated. "Allez. Call in your helicopter."

Sawyer looked around at the soldiers.

"Will two hours be enough time for you to get all your men out of here?"

"But yes. And you will report our interest in U.S. assistance, will you not? An invasion can still be mounted," he added ominously.

Sawyer spat in the dust. He still had enough saliva for that.

"Haven't you had enough fighting?"

"We've been at war for over forty years now, mon vieux. It's all we know."

Sawyer grimaced. "They won't believe me, but I'll tell them."

"Why not?"

"They won't go for it, Lu. You don't understand us any more than we do you. We haven't paid blackmail since the days of the Barbary pirates."

"But it is more logical. And also pour l'humanité—and so much cheaper than a war in Asia."

"Okay, have it your way." Sawyer made a face. "That's none of my affair. Politics is out of my line."

"Mon cher Jack," General Lu said, laughing, holding his quivering belly, "you are still lying to yourself. What do you think you have been involved with all this time if not the politics?" Then more seriously, looking over at Suong, "What will you do with her?"

"I don't know."

General Lu looked into Sawyer's eyes. The glass eye had gotten slightly turned so it stared off to one side. It was very disconcerting. It made Sawyer look as though his thoughts, like a madman's, were always elsewhere. General Lu forced himself to concentrate on Sawyer's good eye. He decided that Sawyer was lying, as usual.

As his men were getting ready to leave, one of them brought

Sawyer's Ingram over to General Lu. He handed it to Sawyer, who checked it over to make sure it was working and loaded.

"With that one, you may need this," General Lu said, indicating Suong.

Sawyer pointed the Ingram at the sky and fired a few rounds. At the sound of the shots, the soldiers froze. Even the jungle birds were silenced momentarily. Then there was a clang of metal as someone picked something up and everything went on as before.

"Don't forget, Jack. For us Asians, America is like a rich, somewhat vulgar uncle. Better that he hate us than that he ignore us—and even what he throws away as garbage is of value to us," General Lu said.

Sawyer nodded, then turned and scrambled up on the head of Buddha, across from Suong. General Lu's aide came up and Lu barked the order for them to pull out. The rumble of truck engines filled the hot afternoon. General Lu looked back one last time as his truck pulled down the dusty road, bordered by those endlessly smiling stone heads. He watched the two figures shrink in the distance.

That was how he left them. Sawyer and the woman. They were still sitting facing each other on the tumbled head of an ancient god, nothing between them but the Ingram submachine gun, waiting for the Americans.

26

Heaven within the mountain.
The superior man stores within his mind
the words and deeds of history,
in order to know what is right.

T HERE were two of them. They were dressed in black that made them almost invisible in the darkness. They were good, moving cautiously down the rain-deserted wharf, using the stacks of rice bags for cover. From his vantage behind a capstan on the freighter's deck, Sawyer watched them approach. They didn't look behind them and that worried Sawyer because there should be more of them and if one of Mith Yon's men opened up too soon— Don't think about that, he told himself.

He blinked the rain out of his eye and lost them for a moment. They had disappeared behind a big rice stack near the gangplank. He eased the Ingram's safety off. He had to force himself to breathe slowly, praying that some trigger-happy ape didn't open up too soon. They had to let them come on board first and signal that it was clear. He had gone over and over that with Mith Yon. They had to wait at least until Vasnasong was on the gangplank before they opened up. That way, whatever additional men Vasnasong had brought would be boxed in. If it worked, even if they missed, the shooting should drive Vasnasong on board, straight into Sawyer's field of fire.

The heavy monsoon rain hammered on the metal deck. A tall palm swayed as the wind swept the rain along the wharf like a giant broom. Drops skimmed across the slick deck. The air smelled of wet rice. Sawyer scanned the wharf for more of them, but all he could make out was the outline of the warehouse on the quay. The rain made the surface of the river choppy, shattering the reflections of the city lights into a billion fragments.

Why are you doing this, sir? Captain Henderson of the Delta team had asked him when Sawyer had put the Ingram to his head on the ride in from U–Tapao air base.

Just get the goddamn message to Harris, Sawyer had replied.

I don't believe you'll shoot me, Henderson had said.

I will, Sawyer said, cocking the Ingram.

Henderson looked into Sawyer's eye. It was red rimmed and bloodshot, and whatever he saw there, he ordered his sergeant driver to pull the car over. Sawyer left the two of them standing on the side of the road just outside Chon Buri. The two army jeeps that had been following them in convoy immediately took up the chase, but it wasn't that hard to lose them in the traffic detouring through the slums around Bangkok.

What you do with me now, So-yah? Suong had asked him just before she made the call to Vasnasong.

He held the receiver in one hand, the Ingram in the other.

No mistakes this time. Tell him you have the morphine and to meet you tonight aboard the Siam Star. *Tell him I'm dead.*

Maybe he not want to come.

Make him come. You know how to make men do things.

Oh, So-yah. You not understand.

Understand what?

You my country now, she said, her eyes shiny like the lights of the city in the rain.

Sawyer glanced back up at the bridge, but he could see nothing of the Swatowese captain, or Mith Yon's man, crouching out of sight, his gun aimed at the captain's back. The rest of the crew were tied up down in the aft hold. From here on deck, Sawyer could see only the rain slanting through the golden haze cast by the freighter's running lights.

The rain was so loud that he sensed the weight of them stepping onto the gangplank before he heard them. They were moving faster now, the gangplank their point of greatest vulnerability.

The metallic scrape of footsteps seemed very near as they came on board. He could see them clearly now. They looked young and tough, crouched over their Uzis. One of them passed on the other side of the capstan, close enough for Sawyer to hear his breathing. Sawyer tried to shrink inside the shadow of the capstan.

The Ingram's magazine grip was wet in Sawyer's hand. He was sure it was going to slip the second he pulled the trigger, but there was no way to wipe it dry. His clothes were soaked anyway, and he couldn't afford to make the slightest sound. He could sense that the man on the other side of the capstan had stopped and was listening intently. The man said something in what sounded like Cambodian and the other flicked on a flashlight. He signaled to someone back on the wharf and a bulky shape that could have been Vasnasong, followed by two others, emerged from the shadows. Vasnasong carried something that looked like an umbrella. The others had guns.

It's going to work, Sawyer thought exultantly. He took a long breath to clear his mind, reminding himself to make sure of the first shot, when all hell broke loose.

There were sudden flashes all over the wharf as heavy gunfire erupted from Mith Yon's positions. It's too soon, Sawyer agonized. Too soon! Vasnasong's men hit the ground as Vasnasong himself scuttled behind a rice bale. The two Cambodians on deck whirled and, ducking behind the railing, began firing back at the muzzle flashes. Sawyer saw one of Mith Yon's men topple from the top of the warehouse down to the wet concrete wharf.

It would be easy to take the two men on deck, Sawyer thought. They had their backs to him and probably wouldn't hear him in all the commotion till it was too late. But then he would have revealed his position to Vasnasong and it would have all been for nothing. Gritting his teeth, he forced himself to hold his fire, hoping to God he didn't get hit by a stray shot from one of Mith Yon's men.

Suddenly he saw Vasnasong peering up at the freighter from behind the rice bale. Vasnasong hesitated for the briefest instant, trying to decide which way to break. Come on, you bastard, Sawyer prayed. It's nice and quiet on the ship and your own men have signaled that it's safe. Come on, come on, said the spider to the fly.

Bullets stitched into the bags of rice near Vasnasong's head and he ducked back. Rice poured out of the bags. Sawyer watched it form a tiny mountain of rice that, even as it formed, was washed away by the rain. For some reason it reminded him of Pranh talking about water and the ancient Khmer rice harvests. He stared blankly at the firefight and the warehouse and its big sign: SOUTH-EAST ASIA RICE AND TRADING COMPANY. His breathing was coming fast now. Maybe because he had almost died in that warehouse, where Suong—*my father was a French rice merchant*—or maybe . . . All at once he remembered sitting in Vasnasong's office, looking at the picture of Vasnasong being greeted by Chou En Lai behind the desk. Christ! What an idiot he had been! It had been staring him in the face all the time. He had been right to get away from Henderson's Delta team and out from under Company control. If only Vasnasong—come on, you bastard!

As if he had somehow heard Sawyer's thoughts, Vasnasong peeked out once, then broke for the gangplank. The two men on deck gave him covering fire, but there was heavy shooting from the direction of the warehouse. Ricochets pinged off the railing. Arms flailing, Vasnasong went down on the gangplank. There was no way to tell if he had been hit or had fallen. All Sawyer could do was wait. Not now, he thought, barely able to restrain himself from an insane try for the gangplank, when Vasnasong suddenly crawled onto the deck on all fours and rolled heavily behind a big metal storage box bolted to the deck.

One of the men on deck started over toward him, but Vasnasong, chest heaving, waved him back. The man turned and fired his Uzi again back at the wharf.

Now, Sawyer thought. Now—moving out from behind the capstan and getting set in the squat position, no longer conscious of the rain or his breathing or anything except telling himself to make it slow and sure. His first burst caught the man farthest away full in the back. The man hadn't even time to arch his back before Sawyer was firing at the second man, already whirling around, the Uzi sweeping toward Sawyer. There was the briefest instant when their eyes locked, and then the Ingram's bullets smashed into the side of his face and the Cambodian went down.

Sawyer ran toward Vasnasong, almost falling on the rain-slick deck. Vasnasong was fumbling with something caught in his umbrella. He wasn't going to make it, Sawyer thought. But Vasnasong couldn't free the umbrella. Vasnasong looked up just as

Sawyer raised the Ingram. With a grunt, he smashed the Ingram into Vasnasong's head. Vasnasong fell to the deck.

A savage joy flooded Sawyer. It felt so good hitting Vasnasong, it took every bit of will he had to keep from pounding Vasnasong's head to mush. Instead, he twisted the umbrella out of Vasnasong's hand and flung it into the river. He hauled Vasnasong to his feet and, using the Ingram as a prod, marched Vasnasong up a ladder on the river side and into a small mess room. Sawyer slammed the heavy metal door behind him, shutting out the rain and the sounds of shooting. He had to hurry. There wasn't much time.

The cabin stank of diesel oil and fish. It was lit by a single dangling bulb. Sitting tied up in a corner was Suong. The three of them just stared at each other. Sawyer tried not to look at Suong's face, because every time he did, he could feel his throat tighten as though a big hand was squeezing it.

"I was right, Sawyer-khrap. You are dangerous man," Vasnasong managed, panting to catch his breath. He steadied himself on the table. There was a red welt on the side of his face where Sawyer had hit him.

Sawyer popped a new clip into the Ingram. The sound of it slamming home was very loud in the small cabin. Sawyer steadied the Ingram with both hands. At this range it was impossible to miss.

"No, So-yah, no," Suong cried out, squirming desperately in the corner.

"You make terrible mistake, Sawyer-khrap," Vasnasong wheezed. His face was waxen in the smoky yellow light.

"Not this time," Sawyer said, gritting his teeth so tightly they could see the line of his jaw throbbing.

"We are on same side, Sawyer-khrap," Vasnasong gasped.

Sawyer pointed the Ingram straight at Vasnasong's belly. They could see Sawyer's face working, trying to hold the rage in.

"How?" Sawyer managed to say. "When the Khmer Rouge was running things in Cambodia, how did they manage to get the rice from the killing fields to Red China?"

Vasnasong didn't answer. His mouth twisted. He looked like he was about to throw up. Suong was barely breathing.

"The Khmer Rouge traded rice to China for arms to use against the Vietnamese. The land routes through Laos and Vietnam were controlled by the Vietnamese, so they would have had to ship it by boat. Maybe even this very boat," Sawyer said, his eyes darting back and forth between them. He didn't wait for an answer. It was written plainly enough in their faces.

"Suong's father was a rice merchant," Sawyer went on. "She didn't just call you. You were in the same business. You knew each other all the time. I should have guessed from that picture of Chou En Lai in your office. You're the link to China, Vasnasong-khrap. And Suong was your pipeline to the Khmer Rouge. This whole thing," Sawyer gestured vaguely with the Ingram, "was being run from Beijing."

A gleam came into Vasnasong's eye. His fleshly lips worked as though he was about to eat something.

"Do you see, Sawyer One-Eye? Do you finally see?"

"And all that bullshit about the British. MI6 only thought they were using you. In reality, you were spoon-feeding them. Christ, you must have strained a gut pretending you didn't know anything whenever Countess Dracula came calling."

"Sometime very difficult. I must use most incompetent agent in Hong Kong to follow MI6 men to convince London of authenticity of coded messages without interfering with information getting through," Vasnasong admitted.

"And the men you sent against me were all Khmer Rouge. That's why they didn't know how Buddhists behave. Under angkar, religion was outlawed in Cambodia. My God." Sawyer shook his head. "Thanks to you and Suong, everyone was dancing to Beijing's tune and didn't even know it."

Vasnasong straightened. His face had begun to lose its waxy look.

"So you see, you cannot kill me, Sawyer-khrap. We are on same side. America and China allies on this."

"What about her? What about the killing?" Sawyer demanded gesturing toward Suong with the Ingram.

Vasnasong splayed his pudgy fingers in a helpless gesture.

"She did it for her country."

"So did Hitler."

"She is for you, Sawyer-khrap. Can you not see?"

A look passed between Vasnasong and Suong. There was something very intimate about it and Sawyer's throat tightened. Vasnasong was just trying to save her, Sawyer told himself, wondering why Vasnasong didn't try to sacrifice her to save himself.

Unless . . . there was more in the look than that. It was the kind of look . . .

"You seduced her, you bastard," Sawyer hissed, aiming the Ingram almost point-blank at Vasnasong's face. "You knew her father, didn't you? Maybe you even ran him. How old was she when you fucked her? How old?"

Vasnasong's mouth opened but nothing came out. He looked sick. Sawyer turned toward Suong.

"He forced you, didn't he? How old were you?"

Her eyes brimmed over. She shook her head wildly.

"Please, So-yah. It was so long ago. It makes nothing now."

Sawyer whirled back to Vasnasong.

"You forced her, you miserable bastard. She was only a little girl and you raped her."

Vasnasong looked at him strangely.

"I fear you not understand women after all, Sawyer-khrap. I was not always old. Before twenty years I was handsome man. Rich. Powerful. And Suong no ordinary young girl."

"So?"

Despite the fear, there was contempt in Vasnasong's face.

"I did not seduce Suong. It was she who seduces me."

Sawyer didn't have to look at Suong's face to know it was true. Then he did look at her and it burst out of him.

"Jesus! Is there anybody you haven't fucked?"

The Ingram hung lifelessly down at his side. Vasnasong brushed himself off and started confidently for the door. Sawyer looked at him.

"I go now. There is no more here. We are allies, yes? You do not have to love your ally, Sawyer-khrap, only not to kill him," Vasnasong said.

"You're forgetting Parker. You set him up," Sawyer said. His voice was toneless. It might have been a dead man talking.

Vasnasong stopped. He looked back at both of them.

"Your Parker was stupid greedy man. He was warned of danger." Vasnasong shrugged. "In Asia many die. Asia is most dangerous place," Vasnasong said, turning toward the door.

The first rounds of the Ingram took off the back of Vasnasong's head. Vasnasong sprawled facedown on the metal floor. The cabin smelled of gunpowder and the faint salt scent of blood. Sawyer came close to Suong. Her eyes were black as death.

"Why you do this? Now you will be stranger in your own country," she whispered.

His face worked. He was holding himself together the way a wounded soldier trying to make it back to his own lines holds himself together.

"We were friends in Vietnam," Sawyer said. "After a while, that was all that mattered. Not big words, not bullshit about God and country, just each other. I never really liked Parker that much, but he was all that was left. At that, he died better than he lived, so maybe there's hope for the rest of us yet. There's got to be something."

Suong pressed her breast against the still-warm muzzle of the Ingram. Sawyer jerked it away as though she had touched it with a torch.

"There is something, my So-yah. I know what men really want. Their deepest desire"—pressing her thighs together as if imagining him between them. Her voice, with its strange three-in-the-morning timbre, caught at him. His throat tightened. "I do anything for you, So-yah. We are both without country. I make you my country. You will be everything for me. I will bring you other women and we will do such things. Nothing is forbidden. Nothing!" she whispered.

"No," he said, backing away from her.

"You want me. I know you want me."

Having her hands tied behind her made her breasts more prominent. He watched her breasts heaving, the nipples poking against the fabric of her blouse, as she came closer.

"Touch me one last time. My hands tied. I can't stop you. Please," she said, kneeling at his feet. He could feel her breath, warm on his wet trousers. "You know you want to."

"No," he lied, feeling himself harden like steel.

She looked up at him. He couldn't stop looking at her, at her breasts and the line of her chin where it came under her ear, at the shining black sweep of her hair, at her eyes and the way her lips parted. She was so beautiful it hurt to look at her.

"Then what you do with me, So-yah?"

"I don't know," he whispered, the tightness in his throat almost choking him.

"Don't be fool, So-yah. Most emotion never truly felt. Most time we only pretend to feel, even to ourself. But with us is no pretend. If you lose me, you not feel again. We both know this, my So-yah. Destroy Suong, destroy you'self."

The door burst open. Mith Yon came in, gun first. His eyes still had the unfocused look that comes with killing. He almost stumbled over Vasnasong's body and just caught his balance against the bulkhead. He looked at both of them. Wind whipped the rain into the room. Water streamed down Mith Yon's face to drip into the puddle of blood spreading on the floor.

The floor began to tremble. Raindrops danced along the floor as a loud rumble filled the silence, followed by a sensation of motion. The *Siam Star* had begun to move.

"What you do now, my So-yah?" Suong whispered, her eyes catching the light like black diamonds. "What you do now?"

EPILOGUE

O N the night of the full moon after the monsoon rains have ended is the festival of the Loy Krathong. As darkness falls, the people gather on the banks of rivers and klongs throughout Thailand to sail tiny boats made of banana leaves. Every boat carries a single burning candle, and there is great excitement, especially among the children, as one by one, each member of the family launches his boat. Wide-eyed, they watch the current carry their boats away to join the thousands of flickering lights already floating in the darkness.

The Loy Krathong is a happy time, and there is much singing and dancing and the night resounds with firecrackers along the shores. No one knows the origin of the festival, for it comes from the time of the ancients. There are those who say the floating lights are an offering to the river dragons. Others say it is a celebration of the end of the monsoon waters that have ensured the fertility of the land. Among the common people it is believed that they are casting their sins upon the waters. Some more cynical types suggest that the lights are a way of apologizing to the Mother of Waters, as the Chao Phraya River is known, for all the pollution the people pour into her. Whatever the origin, everyone knows that most of the waters of Thailand feed into the Chao Phraya and that the view of the river at midnight, with its galaxies of candles floating by in the darkness, is spectacular.

In Bangkok, where the spectacle is at its height and the klongs and riverbanks are noisy till dawn with merrymaking, it is generally conceded that the most prestigious place for viewing is from the upper terrace of the Royal Palace. There, two men stood apart from His Majesty's other guests, gazing down over the parapet at the klongs and the river, delineated by the myriad dots of light like iridescent veins in a vast dark body.

The two men were utterly dissimilar in appearance. One was tall, fair haired, obviously a Westerner. He wore a superbly cut light tropical suit with an air of casual elegance that professional models have to work a long time to perfect. The other was small, bent, Asian. He was very old. He wore a gold-braided black military uniform that sagged and wrinkled and seemed several sizes too big for him. Seen from behind, they looked like a man and his pet monkey. Yet it was because of the little Asian and not the tall Westerner that no one—not even from the royal party— dared approach the two men.

"So the Vietnamese never intended to attack. Only to trap Son Lot and perhaps the opium of Bhun Sa also," Bhamornprayoon said.

"And to send us a warning, your Excellency," Harris replied.

The old man looked shrewdly up at Harris.

"Interesting. That you see the threat but not the offer, Harris-khrap. You of the West are most curious."

Harris made a gesture of dismissal.

"The offer is meaningless, Excellency. No president could ever approach Congress to ask for aid to Communist Vietnam under present circumstances. That Sawyer even mentioned it shows how politically naive he was."

"And the opium of Bhun Sa?"

"Destroyed, it seems. It was all for nothing."

The old man looked up suspiciously, his sharp eyes almost disappearing in a nest of wrinkles.

"Is this certain?"

"It seems so, Excellency" Harris said. "In any case, we have no way of ever finding out for sure. Unfortunately, this agent, Sawyer, managed to give our people the slip."

"Has he?" Bhamornprayoon said, in a tone of voice that left little doubt in Harris' mind that he'd already heard about Sawyer's disappearance from his own sources.

There was nothing to say to that so Harris just looked out over the city and the countless lights twinkling on the river. Behind him, the gold-covered spires of the chedis and mondhops and the phallic golden prangs of the Royal Palace glowed in the floodlights set up for the festival like a fairy-tale castle. In Chinatown, an enormous dragon's tail of firecrackers went off. It sounded almost like a machine gun. There were loud cheers in the streets that could be heard even up here.

"What happened to the woman? This Suong?"

"He took her with him," Harris said, an edge in his voice.

"They were lovers, then?"

"I don't know what they were," Harris snapped, unable to conceal the bitterness. There were lines around his handsome mouth, and all at once, Bhamornprayoon was able to see very clearly what Harris would look like as an old man.

"You blame yourself?" Bhamornprayoon asked quietly.

"Sawyer was out there alone too long. It was my mission. I should have seen it. He suckered us all the way," Harris said sternly.

"Mai pen rai." The old man shrugged. "Why must you Americans see all things only as success or failure. There is no invasion. There will be no war for this year. That is at least something. It has fallen, as the proverb says, on one horn of the buffalo but not the other. The rest"—he shrugged again—"is karma."

"It couldn't have happened if Sawyer hadn't slipped one over on us. That one-eyed bastard pulled a gun on the way in from U-Tapao, and the next thing we knew, they had both gone to ground. It wasn't until later, after the Bangkok police fished Vasnasong's body out of one of the klongs, that we were able to piece together what happened."

"Who killed Vasnasong? So-yah?"

"Don't you know?" Harris asked, elaborately affecting an air of surprise.

"Vasnasong play many sides. In Bangkok, Hong Kong, many sides. Our eminent chief police have theory maybe Vasnasong killed by Western drug smuggler. The men of the drug trade are said to be of desperate character." Bhamornprayoon smiled.

"No doubt that is what happened." Harris smiled back.

"But we forget the woman. What of her?"

A furtive look came into Harris' eyes. At first, Bhamornprayoon thought that Harris was about to lie, and then he saw that it was something else. Harris was confused, almost fearful. For a man like Harris, anything other than absolute certainty had to be a special kind of purgatory, Bhamornprayoon thought.

"Somehow Sawyer managed to spirit the woman Suong onto this rusty old freighter Vasnasong had waiting to take the morphine cargo. One of the Cambodian resistance groups, headed by a certain Mith Yon, had taken over the ship and they all sailed south into the Gulf of Thailand. Apparently, Sawyer had suspected something and set it up with Mith Yon even before he went into Cambodia. The son of a bitch was good, you know. I told you he was good."

"But you say the morphine destroyed. Why he do this?"

Harris looked at the wizened old man, at the deep fissures under his cheeks that made him look both sad and wise, the broad Asian nose, the black buttons that were his eyes. He didn't know how to explain it to Bhamornprayoon. He didn't know how to explain it to himself.

"It wasn't about the dope for them. For Sawyer and Mith Yon. It was about her. Suong."

"I am not understand."

"She was, together with Son Lot and Pol Pot, one of the guiding spirits of the Khmer Rouge and their death camps in Cambodia. Mith Yon and his followers were her victims. Don't you see?" Harris said in a hushed voice. "He was bringing her to trial."

"What happen?" Bhamornprayoon asked gently. From Harris' tone he could tell they were almost there.

Harris' shoulders slumped. He suddenly looked smaller, less sure of himself.

"We've got two versions from two separate sources. But they're both almost the same," he whispered, as though he was ashamed of something. "According to one, Sawyer turned the woman over to Mith Yon, telling him they could do anything they wanted, but not to spill even a single drop of her blood. That all sounds a bit too Shakespearean for me," Harris said, making a face.

"It is an old saying here. But mai pen rai, only say what is known," Bhamornprayoon ordered, his eyes searching Harris' face as if he were trying to see Sawyer's behind it.

"The other version is simpler. Sawyer just turned the woman over to the Cambodians and took off when the ship was somewhere off the coast of the southern peninsula. Or maybe it was one of the islands. I don't know." Harris shrugged. "Nobody's seen him since."

"And the woman?"

"Yeah. The woman. It seems they anchored or drifted—who the hell knows—out in the middle of the gulf. I don't know if they had a trial or what. But they didn't spill a drop of her blood, if that matters.

"Anyway, I can't get the picture out of my mind. The bunch of them on this rusty old hulk drifting nowhere on an empty blue sea under an empty blue sky, the sun blazing down on them. You know what the sun is like in those latitudes. It's unbelievably hot here in Bangkok, but down there, my God!

"There was a big iron box on deck. Maybe it was used to store tools or something at one time. They locked her inside it. It must have been unbelievably hot, worse than an oven," he said, going faster now. "But that wasn't enough. They got aluminum foil or strips from somewhere and made reflectors around the box. It must have been hundreds of degrees in there. They say her hammering and screaming went on for two days."

From across the river on the Thonburi side, they could hear the crash of gongs and the whining tones of festival songs.

"She must to go insane after some hours like that," Bhamornprayoon said finally.

"Probably," Harris agreed. "Most probably."

Behind them the soft murmur of conversation gave way to "oohs" and "aahs" as new arrivals crowded the parapet on the far side of the terrace near the royal box.

"What was she like, this woman?"

Harris paused.

"I never met her. They say she was very pretty."

"Ah," Bhamornprayoon said, as if that explained a great deal. He looked up at Harris.

"A terrible death," he said, clicking his tongue. "No matter what she did. To be burned alive like that."

"No! Don't you understand!" Harris said suddenly, a sick look on his face. "She wasn't burnt. She was cooked! They said when they finally took the body out, the meat was so tender it literally fell off the bones!"

The two men looked away from each other. They stood there for a long time. They looked down over the millions of lights shining on the dark water and just watched and didn't say anything at all.

Below them the Chao Phraya flowed on in the night, a river of stars carrying the sins of men to the sea.